616.0754 D553m 2011 238476
Dhawan, Atam P.
Medical image analysis

COMMUNITY COLLEGE OF PHILADELPHIA
PHILADELPHIA, PENNSYLVANIA

MEDICAL IMAGE ANALYSIS

IEEE Press
445 Hoes Lane
Piscataway, NJ 08854

IEEE Press Editorial Board
Lajos Hanzo, *Editor in Chief*

R. Abari	M. El-Hawary	S. Nahavandi
J. Anderson	B. M. Hammerli	W. Reeve
F. Canavero	M. Lanzerotti	T. Samad
O. Malik	G. Zobrist	T. G. Croda

Kenneth Moore, *Director of IEEE Book and Information Services (BIS)*

SECOND EDITION

MEDICAL IMAGE ANALYSIS

ATAM P. DHAWAN

IEEE Engineering in Medicine and Biology Society, *Sponsor*

IEEE Press Series in Biomedical Engineering
Metin Akay, *Series Editor*

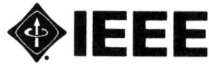

IEEE PRESS

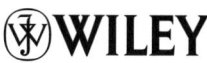

A JOHN WILEY & SONS, INC., PUBLICATION

Copyright © 2011 by the Institute of Electrical and Electronics Engineers, Inc.

Published by John Wiley & Sons, Inc., Hoboken, New Jersey
Published simultaneously in Canada

No part of this publication may be reproduced, stored in a retrieval system, or transmitted in any form or by any means, electronic, mechanical, photocopying, recording, scanning, or otherwise, except as permitted under Section 107 or 108 of the 1976 United States Copyright Act, without either the prior written permission of the Publisher, or authorization through payment of the appropriate per-copy fee to the Copyright Clearance Center, Inc., 222 Rosewood Drive, Danvers, MA 01923, (978) 750-8400, fax (978) 750-4470, or on the web at www.copyright.com. Requests to the Publisher for permission should be addressed to the Permissions Department, John Wiley & Sons, Inc., 111 River Street, Hoboken, NJ 07030, (201) 748-6011, fax (201) 748-6008, or online at http://www.wiley.com/go/permission.

Limit of Liability/Disclaimer of Warranty: While the publisher and author have used their best efforts in preparing this book, they make no representations or warranties with respect to the accuracy or completeness of the contents of this book and specifically disclaim any implied warranties of merchantability or fitness for a particular purpose. No warranty may be created or extended by sales representatives or written sales materials. The advice and strategies contained herein may not be suitable for your situation. You should consult with a professional where appropriate. Neither the publisher nor author shall be liable for any loss of profit or any other commercial damages, including but not limited to special, incidental, consequential, or other damages.

For general information on our other products and services or for technical support, please contact our Customer Care Department within the United States at (800) 762-2974, outside the United States at (317) 572-3993 or fax (317) 572-4002.

Wiley also publishes its books in a variety of electronic formats. Some content that appears in print may not be available in electronic formats. For more information about Wiley products, visit our web site at www.wiley.com.

Library of Congress Cataloging-in-Publication Data is available.

ISBN 978-0-470-622056

Printed in Singapore

oBook: 978-0-470-91854-8
eBook: 978-0-470-91853-1
ePub: 978-0-470-92289-7

10 9 8 7 6 5 4 3 2 1

To my father
Chandar Bhan Dhawan

It is a devotion!

CONTENTS

PREFACE TO THE SECOND EDITION   xiii

CHAPTER 1   **INTRODUCTION**   1

1.1. Medical Imaging: A Collaborative Paradigm   2
1.2. Medical Imaging Modalities   3
1.3. Medical Imaging: from Physiology to Information Processing   6
     1.3.1 Understanding Physiology and Imaging Medium   6
     1.3.2 Physics of Imaging   7
     1.3.3 Imaging Instrumentation   7
     1.3.4 Data Acquisition and Image Reconstruction   7
     1.3.5 Image Analysis and Applications   8
1.4. General Performance Measures   8
     1.4.1 An Example of Performance Measure   10
1.5. Biomedical Image Processing and Analysis   11
1.6. Matlab Image Processing Toolbox   14
     1.6.1 Digital Image Representation   14
     1.6.2 Basic MATLAB Image Toolbox Commands   16
1.7. Imagepro Interface in Matlab Environment and Image Databases   19
     1.7.1 Imagepro Image Processing Interface   19
     1.7.2 Installation Instructions   20
1.8. Imagej and Other Image Processing Software Packages   20
1.9. Exercises   21
1.10. References   22
1.11. Definitions   22

CHAPTER 2   **IMAGE FORMATION**   23

2.1. Image Coordinate System   24
     2.1.1 2-D Image Rotation   25
     2.1.2 3-D Image Rotation and Translation Transformation   26
2.2. Linear Systems   27
2.3. Point Source and Impulse Functions   27
2.4. Probability and Random Variable Functions   29
     2.4.1 Conditional and Joint Probability Density Functions   30
     2.4.2 Independent and Orthogonal Random Variables   31
2.5. Image Formation   32
     2.5.1 PSF and Spatial Resolution   35
     2.5.2 Signal-to-Noise Ratio   37
     2.5.3 Contrast-to-Noise Ratio   39

viii CONTENTS

2.6. Pin-hole Imaging 39
2.7. Fourier Transform 40
    2.7.1 Sinc Function 43
2.8. Radon Transform 44
2.9. Sampling 46
2.10. Discrete Fourier Transform 50
2.11. Wavelet Transform 52
2.12. Exercises 60
2.13. References 62

CHAPTER 3 INTERACTION OF ELECTROMAGNETIC RADIATION WITH MATTER IN MEDICAL IMAGING 65

3.1. Electromagnetic Radiation 65
3.2. Electromagnetic Radiation for Image Formation 66
3.3. Radiation Interaction with Matter 67
    3.3.1 Coherent or Rayleigh Scattering 67
    3.3.2 Photoelectric Absorption 68
    3.3.3 Compton Scattering 69
    3.3.4 Pair Production 69
3.4. Linear Attenuation Coefficient 70
3.5. Radiation Detection 70
    3.5.1 Ionized Chambers and Proportional Counters 70
    3.5.2 Semiconductor Detectors 72
    3.5.3 Advantages of Semiconductor Detectors 73
    3.5.4 Scintillation Detectors 73
3.6. Detector Subsystem Output Voltage Pulse 76
3.7. Exercises 78
3.8. References 78

CHAPTER 4 MEDICAL IMAGING MODALITIES: X-RAY IMAGING 79

4.1. X-Ray Imaging 80
4.2. X-Ray Generation 81
4.3. X-Ray 2-D Projection Imaging 84
4.4. X-Ray Mammography 86
4.5. X-Ray CT 88
4.6. Spiral X-Ray CT 92
4.7. Contrast Agent, Spatial Resolution, and SNR 95
4.8. Exercises 96
4.9. References 97

CHAPTER 5 MEDICAL IMAGING MODALITIES: MAGNETIC RESONANCE IMAGING 99

5.1. MRI Principles 100
5.2. MR Instrumentation 110
5.3. MRI Pulse Sequences 112
    5.3.1 Spin-Echo Imaging 114
    5.3.2 Inversion Recovery Imaging 118

CONTENTS **ix**

        5.3.3   Echo Planar Imaging **119**
        5.3.4   Gradient Echo Imaging **123**
5.4.   Flow Imaging **125**
5.5.   fMRI **129**
5.6.   Diffusion Imaging **130**
5.7.   Contrast, Spatial Resolution, and SNR **135**
5.8.   Exercises **137**
5.9.   References **138**

CHAPTER 6   *NUCLEAR MEDICINE IMAGING MODALITIES*   **139**

6.1.   Radioactivity **139**
6.2.   SPECT **140**
        6.2.1   Detectors and Data Acquisition System **142**
        6.2.2   Contrast, Spatial Resolution, and Signal-to-Noise Ratio in SPECT Imaging **145**
6.3.   PET **148**
        6.3.1   Detectors and Data Acquisition Systems **150**
        6.3.2   Contrast, Spatial Resolution, and SNR in PET Imaging **150**
6.4.   Dual-Modality Spect–CT and PET–CT Scanners **151**
6.5.   Exercises **154**
6.6.   References **155**

CHAPTER 7   *MEDICAL IMAGING MODALITIES: ULTRASOUND IMAGING*   **157**

7.1.   Propagation of Sound in a Medium **157**
7.2.   Reflection and Refraction **159**
7.3.   Transmission of Ultrasound Waves in a Multilayered Medium **160**
7.4.   Attenuation **162**
7.5.   Ultrasound Reflection Imaging **163**
7.6.   Ultrasound Imaging Instrumentation **164**
7.7.   Imaging with Ultrasound: A-Mode **166**
7.8.   Imaging with Ultrasound: M-Mode **167**
7.9.   Imaging with Ultrasound: B-Mode **168**
7.10.   Doppler Ultrasound Imaging **169**
7.11.   Contrast, Spatial Resolution, and SNR **170**
7.12.   Exercises **171**
7.13.   References **172**

CHAPTER 8   *IMAGE RECONSTRUCTION*   **173**

8.1.   Radon Transform and Image Reconstruction **174**
        8.1.1   The Central Slice Theorem **174**
        8.1.2   Inverse Radon Transform **176**
        8.1.3   Backprojection Method **176**
8.2.   Iterative Algebraic Reconstruction Methods **180**
8.3.   Estimation Methods **182**
8.4.   Fourier Reconstruction Methods **185**
8.5.   Image Reconstruction in Medical Imaging Modalities **186**
        8.5.1   Image Reconstruction in X-Ray CT **186**

        8.5.2   Image Reconstruction in Nuclear Emission Computed
                Tomography: SPECT and PET   **188**
                8.5.2.1   A General Approach to ML–EM Algorithms   **189**
                8.5.2.2   A Multigrid EM Algorithm   **190**
        8.5.3   Image Reconstruction in Magnetic Resonance Imaging   **192**
        8.5.4   Image Reconstruction in Ultrasound Imaging   **193**
8.6.   Exercises   **194**
8.7.   References   **195**

CHAPTER 9   IMAGE PROCESSING AND ENHANCEMENT   **199**

9.1.   Spatial Domain Methods   **200**
        9.1.1   Histogram Transformation and Equalization   **201**
        9.1.2   Histogram Modification   **203**
        9.1.3   Image Averaging   **204**
        9.1.4   Image Subtraction   **204**
        9.1.5   Neighborhood Operations   **205**
                9.1.5.1   Median Filter   **207**
                9.1.5.2   Adaptive Arithmetic Mean Filter   **207**
                9.1.5.3   Image Sharpening and Edge Enhancement   **208**
                9.1.5.4   Feature Enhancement Using Adaptive Neighborhood
                          Processing   **209**
9.2.   Frequency Domain Filtering   **212**
        9.2.1   Wiener Filtering   **213**
        9.2.2   Constrained Least Square Filtering   **214**
        9.2.3   Low-Pass Filtering   **215**
        9.2.4   High-Pass Filtering   **217**
        9.2.5   Homomorphic Filtering   **217**
9.3.   Wavelet Transform for Image Processing   **220**
        9.3.1   Image Smoothing and Enhancement Using Wavelet
                Transform   **223**
9.4.   Exercises   **226**
9.5.   References   **228**

CHAPTER 10   IMAGE SEGMENTATION   **229**

10.1.   Edge-Based Image Segmentation   **229**
        10.1.1   Edge Detection Operations   **230**
        10.1.2   Boundary Tracking   **231**
        10.1.3   Hough Transform   **233**
10.2.   Pixel-Based Direct Classification Methods   **235**
        10.2.1   Optimal Global Thresholding   **237**
        10.2.2   Pixel Classification Through Clustering   **239**
                10.2.2.1   Data Clustering   **239**
                10.2.2.2   k-Means Clustering   **241**
                10.2.2.3   Fuzzy c-Means Clustering   **242**
                10.2.2.4   An Adaptive FCM Algorithm   **244**
10.3.   Region-Based Segmentation   **245**
        10.3.1   Region-Growing   **245**
        10.3.2   Region-Splitting   **247**

10.4. Advanced Segmentation Methods 248
    10.4.1 Estimation-Model Based Adaptive Segmentation 249
    10.4.2 Image Segmentation Using Neural Networks 254
        10.4.2.1 Backpropagation Neural Network for Classification 255
        10.4.2.2 The RBF Network 258
        10.4.2.3 Segmentation of Arterial Structure in Digital Subtraction Angiograms 259
10.5. Exercises 261
10.6. References 262

CHAPTER 11 IMAGE REPRESENTATION, ANALYSIS, AND CLASSIFICATION 265

11.1. Feature Extraction and Representation 268
    11.1.1 Statistical Pixel-Level Features 268
    11.1.2 Shape Features 270
        11.1.2.1 Boundary Encoding: Chain Code 271
        11.1.2.2 Boundary Encoding: Fourier Descriptor 273
        11.1.2.3 Moments for Shape Description 273
        11.1.2.4 Morphological Processing for Shape Description 274
    11.1.3 Texture Features 280
    11.1.4 Relational Features 282
11.2. Feature Selection for Classification 283
    11.2.1 Linear Discriminant Analysis 285
    11.2.2 PCA 288
    11.2.3 GA-Based Optimization 289
11.3. Feature and Image Classification 292
    11.3.1 Statistical Classification Methods 292
        11.3.1.1 Nearest Neighbor Classifier 293
        11.3.1.2 Bayesian Classifier 293
    11.3.2 Rule-Based Systems 294
    11.3.3 Neural Network Classifiers 296
        11.3.3.1 Neuro-Fuzzy Pattern Classification 296
    11.3.4 Support Vector Machine for Classification 302
11.4. Image Analysis and Classification Example: "Difficult-To-Diagnose" Mammographic Microcalcifications 303
11.5. Exercises 306
11.6. References 307

CHAPTER 12 IMAGE REGISTRATION 311

12.1. Rigid-Body Transformation 314
    12.1.1 Affine Transformation 316
12.2. Principal Axes Registration 316
12.3. Iterative Principal Axes Registration 319
12.4. Image Landmarks and Features-Based Registration 323
    12.4.1 Similarity Transformation for Point-Based Registration 323
    12.4.2 Weighted Features-Based Registration 324
12.5. Elastic Deformation-Based Registration 325
12.6. Exercises 330
12.7. References 331

CHAPTER 13 IMAGE VISUALIZATION — 335

- 13.1. Feature-Enhanced 2-D Image Display Methods 336
- 13.2. Stereo Vision and Semi-3-D Display Methods 336
- 13.3. Surface- and Volume-Based 3-D Display Methods 338
    - 13.3.1 Surface Visualization 339
    - 13.3.2 Volume Visualization 344
- 13.4. VR-Based Interactive Visualization 347
    - 13.4.1 Virtual Endoscopy 349
- 13.5. Exercises 349
- 13.6. References 350

CHAPTER 14 CURRENT AND FUTURE TRENDS IN MEDICAL IMAGING AND IMAGE ANALYSIS — 353

- 14.1. Multiparameter Medical Imaging and Analysis 353
- 14.2. Targeted Imaging 357
- 14.3. Optical Imaging and Other Emerging Modalities 357
    - 14.3.1 Optical Microscopy 358
    - 14.3.2 Optical Endoscopy 360
    - 14.3.3 Optical Coherence Tomography 360
    - 14.3.4 Diffuse Reflectance and Transillumination Imaging 362
    - 14.3.5 Photoacoustic Imaging: An Emerging Technology 363
- 14.4. Model-Based and Multiscale Analysis 364
- 14.5. References 366

INDEX — 369

PREFACE TO THE SECOND EDITION

Radiological sciences in the last two decades have witnessed a revolutionary progress in medical imaging and computerized medical image processing. The development and advances in multidimensional medical imaging modalities such as X-ray mammography, X-ray computed tomography (X-ray CT), single photon computed tomography (SPECT), positron emission tomography (PET), ultrasound, magnetic resonance imaging (MRI), and functional magnetic resonance imaging (fMRI) have provided important radiological tools in disease diagnosis, treatment evaluation, and intervention for significant improvement in health care. The development of imaging instrumentation has inspired the evolution of new computerized methods of image reconstruction, processing, and analysis for better understanding and interpretation of medical images. Image processing and analysis methods have been used to help physicians to make important medical decisions through physician–computer interaction. Recently, intelligent or model-based quantitative image analysis approaches have been explored for computer-aided diagnosis to improve the sensitivity and specificity of radiological tests involving medical images.

Medical imaging in diagnostic radiology has evolved as a result of the significant contributions of a number of disciplines from basic sciences, engineering, and medicine. Computerized image reconstruction, processing, and analysis methods have been developed for medical imaging applications. The application-domain knowledge has been used in developing models for accurate analysis and interpretation.

In this book, I have made an effort to cover the fundamentals of medical imaging and image reconstruction, processing, and analysis along with brief descriptions of recent developments. Although the field of medical imaging and image analysis has a wide range of applications supported by a large number of advanced methods, I have tried to include the important developments with examples and recent references. The contents of the book should enable a reader to establish basic as well as advanced understanding of major approaches. The book can be used for a senior undergraduate or graduate-level course in medical image analysis and should be helpful in preparing the reader to understand the research issues at the cutting edge. Students should have some knowledge of probability, linear systems, and digital signal processing to take full advantage of the book. References are provided at the end of each chapter. Laboratory exercises for implementation in the MATLAB environment are included. A library of selected radiological images and MATLAB programs demonstrating medical image processing and analysis tasks can be obtained from the following ftp site:

ftp://ftp.wiley.com/public/sci_tech_med/medical_image/

Readers can download Imagepro MATLAB interface files to be installed with MATLAB software to provide a Graphical User Interface (GUI) to perform several image processing functions and exercises described in this book. This ftp site also contains several medical image databases with X-ray mammography, X-ray CT, MRI, and PET images of the brain or full body scans of human patients. Figures included in this book with color or black-and-white illustrations are provided in a separate folder. Additional supporting material includes Microsoft Power-Point slides for sample lectures. Thanks to Wiley-IEEE Press for providing and maintaining the ftp site for this book.

I am pleased that the first edition of this book, published in 2003, was very well received and used as a textbook in many universities worldwide. I have carefully revised and expanded the second edition with several new sections and additional material to provide a stronger and broader foundation to readers and students. Chapter 4 of the first edition, which included all four major medical imaging modalities (X-ray, MRI, nuclear medicine, and ultrasound), is now expanded into four individual chapters focused on each modality in greater detail. Several new sections with more details on principles of feature selection and classification have been added in chapters covering the image processing and analysis part of the book.

Chapter 1 presents an overview of medical imaging modalities and their role in radiology and medicine. It introduces the concept of a multidisciplinary paradigm in intelligent medical image analysis. Medical imaging modalities are presented according to the type of signal used in image formation.

Chapter 2 describes the basic principles of image formation and reviews the essential mathematical foundation and transforms. Additional methods such as wavelet transforms and neural networks are not described in this chapter but are explained in later chapters with applications to medical image enhancement, segmentation, and analysis.

Chapter 3 provides an overview of electromagnetic (EM) interaction of energy particles with matter and presents basic principles of detection and measurements in medical imaging.

Chapter 4 describes the principles, instrumentation, and data acquisition methods of X-ray imaging modalities including X-ray radiograph imaging, X-ray mammography, and X-ray CT.

Chapter 5 provides a complete spectrum of MRI modalities including fMRI and diffusion tensor imaging (DTI). Instrumentation and imaging pulse sequences are discussed.

Chapter 6 discusses nuclear medicine imaging modalities including SPECT and PET with more details on detectors and data acquisition systems.

Chapter 7 provides ultrasound imaging principles and methods for real-time imaging. Data acquisition and instrumentation control systems for ultrasound imaging are discussed with dynamic medical imaging applications.

Chapter 8 presents various image reconstruction algorithms used and investigated in different imaging modalities. It starts with the introduction of two-dimensional and three-dimensional image reconstruction methods using the Radon transform. The chapter then continues with the iterative and model-based reconstruction methods.

Chapter 9 starts with the preliminaries in image processing and enhancements. Various methods for image smoothing and enhancement, to improve image quality for visual examination as well as computerized analysis, are described.

Chapter 10 presents the image segmentation methods for edge and region feature extraction and representation. Advanced and model-based methods for image segmentation using wavelet transform and neural networks are described.

Chapter 11 presents feature extraction and analysis methods for qualitative and quantitative analysis and understanding. The role of using a priori knowledge in adaptive, model-based, and interactive medical image processing methods is emphasized. These methods are discussed for classification, quantitative analysis, and interpretation of radiological images. Recent approaches with neural network-based image analysis and classification are also presented.

Chapter 12 describes recent advances in multimodality medical image registration and analysis. Emphasis is given on model-based and interactive approaches for better performance in registering multidimensional multimodality brain images. Registration of brain images is discussed in detail as an example of image registration methods.

Chapter 13 describes multidimensional methods for image visualization. Feature-based surface and volume rendering methods as well as intelligent adaptive methods for dynamic visualization are presented. Recent advances in multiparameter visualization with virtual reality-based navigation are also presented.

Chapter 14 presents some remarks on current and future trends in medical imaging, processing, analysis, and interpretation and their role in computer-aided-diagnosis, image-guided surgery, and other radiological applications. Recent advances in multispectral optical imaging are also introduced.

I would like to thank Metin Akay for his support, encouragement, and comments on the book. I would also like to thank my previous graduate students, M.V. Ranganath, Louis Arata, Thomas Dufresne, Charles Peck, Christine Bonasso, Timothy Donnier, Anne Sicsu, Prashanth Kini, Aleksander Zavaljevski, Sven Loncaric, Alok Sarwal, Amar Raheja, Shuangshuang Dai, and Brian D'Alssandro. Some of the material included in this book is based on the dissertation work done by graduate students under my supervision. Thanks are also due to Sachin Patwardhan, who conducted laboratory exercises in the MATLAB environment. Special thanks to Dr. Kuo-Sheng Cheng for his valuable comments and reviews. I would also like to thank Mary Mann from John Wiley & Sons, Inc., and Naomi Fernandez from Mathworks for their support during the entire writing of this book.

I thank my wife, Nilam, and my sons, Anirudh and Akshay, for their support and patience during the weekends and holidays when I was continuously writing to finish this book.

ATAM P. DHAWAN

Newark, New Jersey
July 2010

CHAPTER 1

INTRODUCTION

The last two decades have witnessed significant advances in medical imaging and computerized medical image processing. These advances have led to new two-, three-, and multidimensional imaging modalities that have become important clinical tools in diagnostic radiology. The clinical significance of radiological imaging modalities in diagnosis and treatment of diseases is overwhelming. While planar X-ray imaging was the only radiological imaging method in the early part of the last century, several modern imaging modalities are in practice today to acquire anatomical, physiological, metabolic, and functional information from the human body. Commonly used medical imaging modalities capable of producing multidimensional images for radiological applications are X-ray computed tomography (X-ray CT), magnetic resonance imaging (MRI), single photon emission computed tomography (SPECT), positron emission tomography (PET), and ultrasound. It should be noted that these modern imaging methods involve sophisticated instrumentation and equipment using high-speed electronics and computers for data collection and image reconstruction and display. Simple planar radiographic imaging methods such as chest X rays and mammograms usually provide images on a film that is exposed during imaging through an external radiation source (X ray) and then developed to show images of body organs. These planar radiographic imaging methods provide high-quality analog images that are shadows or two-dimensional (2-D) projected images of three-dimensional (3-D) organs. Recent complex medical imaging modalities such as X-ray CT, MRI, SPECT, PET, and ultrasound heavily utilize computer technology for creation and display of digital images. Using the computer, multidimensional digital images of physiological structures can be processed and manipulated to visualize hidden characteristic diagnostic features that are difficult or impossible to see with planar imaging methods. Further, these features of interest can be quantified and analyzed using sophisticated computer programs and models to understand their behavior to help with a diagnosis or to evaluate treatment protocols. Nevertheless, the clinical significance of simple planar imaging methods such as X-ray radiographs (e.g., chest X ray and mammograms) must not be underestimated as they offer cost-effective and reliable screening tools that often provide important diagnostic information sufficient to make correct diagnosis and judgment about the treatment.

However, in many critical radiological applications, the multidimensional visualization and quantitative analysis of physiological structures provide unprecedented clinical information extremely valuable for diagnosis and treatment.

Medical Image Analysis, Second Edition, by Atam P. Dhawan
Copyright © 2011 by the Institute of Electrical and Electronics Engineers, Inc.

Computerized processing and analysis of medical imaging modalities provides a powerful tool to help physicians. Thus, computer programs and methods to process and manipulate the raw data from medical imaging scanners must be carefully developed to preserve and enhance the real clinical information of interest rather than introducing additional artifacts. The ability to improve diagnostic information from medical images can be further enhanced by designing computer processing algorithms intelligently. Often, incorporating relevant knowledge about the physics of imaging, instrumentation, and human physiology in computer programs provides outstanding improvement in image quality as well as analysis to help interpretation. For example, incorporating knowledge about the geometrical location of the source, detector, and patient can reduce the geometric artifacts in the reconstructed images. Further, the use of geometrical locations and characteristic signatures in computer-aided enhancement, identification, segmentation, and analysis of physiological structures of interest often improves the clinical interpretation of medical images.

1.1. MEDICAL IMAGING: A COLLABORATIVE PARADIGM

As discussed above, with the advent and enhancement of modern medical imaging modalities, intelligent processing of multidimensional images has become crucial in conventional or computer-aided interpretation for radiological and diagnostic applications. Medical imaging and processing in diagnostic radiology has evolved with significant contributions from a number of disciplines including mathematics, physics, chemistry, engineering, and medicine. This is evident when one sees a medical imaging scanner such as an MRI or PET scanner. The complexity of instrumentation and computer-aided data collection and image reconstruction methods clearly indicates the importance of system integration as well as a critical understanding of the physics of imaging and image formation. Intelligent interpretation of medical images requires understanding the interaction of the basic unit of imaging (such as protons in MRI, or X-ray photons in X-ray CT) in a biological environment, formation of a quantifiable signal representing the biological information, detection and acquisition of the signal of interest, and appropriate image reconstruction. In brief, intelligent interpretation and analysis of biomedical images require an understanding of the acquisition of images.

A number of computer vision methods have been developed for a variety of applications in image processing, segmentation, analysis, and recognition. However, medical image reconstruction and processing requires specialized knowledge of the specific medical imaging modality that is used to acquire images. The character of the collected data in the application environment (such as imaging the heart through MRI) should be properly understood for selecting or developing useful methods for intelligent image processing, analysis, and interpretation. The use of application domain knowledge can be useful in selecting or developing the most appropriate image reconstruction and processing methods for accurate analysis and interpretation.

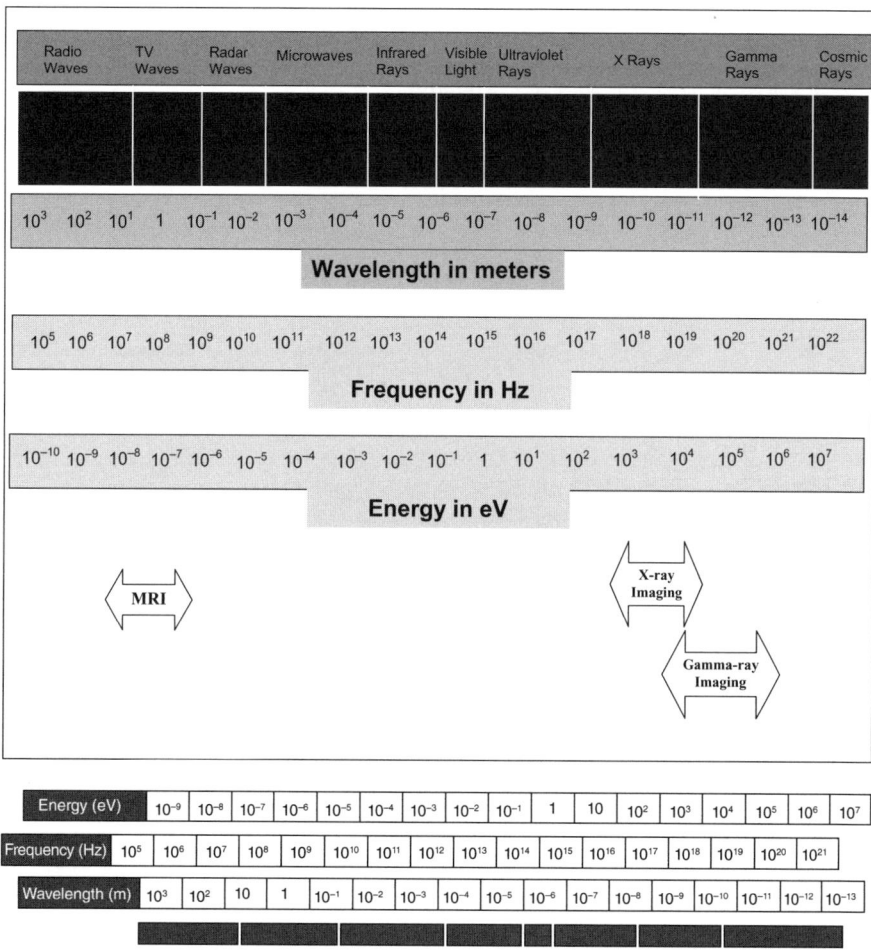

Figure 1.1 Energy sources for different medical imaging modalities.

1.2. MEDICAL IMAGING MODALITIES

The field of medical imaging and image analysis has evolved due to the collective contributions from many areas of medicine, engineering, and basic sciences. The overall objective of medical imaging is to acquire useful information about the physiological processes or organs of the body by using external or internal sources of energy (1–3). Figure 1.1 classifies energy sources for different medical imaging modalities. Imaging methods available today for radiological applications may use external, internal or a combination of energy sources (Fig. 1.2). In most commonly used imaging methods, ionized radiation such as X rays is used as an external energy source primarily for anatomical imaging. Such anatomical imaging modalities are based on the attenuation coefficient of radiation passing through the body. For

4 CHAPTER 1 INTRODUCTION

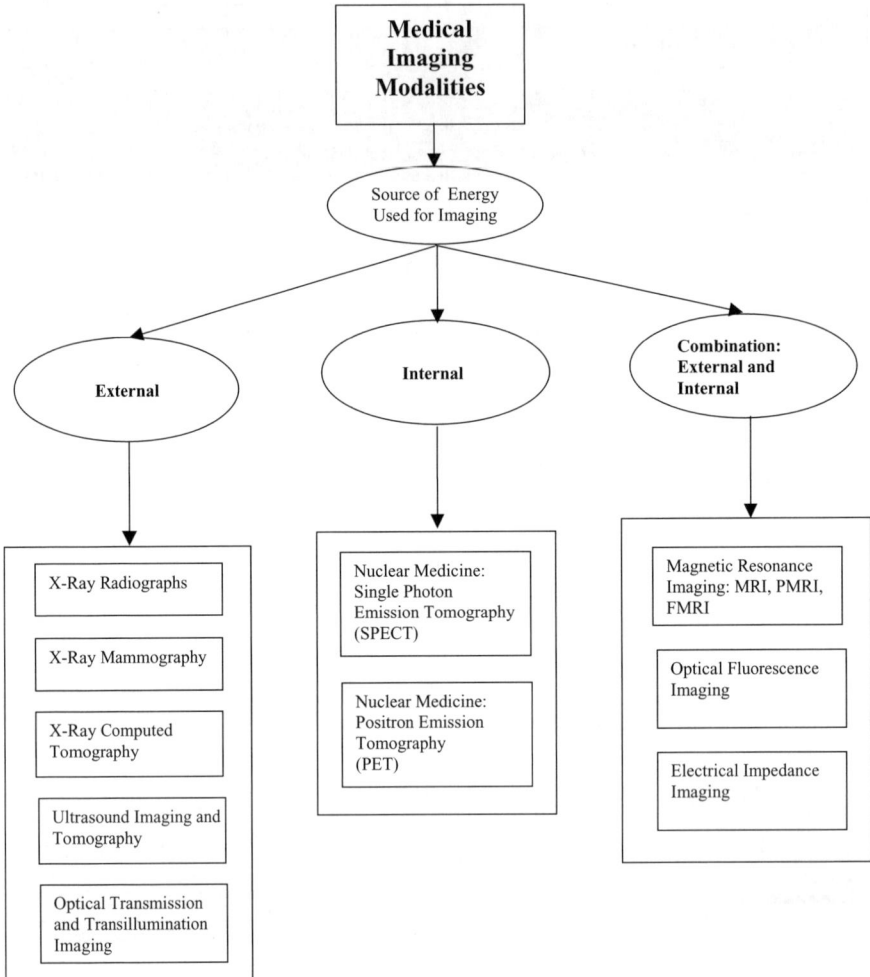

Figure 1.2 A classification of different medical imaging modalities with respect to the type of energy source used for imaging.

example, X-ray radiographs and X-ray CT imaging modalities measure attenuation coefficients of X ray that are based on the density of the tissue or part of the body being imaged. The images of chest radiographs show a spatial distribution of X-ray attenuation coefficients reflecting the overall density variations of the anatomical parts in the chest. Another example of external energy source-based imaging is ultrasound or acoustic imaging. Nuclear medicine imaging modalities use an internal energy source through an emission process to image the human body. For emission imaging, radioactive pharmaceuticals are injected into the body to interact with selected body matter or tissue to form an internal source of radioactive energy that is used for imaging. The emission imaging principle is applied in SPECT and PET. Such types of nuclear medicine imaging modalities provide useful metabolic information about the physiological functions of the organs. Further, a clever combination of external stimulation on internal energy sources can be used in medical imaging to acquire more accurate information about the tissue material and physiological responses and functions. MRI uses external magnetic energy to stimulate selected atomic nuclei such as hydrogen protons. The excited nuclei become the internal source of energy to provide electromagnetic signals for imaging through the process of relaxation. MRI of the human body provides high-resolution images of the human body with excellent soft-tissue characterization capabilities. Recent advances in MRI have led to perfusion and functional imaging aspects of human tissue and organs (3–6). Another emerging biophysiological imaging modality is fluorescence imaging, which uses an external ultraviolet energy source to stimulate the internal biological molecules of interest, which absorb the ultraviolet energy, become internal sources of energy, and then emit the energy at visible electromagnetic radiation wavelengths (7).

Before a type of energy source or imaging modality is selected, it is important to understand the nature of physiological information needed for image formation. In other words, some basic questions about the information of interest should be answered. What information about the human body is needed? Is it anatomical, physiological, or functional? What range of spatial resolution is acceptable? The selection of a specific medical imaging modality often depends on the type of suspected disease or localization needed for proper radiological diagnosis. For example, some neurological disorders and diseases demand very high resolution brain images for accurate diagnosis and treatment. On the other hand, full-body SPECT imaging to study metastasizing cancer does not require submillimeter imaging resolution. The information of interest here is cancer metastasis in the tissue, which can be best obtained from the blood flow in the tissue or its metabolism. Breast imaging can be performed using X rays, magnetic resonance, nuclear medicine, or ultrasound. But the most effective and economical breast imaging modality so far has been X-ray mammography because of its simplicity, portability, and low cost. One important source of radiological information for breast imaging is the presence and distribution of microcalcifications in the breast. This anatomical information can be obtained with high resolution using X rays.

There is no perfect imaging modality for all radiological applications and needs. In addition, each medical imaging modality is limited by the corresponding physics of energy interactions with human body (or cells), instrumentation, and often physiological constraints. These factors severely affect the quality and resolution of images, sometimes making the interpretation and diagnosis difficult. The performance of an imaging modality for a specific test or application is characterized by sensitivity and specificity factors. Sensitivity of a medical imaging test is defined primarily by its ability to detect true information. Let us suppose we have an X-ray imaging scanner for mammography. The sensitivity for imaging microcalcifications for a mammography scanner depends on many factors including the X-ray wavelength used in the beam, intensity, and polychromatic distribution of the input radiation beam, behavior of X rays in breast tissue such as absorption and scattering coefficients, and film/detector efficiency to collect the output radiation. These factors eventually affect the overall signal-to-noise ratio leading to the loss of sensitivity of detecting microcalcifications. The specificity for a test depends on its ability to not detect information when it is truly not there.

1.3. MEDICAL IMAGING: FROM PHYSIOLOGY TO INFORMATION PROCESSING

From physiology to image interpretation and information retrieval, medical imaging may be defined as a five-step paradigm (see Fig. 1.3). The five-step paradigm allows acquisition and analysis of useful information to understand the behavior of an organ or a physiological process.

1.3.1 Understanding Physiology and Imaging Medium

The imaged objects (organs, tissues, and specific pathologies) and associated physiological properties that could be used for obtaining signals suitable for the formation of an image must be studied for the selection of imaging instrumentation. This information is useful in designing image processing and analysis techniques for correct interpretation. Information about the imaging medium may involve static or dynamic properties of the biological tissue. For example, tissue density is a static property that causes attenuation of an external radiation beam in X-ray imaging modality. Blood flow, perfusion, and cardiac motion are examples of dynamic physiological properties that may alter the image of a biological entity. Consideration of the dynamic behavior of the imaging medium is essential in designing compensation methods needed for correct image reconstruction and analysis. Motion artifacts pose serious limitations on data collection time and resolution in medical imaging instrumentation and therefore have a direct effect on the development of image processing methods.

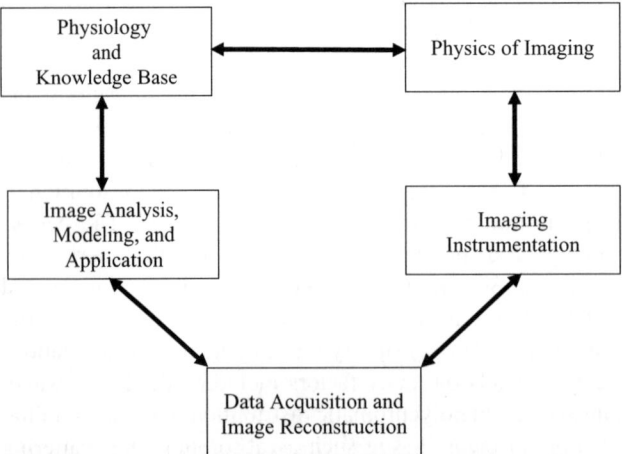

Figure 1.3 A collaborative multidisciplinary paradigm of medical imaging research and applications.

1.3.2 Physics of Imaging

The next important consideration is the principle of imaging to be used for obtaining the data. For example, X-ray imaging modality uses transmission of X rays through the body as the basis of imaging. On the other hand, in the nuclear medicine modality, SPECT uses the emission of gamma rays resulting from the interaction of a radiopharmaceutical substance with the target tissue. The emission process and the energy range of gamma rays cause limitations on the resolution and data acquisition time for imaging. The associated methods for image formation in transmission and emission imaging modalities are so different that it is difficult to see the same level of anatomical information from both modalities. SPECT and PET provide images that are poor in contrast and anatomical details, while X-ray CT provides sharper images with high-resolution anatomical details. MRI provides high-resolution anatomical details with excellent soft-tissue contrast (6, 7).

1.3.3 Imaging Instrumentation

The instrumentation used in collecting the data is one of the most important factors defining the image quality in terms of signal-to-noise ratio, resolution, and ability to show diagnostic information. Source specifications of the instrumentation directly affect imaging capabilities. In addition, detector responses such as nonlinearity, low efficiency, long decay time, and poor scatter rejection may cause artifacts in the image. An intelligent image formation and processing technique should be the one that provides accurate and robust detection of features of interest without any artifacts to help diagnostic interpretation.

1.3.4 Data Acquisition and Image Reconstruction

The data acquisition methods used in imaging play an important role in image formation. Optimized with the imaging instrumentation, the data collection methods become a decisive factor in determining the best temporal and spatial resolution. It is also crucial in developing strategies to reduce image artifacts through active filtering or postprocessing methods. For example, in X-ray CT, the spatially distributed signal is based on the number of X-ray photons reaching the detector within a time interval. The data for 3-D imaging may be obtained using a parallel-, cone-, or spiral-beam scanning method. Each of these scanning methods causes certain constraints on the geometrical reconstruction of the object under imaging. Since the scanning time in each method may be different, spatial resolution has to be balanced by temporal resolution. This means that a faster scan would result in an image with a lower spatial resolution. On the other hand, a higher spatial resolution method would normally require longer imaging time. In dynamic studies where information about blood flow or a specific functional activity needs to be acquired, the higher resolution requirement is usually compromised. Image reconstruction algorithms such as backprojection, iterative, and Fourier transform methods are tailored to incorporate specific information about the data collection methods and scanning geometry. Since the image quality may be affected by the data collection methods, the image reconstruction and processing methods should be designed to optimize the representation of diagnostic information in the image.

1.3.5 Image Analysis and Applications

Image processing and analysis methods are aimed at the enhancement of diagnostic information to improve manual or computer-assisted interpretation of medical images. Often, certain transformation methods improve the visibility and quantification of features of interest. Interactive and computer-assisted intelligent medical image analysis methods can provide effective tools to help the quantitative and qualitative interpretation of medical images for differential diagnosis, intervention, and treatment monitoring. Intelligent image processing and analysis tools can also help in understanding physiological processes associated with the disease and its response to a treatment.

1.4. GENERAL PERFORMANCE MEASURES

Let us define some measures often used in the evaluation of a medical imaging or diagnostic test for detecting an object such as microcalcifications or a physiological condition such as cancer. A "positive" observation in an image means that the object was observed in the test. A "negative" observation means that the object was not observed in the test. A "true condition" is the actual truth, while an observation is the outcome of the test. Four basic measures are defined from the set of true conditions and observed information as shown in Figure 1.4. These basic measures are true positive, false positive, false negative, and true negative rates or fractions. For example, an X-ray mammographic image should show only the regions of pixels with bright intensity (observed information) corresponding to the microcalcification areas (true condition when the object is present). Also, the mammographic image should not show similar regions of pixels with bright intensity corresponding to the

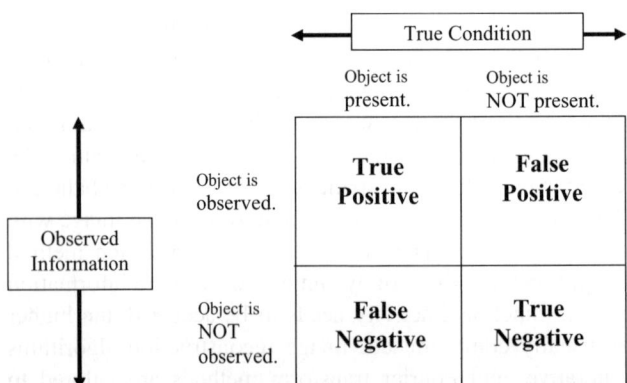

Figure 1.4 A conditional matrix for defining four basic performance measures of receiver operating characteristic curve (ROC) analysis.

1.4. GENERAL PERFORMANCE MEASURES

areas where there is actually no microcalcification (true condition when the object is not present).

Let us assume the total number of examination cases to be N_{tot}, out of which N_{tp} cases have positive true condition with the actual presence of the object and the remaining cases, N_{tn}, have negative true condition with no object present. Let us suppose these cases are examined via the test for which we need to evaluate accuracy, sensitivity, and specificity factors. Considering the observer does not cause any loss of information or misinterpretation, let N_{otp} (true positive) be the number of positive observations from N_{tp} positive true condition cases and N_{ofn} (false negative) be the number of negative observations from N_{tp} positive true condition cases. Also, let N_{otn} (true negative) be the number of negative observations from N_{tn} negative true condition cases and N_{ofp} (false positive) be the number of positive observations from N_{tn} negative true condition cases.

Thus,

$$N_{tp} = N_{otp} + N_{ofn} \quad \text{and} \quad N_{tn} = N_{ofp} + N_{otn}.$$

1. True positive fraction (TPF) is the ratio of the number of positive observations to the number of positive true condition cases.

$$\text{TPF} = N_{otp}/N_{tp}. \tag{1.1}$$

2. False negative fraction (FNF) is the ratio of the number of negative observations to the number of positive true condition cases.

$$\text{FNF} = N_{ofn}/N_{tp} \tag{1.2}$$

3. False positive fraction (FPF) is the ratio of the number of positive observations to the number of negative true condition cases.

$$\text{FPF} = N_{ofp}/N_{tn} \tag{1.3}$$

4. True negative fraction (TNF) is the ratio of the number of negative observations to the number of negative true condition cases.

$$\text{TNF} = N_{otn}/N_{tn} \tag{1.4}$$

It should be noted that

$$\text{TPF} + \text{FNF} = 1$$
$$\text{TNF} + \text{FPF} = 1. \tag{1.5}$$

A graph between TPF and FPF is called a receiver operating characteristic (ROC) curve for a specific medical imaging or diagnostic test for detection of an object. Various points on the ROC curves shown in Figure 1.5 indicate different decision thresholds used for classification of the examination cases into positive and negative observations, and therefore defining specific sets of paired values of TPF and FPF. It should also be noted that statistical random trials with equal probability of positive and negative observations would lead to the diagonally placed straight line as the ROC curve. Different tests and different observers may lead to different ROC curves for the same object detection.

TPF

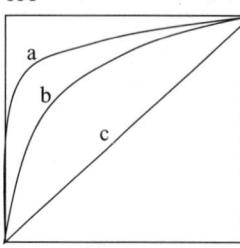

FPF

Figure 1.5 ROC curves, with "a" indicating better classification ability than "b," and "c" showing the random probability.

True positive fraction is also called the sensitivity while the true negative fraction is known as specificity of the test for detection of an object. Accuracy of the test is given by a ratio of correct observation to the total number of examination cases. Thus,

$$\text{Accuracy} = (N_{otp} + N_{otn})/N_{tot}. \tag{1.6}$$

The positive predictive value (PPV) considered to be the same as precision of a diagnostic test is measured as

$$\text{PPV} = N_{otp}/(N_{otp} + N_{ofp}). \tag{1.7}$$

In other words, different imaging modalities and observers may lead to different accuracy, PPV, sensitivity, and specificity levels.

The accuracy, sensitivity, and specificity factors are given serious consideration when selecting a modality for radiological applications. For example, X-ray mammography is so successful in breast imaging because it provides excellent sensitivity and specificity for imaging breast calcifications. In neurological applications requiring a demanding soft-tissue contrast, however, MRI provides better sensitivity and specificity factors than X-ray imaging.

1.4.1 An Example of Performance Measure

Let us assume that 100 female patients were examined with X-ray mammography. The images were observed by a physician to classify into one of the two classes: normal and cancer. The objective here is to determine the basic performance measures of X-ray mammography for detection of breast cancer. Let us assume that all patients were also tested through tissue-biopsy examination to determine the true condition. If the result of the biopsy examination is positive, the cancer (object) is present as the true condition. If the biopsy examination is negative, the cancer (object) is not present as the true condition. If the physician diagnoses the cancer from X-ray mammography, the object (cancer) is observed. Let us assume the following distribution of patients with respect to the true conditions and observed information:

1. Total number of patients = $N_{tot} = 100$
2. Total number of patients with biopsy-proven cancer (true condition of object present) = $N_{tp} = 10$
3. Total number of patients with biopsy-proven normal tissue (true condition of object NOT present) = $N_{tn} = 90$
4. Of the patients with cancer N_{tp}, the number of patients diagnosed by the physician as having cancer = number of true positive cases = $N_{otp} = 8$
5. Of the patients with cancer N_{tp}, the number of patients diagnosed by the physician as normal = number of false negative cases = $N_{ofn} = 2$
6. Of the normal patients N_{tn}, the number of patients rated by the physician as normal = number of true negative cases = $N_{otn} = 85$
7. Of the normal patients N_{tn}, the number of patients rated by the physician as having cancer = number of false positive cases = $N_{ofp} = 5$

Now the TPF, FNF, FPF, and TNF can be computed as

$$TPF = 8/10 = 0.8$$
$$FNF = 2/10 = 0.2$$
$$FPF = 5/90 = 0.0556$$
$$TNF = 85/90 = 0.9444$$

This should be noted that the above values satisfy Equation 1.5 as

$$TPF + FNF = 1.0 \quad \text{and} \quad FPF + TNF = 1.0$$

1.5. BIOMEDICAL IMAGE PROCESSING AND ANALYSIS

A general-purpose biomedical image processing and image analysis system must have three basic components: an image acquisition system, a digital computer, and an image display environment. Figure 1.6 shows a schematic block diagram of a biomedical image processing and analysis system.

The image acquisition system usually converts a biomedical signal or radiation carrying the information of interest to a digital image. A digital image is

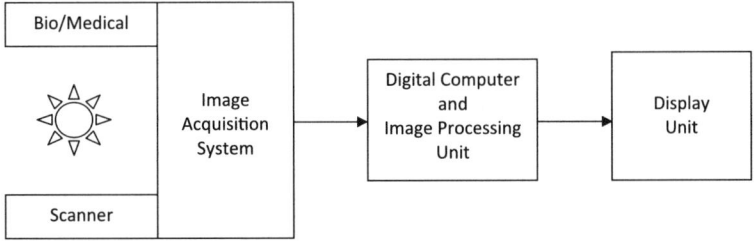

Figure 1.6 A general schematic diagram of biomedical image analysis system.

represented by an array of digital numbers that can be read by the processing computer and displayed as a two-, three-, or multidimensional image. As introduced above, medical imaging modalities use different image acquisition systems as a part of the imaging instrumentation. The design of the image acquisition system depends on the type of modality and detector requirements. In some applications, the output of the scanner may be in analog form, such as a film-mammogram or a chest X-ray radiograph. In such applications, the image acquisition system may include a suitable light source to illuminate the radiograph (the film) and a digitizing camera to convert the analog image into a digital picture. Other means of digitizing an image include several types of microdensitometers and laser scanners. There is a variety of sources of biomedical imaging applications. The data acquisition system has to be modified accordingly. For example, a microscope can be directly hooked up with a digitizing camera for acquisition of images of a biopsy sample on a glass slide. But such a digitizing camera is not needed for obtaining images from an X-ray CT scanner. Thus, the image acquisition system differs across applications.

The second part of the biomedical image processing and analysis system is a computer used to store digital images for further processing. A general-purpose computer or a dedicated array processor can be used for image analysis. The dedicated hardwired image processors may be used for the real-time image processing operations such as image enhancement, pseudo-color enhancement, mapping, and histogram analysis.

A third essential part of the biomedical image processing and analysis system is the image display environment where the output image can be viewed after the required processing. Depending on the application, there may be a large variation in the requirements of image display environment in terms of resolution grid size, number of gray levels, number of colors, split-screen access, and so on. There might be other output devices such as a hard-copy output machine or printer that can also be used in conjunction with the regular output display monitor.

For an advanced biomedical image analysis system, the image display environment may also include a real-time image processing unit that may have some built-in processing functions for quick manipulation. The central image processing unit, in such systems, does the more complicated image processing and analysis only. For example, for radiological applications, the image display unit should have a fast and flexible environment to manipulate the area of interest in the image. This manipulation may include gray-level remapping, pseudo-color enhancement, zoom-in, or split-screen capabilities to aid the attending physician in seeing more diagnostic information right away. This type of real-time image processing may be part of the image-display environment in a modern sophisticated image analysis system that is designed for handling the image analysis and interpretation tasks for biomedical applications (and many others). The display environment in such systems includes one or more pixel processors or point processors (small processing units or single-board computers) along with a number of memory planes, which act as buffers. These buffers or memory planes provide an efficient means of implementing a number of look-up-tables (LUTs) without losing the original image data. The specialized hardwired processing units including dedicated processors are accessed and communicated with by using the peripheral devices such as keyboard, data tablet, mouse, printer, and high-resolution monitors.

There are several image processing systems available today that satisfy the usual requirements (as discussed above) of an efficient and useful biomedical image analysis system. All these systems are based on a special pipeline architecture with an external host computer and/or an array processor allowing parallel processing and efficient communication among various dedicated processors for real-time or near real-time split-screen image manipulation and processing performance. Special-purpose image processing architectures includes array processors, graphic accelerators, logic processors, and field programmable gate arrays (FPGA).

As discussed above, every imaging modality has limitations that affect the accuracy, sensitivity, and specificity factors, which are extremely important in diagnostic radiology. Scanners are usually equipped with instrumentation to provide external radiation or energy source (as needed) and measure an output signal from the body. The output signal may be attenuated radiation or another from of energy carrying information about the body. The output signal is eventually transformed into an image to represent the information about the body. For example, an X-ray mammography scanner uses an X-ray tube to generate a radiation beam that passes through the breast tissue. As a result of the interactions among X-ray photons and breast tissue, the X-ray beam is attenuated. The attenuated beam of X-ray radiation coming out of the breast is then collected on a radiographic film. The raw signals obtained from instrumentation of an imaging device or scanner are usually preprocessed for a suitable transformation to form an image that makes sense from the physiological point of view and is easy to interpret. Every imaging modality uses some kind of image reconstruction method to provide the first part of this transformation for conversions of raw signals into useful images. Even after a good reconstruction or initial transformation, images may not provide useful information with a required localization to help interpretation. This is particularly important when the information about suspect objects is occluded or overshadowed by other parts of the body. Often reconstructed images from scanners are degraded in a way that unless the contrast and brightness are adjusted, the objects of interest may not be easily visualized. Thus, an effective and efficient image processing environment is a vital part of the medical imaging system.

Since the information of interest about biological objects often is associated with characteristic features, it is crucial to use specially designed image processing methods for visualization and analysis of medical images. It is also important to know about the acquisition and transformation methods used for reconstruction of images before appropriate image processing and analysis algorithms are designed and applied. With the new advances in image processing, adaptive learning, and knowledge-based intelligent analysis, the specific needs of medical image analysis to improve diagnostic information for computer-aided diagnosis can be addressed.

Figure 1.7a,b shows an example of feature-adaptive contrast enhancement processing as applied to a part of the mammogram to enhance microcalcification areas. Figure 1.7c shows the result of a standard histogram equalization method commonly used for contrast enhancement in image processing. It is clear that standard image processing algorithms may not be helpful in medical image processing.

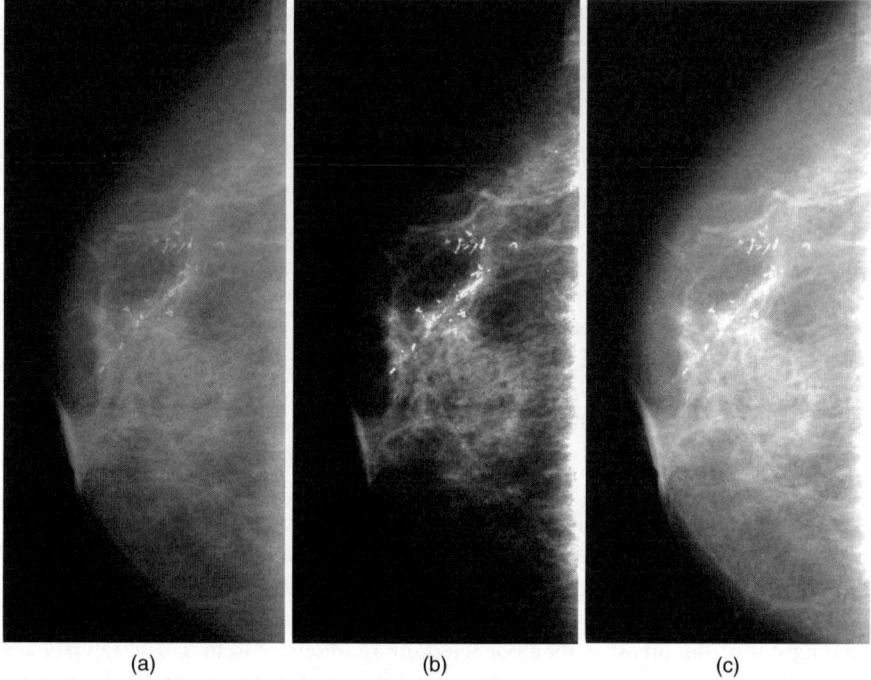

(a) (b) (c)

Figure 1.7   (a) a digital mammogram image; (b) microcalcification enhanced image through feature adaptive contrast enhancement algorithm; and (c) enhanced image through histogram equalization method (see Chapter 9 for details on image enhancement algorithms).

Specific image processing operations are needed to deal with the information of radiological interest. The following chapters will introduce fundamental principles of medical imaging systems and image processing tools. The latter part of the book is dedicated to the design and application of intelligent and customized image processing algorithms for radiological image analysis.

1.6. MATLAB IMAGE PROCESSING TOOLBOX

The MATLAB image processing toolbox is a compilation of a number of useful commands and subroutines for efficient image processing operations. The image processing toolbox provides extensive information with syntax and examples about each command. It is strongly recommended that readers go through the description of commands in the help menu and follow tutorials for various image processing tasks. Some of the introductory commands are described below.

1.6.1   Digital Image Representation

A 2-D digital image of spatial size $M \times N$ pixels (picture elements with M rows and N columns) may be represented by a function $f(x, y)$ where (x, y) is the location of a pixel whose gray level value (or brightness) is given by the function $f(x, y)$ with $x = 1, 2, \ldots, M$; $y = 1, 2, \ldots, N$. The brightness values or gray levels of the function $f(x, y)$ are digitized in a specific resolution such as 8-bit (256 levels), 12-bit (4096 levels), or more. For computer processing, a digital image can be described by a 2-D matrix [F] of elements whose values and locations represents, respectively, the gray levels and location of pixels in the image as

$$F = \begin{bmatrix} f(1,1) & f(1,2) & \cdots & f(1,N) \\ f(2,1) & f(2,2) & & f(2,N) \\ & & & \\ f(M,1) & f(M,2) & & f(M,N) \end{bmatrix}. \tag{1.8}$$

For example, a synthetic image of size 5×5 pixels with "L" letter shape of gray level 255 over a background of gray level 20 may be represented as

$$F = \begin{bmatrix} 20 & 20 & 255 & 20 & 20 \\ 20 & 20 & 255 & 20 & 20 \\ 20 & 20 & 255 & 20 & 20 \\ 20 & 20 & 255 & 20 & 20 \\ 20 & 20 & 255 & 255 & 255 \end{bmatrix}. \tag{1.9}$$

It is clear from the above that a digital image is discrete in both space and gray-level values as pixels are distributed over space locations. Thus, any static image is characterized by (1) spatial resolution (number of pixels in x- and y-directions such as 1024×1024 pixels for 1M pixel image), and (2) gray-level resolution (number of brightness levels such as 256 in 8-bit resolution image). In addition, images can also be characterized by number of dimensions (2-D, 3-D, etc.) and temporal resolution if images are taken as a sequence with regular time interval. A 4-D image data set may include, for example, 3-D images taken with a temporal resolution of 0.1 s.

Images that are underexposed (and look darker) may not utilize the entire gray-level range. For example, an underexposed image with 8-bit gray-level resolution (0–255 gray-level range) may have gray-level values from 0 to 126. Thus, the maximum brightness level in the image appears to be at about half the intensity it could have been if it was stretched to 255. One solution to this problem is to stretch the gray-level range from 0–126 to 0–255 linearly. Such a method is commonly known as gray-level scaling or stretching and can be shown as a linear mapping as

$$g(x, y) = \frac{(d-c)}{(b-a)}(f(x, y) - a) + c \tag{1.10}$$

where an original image $f(x, y)$ with gray-level range (a, b) is scaled linearly to an output image $g(x, y)$ with gray-level range (c, d).

Sometimes an image shows some pixels at the maximum brightness intensity level, yet the rest of the image appears to be quite dark. This may happen if there are some very high values in the image but most of other pixels have very low values. For example, a Fourier transform of an image may have a very high dc value

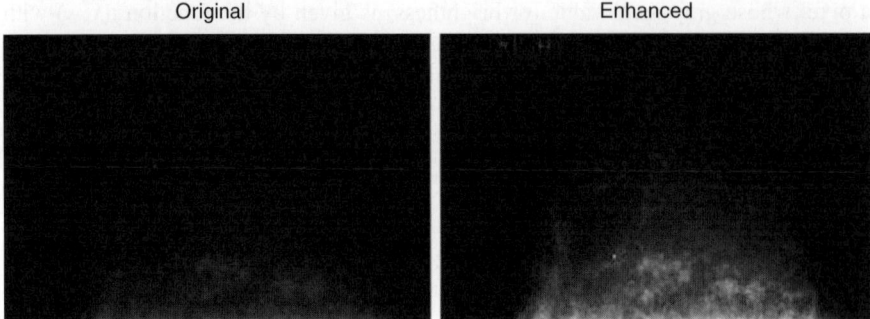

Figure 1.8 An original mammogram image (left) and the gray-level scaled image (right).

```
x = imread(f);
x = rgb2gray(x);
figure('Name', 'Contrast
Enhancement');
subplot(1,2,1)
imshow(x);
title('Original');
subplot(1,2,2)
imshow(x, []);
title('Enhanced');
```

Figure 1.9 M-Script code for the example shown in Figure 1.8.

but other parts of the frequency spectrum carry very low values. In such cases, a nonlinear transformation is used to reduce the wide gap between the low and high values. A commonly used logarithm transformation for displaying images with a wide range of values is expressed as $\log\{abs(f)\}$ or $\log\{1+abs(f)\}$ such that

$$g(x, y) = \log(|f(x, y)|)$$

or

$$g(x, y) = \log(1+|f(x, y)|) \qquad (1.11)$$

Examples of image scaling and log-transformation operations in the MATLAB image processing toolbox are shown in Figures 1.8 and 1.9. More image processing operations are described in Chapter 9.

1.6.2 Basic MATLAB Image Toolbox Commands

In the MATLAB environment, an image can be read and displayed using the image processing toolbox as

≫ *f = imread('filename.format');*

1.6. MATLAB IMAGE PROCESSING TOOLBOX

There are several image storage and compression formats in which the image data is stored and managed. Some of the common formats are JPEG (created by Joint Photography Expert Group), graphical interchange format (GIF), tagged image file format (TIFF); and Windows Bitmap (BMP).

The format could be any of the above allowed formats. The semicolon (;) is added if the program is continued, otherwise the MATLAB displays the results of the operation(s) given in the preceding command. Directory information can be added in the command before the filename such as

\>\> *f = imread('C:\medimages\mribrain1.jpg');*

The size information is automatically taken from the file header but it can be queried using the command *size(f)* that returns the size of the image in M × N format. In addition, *whos(f)* command can also be used to return the information about the image file:

\>\> *whos(f)*

which may provide the following information

Name	Size	Bytes	Class
f	512 × 512	262,144	uint8 array

Grand total is 262,144 elements using 262,144 bytes

To display images, *imshow* command can be used:

\>\> *imshow(f)*

To keep this image and display another image in a spate window, command *figure* can be used:

\>\> *imshow(f), figure, imshow(g)*

Scaling the gray-level range of an image is sometimes quite useful in display. Images with low gray-level utilization (such as dark images) can be displayed with a scaling of the gray levels to full or stretched dynamic range using the *imshow* command:

\>\> *imshow(f, [ ])* or
\>\> *imshow(f, [low high])*

The scaled images are brighter and show better contrast. An example of gray-level scaling of an X-ray mammographic image is shown in Figure 1.8. On the left, the original mammogram image is shown, which is quite dark, while the gray-level scaled image on the right demonstrates the enhanced contrast. M-script commands are shown in Figure 1.9.

To display a matrix [f] as an image, the "scale data and display image object" command can be used through *imagesc* function. This MATLAB function helps in creating a synthetic image from a 2-D matrix of mathematical, raw, or transformed data (such as transformation of red, green, and blue [RGB] to gray-level format can be done using the command *rgb2gray(f)*). The elements of the matrix can be scaled and displayed as an image using *colormap* function as

```
>> imagesc(x, y, f)
```
or
```
>> imagesc(f)
```
and
```
>> colormap(code)
```

In the *imagesc* function format, *x* and *y* values specify the size of data in respective directions. The *imagesc* function creates an image with data set to scaled values with direct or indexed colors (see more details in the MATLAB manual or helpdesk Web site http://www.mathworks.com/access/helpdesk/help/techdoc/ref/imagesc.html). An easier way is follow-up *imagesc* function with a *colormap* function choosing one of the color code palettes built in MATLAB as gray, bone, copper, cool, spring, jet, and so on (more details can be found on the helpdesk Web site http://www.mathworks.com/access/helpdesk/help/techdoc/ref/colormap.html). An example of using *imagesc* and *colormap* functions can be seen in the M-script given in Figure 1.11.

Figure 1.10 (left) shows an image whose Fourier transform is shown in the middle. The Fourier transform image shows bright pixels in the middle representing very high dc value, but the rest of the image is quite dark. The Fourier transformed image after the logarithm transform as described above in Equation 1.11 is shown at the right. M-script is shown in Figure 1.11.

After image processing operation(s), the resultant image can be stored using the *imwrite* command:

```
>> imwrite(f, 'filename', 'format')
```

More generalized *imwrite* syntax with different compression formats are available and can be found in the MATLAB HELP menu.

The MATLAB image processing toolbox supports several types of images including gray-level (intensity), binary, indexed, and RGB images. Care should be taken in identifying data classes and image types and then converting them appropriately as needed before any image processing operation is performed.

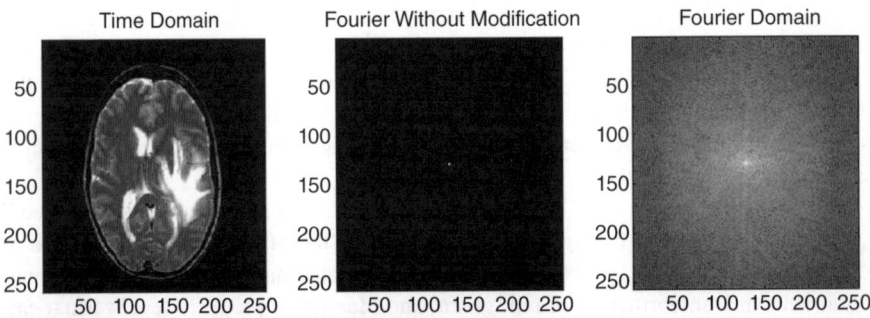

Figure 1.10 An original MR brain image (left), its Fourier transform (middle), and Fourier transformed image after logarithm transformation (right).

```
figure
subplot(1,3,1)
pic=imread(f);
pic=rgb2gray(pic);
imagesc(pic);
title('Time Domain')
colormap(gray)
subplot(1,3,2)
%To show importance of log in image display
imagesc(fftshift(abs(fft2(pic))));
title('Fourier Without Modification');
subplot(1,3,3);
%Now with log
qb=fftshift(log(abs(fft2(pic))));
imagesc(qb);
title('Fourier Domain')
colormap(gray)
```

Figure 1.11   M-script code for the example shown in Figure 1.10.

1.7. IMAGEPRO INTERFACE IN MATLAB ENVIRONMENT AND IMAGE DATABASES

The website for this book (ftp://ftp.wiley.com/public/sci_tech_med/medical_image/) provides access to all figures and images included. In addition, an Imagepro Image Processing Interface in the MATLAB environment and several medical image databases can be downloaded from the Web site to implement image processing tasks described in the book as part of MATLAB exercises.

The image databases include X-ray mammograms, multimodality magnetic resonance–computed tomography (MR–CT) brain images, multimodality positron emission tomography-computed tomography (PET–CT) full-body images, CT brain images of intracerebral brain hemorrhage, and multispectral optical transillumination images of skin lesions. "Readme" instructions are provided in each database folder with a brief description of the images and associated pathologies wherever available.

1.7.1   Imagepro Image Processing Interface

The Imagepro Image Processing Interface provides various image processing functions and tools with a user-friendly graphical user interface (GUI). On the GUI, six buttons corresponding to the six interfaces are provided to include

1. FIR filter interface
2. Morphological operation interface
3. Histogram interface
4. Edge detection interface
5. Noise reduction interface
6. Wavelet interface

An "Info" button is provided in each interface to obtain information about the different controls and abilities. Information about the image processing functions is also provided. Although the purpose of this interface is for demonstration, users can load the image of their choice and see the effects of the different image processing functions on the image.

1.7.2 Installation Instructions

Download all files for the Imagepro MATLAB interface from the Web site* ftp://ftp.wiley.com/publicisei_tech_med/medicalimage/ on your computer in the Impagepro folder in the MATLAB program directory. Open MATLAB and using the "set path" option under the File Menu select "add to path," or current directory selection to open the folder in which Imagepro files are copied.

Once the Imagepro folder is set up as the current directory, just type "imagepro" in the MATLAB command window to open the GUI. Help files are attached on each tool on the respective interface screens.

The software tools and images are intended to be used as an instructional aid for this book. The user needs to have a version of MATLAB to use the full software included in the image database files. Each folder included with the software has a separate "Readme" or Instructions file in text format. These files give information about the images or the interface installation instructions.

1.8. IMAGEJ AND OTHER IMAGE PROCESSING SOFTWARE PACKAGES

There are software packages other than MATLAB that readers can download and install on their personal computers for Windows, MAC, and other operating systems. One of the popular software packages, ImageJ, can be downloaded from the Web site http://rsbweb.nih.gov/ij/index.html. ImageJ software packages can be installed on personal computers with Windows, Mac OS, Mac OS X, and Linux operating systems.

ImageJ software provides a complete spectrum of image processing features with GUI-based functions to display, edit, analyze, process, save, and print 8-bit, 16-bit, and 32-bit images (8). The software reads multiple image formats including TIFF, GIF, JPEG, BMP, DICOM, FITS, and "raw," and supports series of images as "stacks" sharing a single window. It provides sophisticated 3-D image registration image analysis and visualization operations.

Another free open-source software package for image visualization and analysis is 3D Slicer, which can be downloaded from the Web site http://www.slicer.org/. 3D Slicer can be installed on personal computers with Windows, Linux, and Mac Os X operating systems (9). The user-friendly GUI-based 3D Slicer image analysis

---

*All image and textual content included on this site is distributed by IEEE Press and John Wiley & Sons, Inc. All content is to be used for educational and instructional purposes only and may not be reused for commercial purposes.

software package provides a spectrum of image processing functions and features, including multiple image format and DICOM support, 3-D registration, analysis and visualization, fiducial tractography, and tracking analysis for image-guided surgery and therapy.

1.9. EXERCISES

1.1. Is it necessary to understand the physics and instrumentation of medical imaging modality before processing the data for image reconstruction, processing, and interpretation? Give reasons to support your answer.

1.2. What are the measures for evaluation of a medical imaging modality?

1.3. Explain the significance of the receiver operating characteristic (ROC) curve?

1.4. A chest phantom was implanted with different sizes and types of nodular lesions and was imaged with a new X-ray scanner. Let us assume that there are 156 radiographs of the chest phantom screened for detection of nodular lesions. The radiographs showed 44 lesions, out of which four lesions were verified to be false. The radiographs also missed three lesions that could not be seen by an observer. Compute accuracy, sensitivity, and specificity of the X-ray scanner in imaging nodular lesions in the chest.

1.5. A false positive fraction (FPF) or rate is defined and characterized by (choose the best answer)
   a. Number of negative observations divided by number of positive observations.
   b. Number of negative observations divided by number of true positive conditions.
   c. Number of positive observations divided by number of negative observations.
   d. Number of positive observations divided by number of true negative conditions.

1.6. In the evaluation of two imaging scanners, A and B, the following set of TPF and FPF are observed for detection of lung tumors:
   A. TPF = 0.8; FPF = 0.5
   B. TPF = 0.7; FPF = 0.1
   Which of the above scanners would you recommend to use and why?

1.7. Compared with image processing methods used in computer vision, do you think medical image processing methods should be customized based on the physics of imaging and properties of the imaging medium? Explain your answer.

1.8. In the MATLAB environment, display an image of a breast mammogram from the MAMMO database. Apply gray-level scaling, histogram equalization, and an LOG enhancement mask for image enhancement as given below. Compare the enhanced images to original image qualitatively.

LOG enhancement mask to be convolved with the image:

$$\begin{matrix} -1 & -1 & -1 \\ -1 & 9 & -1 \\ -1 & -1 & -1 \end{matrix}$$

1.9. Repeat Exercise 6 for a magnetic resonance image of the brain from the MRI_BRAIN database. Do you see the same type of enhancement effect in each method for two images from different imaging modalities? Look for edge and object definitions in the original and enhanced images. Also, comment on the saturation and noise artifacts in the enhanced images.

1.10. In the MATLAB environment, display an X-ray CT image of the chest and compute its Fourier transform image as logarithmic magnitude folded to display dc value at the center of the image. Use *imagesc* and *colormap* functions to display the Fourier transformed image in gray, spring, and jet color maps built in MATLAB. Compare these displays and comment on the visualization of frequency components in the Fourier transform image.

1.10. REFERENCES

1. H. Barrett and W. Swindell, *Radiological Imaging: The Theory of Image Formation, Detection and Processing*, Volumes 1–2, Academic Press, New York, 1981.
2. J.T. Bushberg, J.A. Seibert, E.M. Leidholdt, and J.M. Boone, *The Essentials of Medical Imaging*, 2nd edition, Williams & Wilkins, Baltimore, MD, 2002.
3. Z.H. Cho, J.P. Jones, and M. Singh, *Fundamentals of Medical Imaging*, John Wiley & Sons, New York, 1993.
4. A.P. Dhawan, "A review on biomedical image processing and future trends," *Comput. Methods Programs Biomed.*, Vol. 31, No. 3–4, pp. 141–183, 1990.
5. Z. Liang and P.C. Lauterbur, *Principles of Magnetic Resonance Imaging*, IEEE Press, Hoboken, NJ, 2000.
6. K.K. Shung, M.B. Smith, and B. Tsui, *Principles of Medical Imaging*, Academic Press, New York, 1992.
7. MATLAB Web site: http://www.mathworks.com/.
8. ImageJ Web site: http://rsbweb.nih.gov/ij/index.html.
9. 3D Slicer Web site: http://www.slicer.org/.

1.11. DEFINITIONS

Accuracy: Accuracy is the ability to measure a quantity with respect to its true value. In normalized sense, this is the difference between measured value and true value divided by true value.

Precision: The precision of a measurement expresses the number of distinguishable values or alternatives from which a given result is selected. Precision makes no comparison with the true value. Therefore, high precision does not mean high accuracy.

Resolution: The smallest incremental quality that can be measured with certainty is the resolution.

Reproducibility: The ability to give the same output for equal inputs applied at different times is called reproducibility or repeatability. Reproducibility does not imply accuracy.

Sensitivity: The sensitivity of a test is the probability of yielding positive results when a given condition is true. This is also provided in terms of true positive fraction (TPF).

Specificity: The specificity of a test is the probability of yielding negative results in patients who do not havNe a disease. This is also provided in terms of true negative fraction (TNF).

CHAPTER 2

IMAGE FORMATION

Two-dimensional (2-D) images can be acquired in several ways. Using optical instrumentation such as a camera or a microscope, a 2-D image of a three-dimensional (3-D) object can be obtained through optical lens geometry. Through medical imaging modalities, 2-D and 3-D images of an organ can be obtained using transmission, emission, reflectance, diffraction, or nuclear resonance methods as outlined in the previous chapter. Most recent advances in medical imaging allow the acquisition of even 4-D time-varying image sequences of 3-D organs such as a beating heart. For example, magnetic resonance imaging (MRI) can be used to obtain time-based image sequences of a beating heart. The sophisticated medical imaging modalities such as 3-D computed tomography (CT) and MRI require multidimensional reconstruction methods to create images. Nevertheless, the basic principles of image formation are utilized throughout the image reconstruction, processing, and display processes. This chapter provides some of the basic principles of image formation that are universally applicable, from general purpose optical camera-based 2-D imaging to more sophisticated multidimensional medical imaging systems.

An analog image is described by the spatial distribution of brightness or gray levels that reflect a distribution of detected energy. The image can be displayed using a medium such as paper or film. A photograph on paper may show a black and white image with gray levels representing grades of brightness from black to white. While black and white images require only one gray level or intensity variable, the color images are produced by using multiple variables. For examples, three basic colors, red, green, and blue (RGB), could be used as three variables for representing color images. When combined together, the RGB intensities can produce a selected color at a spatial location in the image. Thus, a true color image can be represented by three RGB component images with the corresponding gray-level or intensity variables (1–3). Other color image representation schemes can be derived from the basic RGB color representation (1–3). For example, a commonly used color representation scheme is intensity I, saturation S, and hue H, which can be expressed as (3)

Medical Image Analysis, Second Edition, by Atam P. Dhawan
Copyright © 2011 by the Institute of Electrical and Electronics Engineers, Inc.

$$I = \frac{R+G+B}{3}$$

$$S = 1 - \frac{3}{(R+G+B)}(\min(R,G,B))$$

$$H = \begin{cases} \theta & \text{if } B \leq G \\ 2\pi - \theta & \text{if } B > G \end{cases}$$

$$\text{with} \quad \theta = \cos^{-1}\left\{\frac{\frac{1}{2}[(R-G)+(R-B)]}{\left[(R-G)^2+(R-B)(G-B)\right]^{1/2}}\right\} \tag{2.1}$$

where angle θ is measured with respect to the red axis in the *ISH* coordinate space and R, G, and B are, respectively, the red, green, and blue values in the RGB coordinate space.

The advantage of the ISH color representation scheme is that it provides the overall intensity component, which is the average of the RGB values. The RGB color images of skin lesions have been converted into an ISH coordinate system for multichannel intensity and texture-based segmentation (4).

It should be noted that a black and white image can be converted into a pseudo-color image by transforming the original gray levels of the black and white image into the specific components of a color representation scheme (1–3). One simple method of pseudo-color transformation is intensity slicing in which the entire range of gray levels of the black and white image is divided into three subranges. The three subranges are then assigned to the RGB input of the color monitor for pseudo-color visualization. Such a pseudo-color representation often helps visualization of structures in medical images (3, 5, 6).

For a digital image representation suitable for processing on the computer, the image has to be discrete in both spatial and intensity (gray level) domains. A discrete spatial location of finite size with a discrete gray-level value is called a pixel. For example, an image of 1024 × 1024 pixels may be displayed in 8-bit gray-level resolution. This means that each pixel in the image may have any value from 0 to 255 (i.e., a total of 256 gray levels). The pixel dimensions would depend on the spatial sampling. An analog image may be converted into a digital image using image scanners or digitizers. On the other hand, digital images may be acquired directly using an array of discrete detectors or sensors as found in digital cameras or CT medical imaging systems. The pixel dimensions may be carefully correlated with the actual physical dimensions of objects in the real world. For example, if a real-world object is sampled with 1 mm spatial sampling in each direction for image formation, a 2-D image with 1024 × 1024 pixel resolution may represent the actual spatial dimension of 10.24 cm × 10.24 cm.

2.1. IMAGE COORDINATE SYSTEM

In the process of image formation, the object coordinates are mapped into image coordinates. If the image formation system is linear, a simple transformation with

2.1. IMAGE COORDINATE SYSTEM

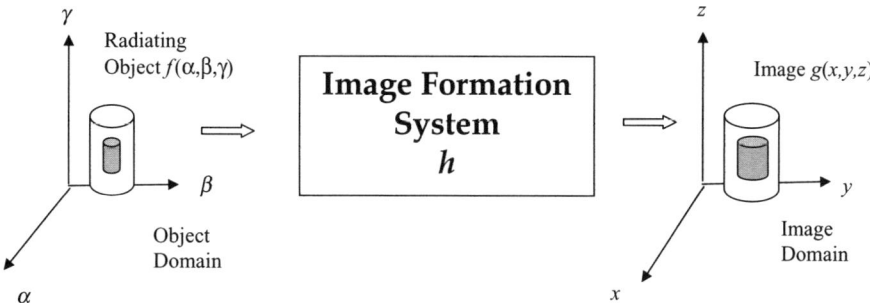

Figure 2.1 The object and image domain coordinates systems.

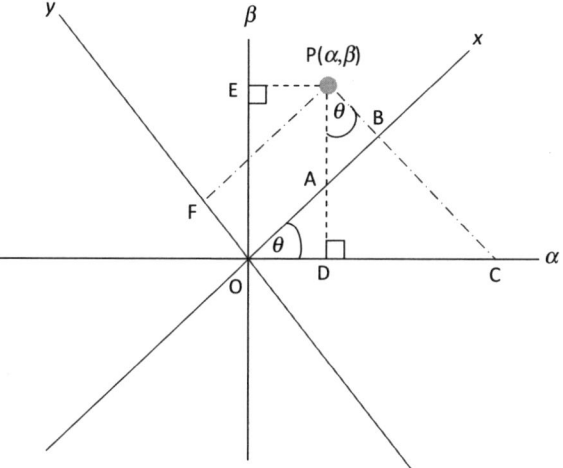

Figure 2.2 A pixel P is projected on the original (α, β) and (x, y) coordinate system rotated by θ.

proper translation, scaling, and rotation can define the correspondence between the coordinate systems of the object and image domains. Such transformation operations may be used to restore real-world features and to establish correspondence among images for registration and interpretation. Figure 2.1 shows the object and image coordinate systems such that the object coordinate system (α, β, γ) is mapped onto the image coordinate system (x, y, z) as output from an image formation system.

2.1.1 2-D Image Rotation

Let us consider rotating a 2-D image $f(\alpha, \beta)$ by an angle θ. Let us assume that (α, β) coordinate system is rotated by angle θ to (x, y) coordinates. Figure 2.2 shows a pixel P in image $f(\alpha, \beta)$ projected on the (x, y) coordinate system.

The pixel P can be projected on (α, β) and (x, y) coordinate systems as

$$\alpha = OD; \quad \beta = PD$$
$$x = OB; \quad y = PB. \qquad (2.2)$$

Considering $\triangle PDC$ and $\triangle OBC$, the following relationships can be observed:

$$x = OB = OC\cos\theta$$
$$x = (OD + DC)\cos\theta$$
$$x = (\alpha + \beta\tan\theta)\cos\theta$$
$$x = \alpha\cos\theta + \beta\sin\theta. \tag{2.3}$$

and

$$y = PA\cos\theta$$
$$y = (PD - AD)\cos\theta$$
$$y = (\beta - \alpha\tan\theta)\cos\theta$$
$$y = \beta\cos\theta - \alpha\sin\theta. \tag{2.4}$$

Thus, a 2-D rotation transformation for output image $g(x, y)$ obtained by rotating $f(\alpha, \beta)$ is given by

$$\begin{bmatrix} x \\ y \end{bmatrix} = \begin{bmatrix} \cos\theta & \sin\theta \\ -\sin\theta & \cos\theta \end{bmatrix} \begin{bmatrix} \alpha \\ \beta \end{bmatrix}. \tag{2.5}$$

2.1.2 3-D Image Rotation and Translation Transformation

If an object $f(\alpha, \beta, \gamma)$ is mapped into an image $g(x, y, z)$ through a linear image formation system h, a transformation involving translation and rotation may be established to define object and image coordinate systems as

$$\mathbf{G} = \mathbf{R}(\mathbf{F} - \mathbf{T}) \tag{2.6}$$

where $\mathbf{G}$ and $\mathbf{F}$ are, respectively, image and object domain coordinate systems denoted as column vectors and $\mathbf{R}$ and $\mathbf{T}$ are, respectively, rotation and translation matrices.

Translation is simply a vector subtraction operation. Scaling is a vector multiplication operation. For rotation in 3-D, three rotations about three axes can be defined in a sequence to define the complete rotation transformation. It can be shown that a rotation transformation can be defined by the following three operations:

1. Rotation of $\mathbf{G}(\alpha, \beta, \gamma)$ about β by an angle θ such that $\mathbf{G}_1(\zeta, \tau, \sigma) = \mathbf{R}_\theta \mathbf{G}(\alpha, \beta, \gamma)$

$$\text{where } R_\theta = \begin{bmatrix} \cos\theta & 0 & \sin\theta \\ 0 & 1 & 0 \\ -\sin\theta & 0 & \cos\theta \end{bmatrix} \tag{2.7}$$

2. Rotation of $\mathbf{G}_1(\zeta, \tau, \sigma)$ about α by an angle ϕ such that $\mathbf{G}_2(\omega, \varepsilon, \nu) = \mathbf{R}_\phi \mathbf{G}_1(\zeta, \tau, \sigma)$

$$\text{where } R_\phi = \begin{bmatrix} 1 & 0 & 0 \\ 0 & \cos\phi & \sin\phi \\ 0 & -\sin\phi & \cos\phi \end{bmatrix} \tag{2.8}$$

3. Rotation of $G_2(\omega, \varepsilon, v)$ about γ by an angle ψ such that $F(x, y, z) = R_\psi G_2(\omega, \varepsilon, v)$

$$\text{where } R_\psi = \begin{bmatrix} \cos\psi & \sin\psi & 0 \\ -\sin\psi & \cos\psi & 0 \\ 0 & 0 & 1 \end{bmatrix}. \tag{2.9}$$

It should be noted that the sequence of rotational operations is important because these operations are not commutative.

2.2. LINEAR SYSTEMS

It is usually desirable for an image formation system to behave like a linear, spatially invariant system. In other words, the response of the imaging system should be consistent, scalable, and independent of the spatial position of the object being imaged. A system is said to be linear if it follows two properties: scaling and superposition. In mathematical representation, it can be expressed as

$$h\{aI_1(x, y, z) + bI_2(x, y, z)\} = ah\{I_1(x, y, z)\} + bh\{I_2(x, y, z)\} \tag{2.10}$$

where a and b are scalar multiplication factors, and $I_1(x, y, z)$ and $I_2(x, y, z)$ are two inputs to the system represented by the response function h.

It should be noted that in real-world situations, it is difficult to find a perfectly linear image formation system. For example, the response of photographic film or X-ray detectors cannot be linear over the entire operating range. Nevertheless, under constrained conditions and limited exposures, the response can be practically linear. Also, a nonlinear system can be modeled with piecewise linear properties under specific operating considerations.

2.3. POINT SOURCE AND IMPULSE FUNCTIONS

The image formation process requires an energy source that is used on the object through an imaging operation, for example, reflection or transmission. As the response of the imaging operation is recorded on a film or array of detectors, an image can be modeled in terms of responses of spatially distributed point sources. As shown later in this chapter, if image formation is considered to be linear, the image can be described in terms of integration of responses of spatially distributed point sources. Thus, an image can be characterized through responses of point sources, also known as point spread functions (PSF).

A point source can be modeled through an impulse or Dirac delta function. To understand the properties of an impulse function, let us first define a 2-D rectangular function with a unit magnitude over a unit area (Fig. 2.3) as

$$rect(x, y) = \begin{cases} 1 & \text{for } |x| \leq \frac{1}{2}, \ |y| \leq \frac{1}{2} \\ 0 & \text{otherwise} \end{cases}. \tag{2.11}$$

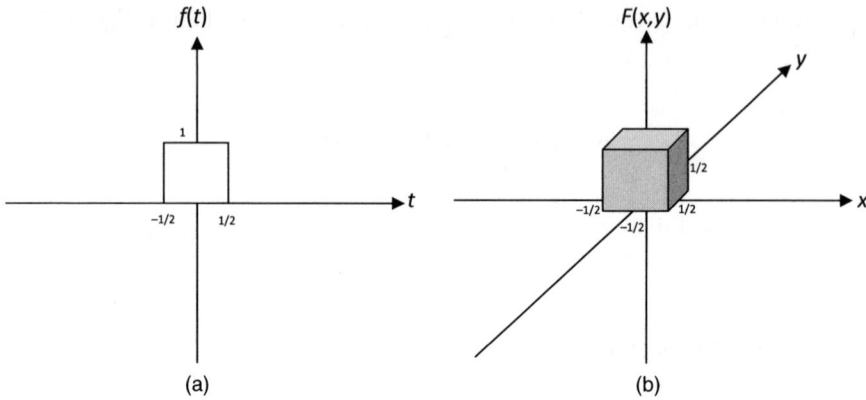

Figure 2.3 (a) One-dimensional unit rectangular function; (b) two-dimensional unit rectangular function.

A family of delta functions can be derived from rectangular functions as

$$\partial_n(x, y) = n^2 \text{rect}(nx, ny)$$

$$= \begin{cases} n^2 & \text{for } |x| \le \dfrac{1}{2n}, \ |y| \le \dfrac{1}{2n} \\ 0 & \text{otherwise} \end{cases} \quad \text{for } n = 1, 2. \quad (2.12)$$

It can be seen from Equation 2.12 that as n increases, the base of the impulse reduces and magnitude increases. For $n \to \infty$, the delta function is zero everywhere except at $(0, 0)$, where its magnitude becomes infinite. This is also called Dirac delta or impulse function. However, the basic constraint remains the same as

$$\int_{-\infty}^{\infty} \int_{-\infty}^{\infty} \partial(x, y) \, dx \, dy = 1. \quad (2.13)$$

The Dirac delta or impulse function can be used in modeling point sources as it has good sifting properties:

$$\int_{-\infty}^{\infty} \int_{-\infty}^{\infty} f(x, y) \partial(x, y) \, dx \, dy = f(0, 0)$$

and

$$\int_{-\infty}^{\infty} \int_{-\infty}^{\infty} f(x, y) \partial(x - \alpha, y - \beta) \, dx \, dy = f(\alpha, \beta). \quad (2.14)$$

The above property can be used to sample a multidimensional function. For example, a 2-D array of impulse functions, called comb function, as shown in Figure 2.4, can be used to sample an image, and can be expressed as

$$\text{comb}(x, y) = \sum_{m=-\infty}^{\infty} \sum_{n=-\infty}^{\infty} \partial(x - m, y - n). \quad (2.15)$$

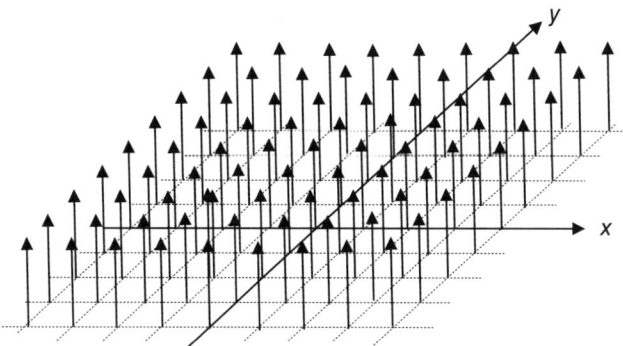

Figure 2.4 A schematic diagram of two-dimensional comb (x, y) function. The vertical arrows represent approaching infinite magnitude in the limiting case as $n \to \infty$ (see text for details).

2.4. PROBABILITY AND RANDOM VARIABLE FUNCTIONS

In any statistical data or experiment, a set of outcomes can be defined as $\Omega = \{\omega_i\}$; $i = 1, \ldots N$ with probability p_i to each outcome ω_i such that

$$p_i \geq 0 \quad \text{and} \quad \sum_{i=1}^{N} p_i = 1. \tag{2.16}$$

Let us define a random variable **f** as a function of the outcome as $\mathbf{f}(\omega_i)$ that is assigned an arbitrary but fixed number z such that for any z, the set $\{\mathbf{f} \leq z\}$ is an event. The probability of the event $\{\mathbf{f} \leq z\}$ is called the distribution function of the random variable **f** and may be denoted as $P_f(z)$. Properties of the distribution function $P_f(z)$ includes (13, 18)

a. $P_f(-\infty) = 0$; $P_f(\infty) = 1$
b. $P_f(z_1) \leq P_f(z_2)$ if $z_1 \leq z_2$
c. Let us denote the probability of random variable **f** within the range $z_1 < \mathbf{f} \leq z_2$ by $Pr\{z_1 < \mathbf{f} \leq z_2\}$ then

$$Pr\{z_1 < \mathbf{f} \leq z_2\} = P_f(z_2) - P_f(z_1)$$

d. $p_f(z) = \dfrac{dP_f(z)}{dz}$ where $P_f(z)$ is called the probability density function of random variable **f**.

It can be noted that

$$Pr\{z_1 < \mathbf{f} \leq z_2\} = \int_{z_1}^{z_2} p_f(z)\, dz. \tag{2.17}$$

The expected or mean value $E(\mathbf{f})$ of a random variable can be defined as

$$E(\mathbf{f}) = \int_{-\infty}^{\infty} z p_f(z)\, dz = \mu_f. \qquad (2.18)$$

The variance σ_f^2 of $\mathbf{f}$ can be defined as

$$\sigma_f^2 = E\{(\mathbf{f} - \mu_f)^2\} = \int_{-\infty}^{\infty} (z - \mu_f)^2 p_f(z)\, dz. \qquad (2.19)$$

A commonly used probability density function in statistical estimation-based image reconstruction, processing, and analysis operations is normal or Gaussian density function given as

$$p_f(z) = \frac{1}{\sigma_f \sqrt{2\pi}} \exp \frac{-(z - \mu_f)^2}{2\sigma_f^2}. \qquad (2.20)$$

2.4.1 Conditional and Joint Probability Density Functions

Conditional probability of an event A when B has occurred is defined by

$$Pr(A/B) = \frac{Pr(A \cap B)}{Pr(B)} = \frac{Pr(AB)}{Pr(B)}. \qquad (2.21)$$

If the two events A and B are said to be independent, then

$$Pr(A/B) = \frac{Pr(AB)}{Pr(B)} = \frac{Pr(A)Pr(B)}{Pr(B)} = Pr(A). \qquad (2.22)$$

If events A and B are not independent, then the Equation 2.21 can be expressed as

$$Pr(AB) = Pr(A/B)Pr(B). \qquad (2.23)$$

Similarly, the conditional probability of event B given that event A has occurred can be given as

$$Pr(B/A) = \frac{Pr(BA)}{Pr(A)} = \frac{Pr(AB)}{Pr(A)}$$

or

$$Pr(AB) = Pr(B/A)Pr(A). \qquad (2.24)$$

From Equations 2.23 and 2.24, it is implied that

$$Pr(A/B)Pr(B) = Pr(B/A)Pr(A). \qquad (2.25)$$

Equation 2.25 yields to Bayes' theorem that the conditional probability of determining event A given B can be expressed in the form of a priori knowledge of class probabilities (18) as

$$Pr(A/B) = \frac{Pr(B/A)}{Pr(B)} Pr(A). \qquad (2.26)$$

A generalized version of Bayes' rule can be used to improve a priori knowledge of A, and the new information gives out the posteriori probability of A given B. In the generalized version, with a set of events A_i; $i = 1, \ldots n$ as

$$Pr(A_i/B) = \frac{Pr(B/A_i)Pr(A_i)}{Pr(B)} = \frac{Pr(B/A_i)Pr(A_i)}{\sum_{i=1}^{n} Pr(B/A_i)Pr(A_i)}. \quad (2.27)$$

The conditional distribution function $P_f(z/B)$ of a random variable **f** while B has occurred, and its expected value, are defined as

$$P_f(z/B) = \frac{Prob(\{\mathbf{f} \le z\} \cap B)}{Prob(B)} \quad (2.28)$$

$$E\{\mathbf{f}/B\} = \int_{-\infty}^{\infty} z p_f(z/B) dz. \quad (2.29)$$

The set $\Omega = \{\omega_i\}$; $i = 1, \ldots N$ of all events can be characterized by the individual probability distribution functions of respective random variables as

$$p_{fi}(z_i) = Prob\{\mathbf{f}_i \le z_i\}; \quad i = 1, 2, \ldots, N. \quad (2.30)$$

The joint probability density function of the random variables $\mathbf{f}_1, \mathbf{f}_2, \ldots, \mathbf{f}_N$ is defined as

$$p_{f1,f2,\ldots,fN}(z_1, z_2, \ldots, z_N) = \frac{\partial^N P_{f1,f2,\ldots,fN}(z_1, z_2, \ldots, z_N)}{\partial z_1 \partial z_2 \ldots \partial z_N} \quad (2.31)$$

where $P_{f1,f2,\ldots,fN}(z_1, z_2, \ldots, z_N) = \text{Prob } \{\mathbf{f}_1 \le z_1, \mathbf{f}_2 \le z_2, \ldots, \mathbf{f}_N \le z_N\}$.

2.4.2 Independent and Orthogonal Random Variables

The random variables $\mathbf{f}_1, \mathbf{f}_2, \ldots, \mathbf{f}_N$ are independent if their joint density function can be expressed as the product of individual density functions as

$$p_{f1,f2,\ldots,fN}(z_1, z_2, \ldots, z_N) = p_{f1}(z_1) p_{f2}(z_2) \ldots p_{fN}(z_N). \quad (2.32)$$

It follows that if random variables $\mathbf{f}_1, \mathbf{f}_2, \ldots, \mathbf{f}_N$ are uncorrelated, their expected values can be explicitly expressed as

$$E\{\mathbf{f}_i \mathbf{f}_j\} = E\{\mathbf{f}_i\} E\{\mathbf{f}_j\} \quad \text{for all } i, j \text{ and } i \ne j. \quad (2.33)$$

The above expression becomes 0 when the random variables $\mathbf{f}_1, \mathbf{f}_2, \ldots, \mathbf{f}_N$ are orthogonal with

$$E\{\mathbf{f}_i \mathbf{f}_j\} = 0 \quad \text{for all } i, j \text{ and } i \ne j. \quad (2.34)$$

Orthogonality is an important property that allows one to design appropriate basis functions for series expansion and several transformations such as wavelet transform for image processing and compression tasks.

In statistical estimation-based image reconstruction and restoration tasks, functions of the random variable are often used. As functions of random variables are also random variables, their joint probability distributions are related to Jacobian transformation. Let us assume random variables $\mathbf{g}_1, \mathbf{g}_2, \ldots, \mathbf{g}_N$ are functions of random variables $\mathbf{f}_1, \mathbf{f}_2, \ldots, \mathbf{f}_N$ defined as (13, 18)

32 CHAPTER 2 IMAGE FORMATION

$$\mathbf{g}_1 = \Psi_1(\mathbf{f}_1, \mathbf{f}_2, \ldots, \mathbf{f}_N)$$
$$\mathbf{g}_2 = \Psi_1(\mathbf{f}_1, \mathbf{f}_2, \ldots, \mathbf{f}_N)$$
$$\ldots$$
$$\mathbf{g}_N = \Psi_1(\mathbf{f}_1, \mathbf{f}_2, \ldots, \mathbf{f}_N). \tag{2.35}$$

Following the above representation, the joint density function of the random variables $\mathbf{g}_1, \mathbf{g}_2, \ldots, \mathbf{g}_N$ can be expressed as

$$p_{g1,g2,\ldots,gN}(x_1, x_2, \ldots, x_N) = \frac{\partial^N P_{g1,g2,\ldots,gN}(x_1, x_2, \ldots, x_N)}{\partial z_1 \partial z_2 \ldots \partial z_N} \tag{2.36}$$

where $P_{g1,g2,\ldots,gN}(x_1, x_2, \ldots, x_N) = \text{Prob } \{\mathbf{g}_1 \leq x_1, \mathbf{g}_2 \leq x_2, \ldots, \mathbf{g}_N \leq x_N\}$.

The probability distribution functions for random variables $\mathbf{g}_1, \mathbf{g}_2, \ldots, \mathbf{g}_N$ and $\mathbf{f}_1, \mathbf{f}_2, \ldots, \mathbf{f}_N$ are thus related by

$$P_{g1,g2,\ldots,gN}(x_1, x_2, \ldots, x_N) = \frac{P_{f1,f2,\ldots,fN}(z_1, z_2, \ldots, z_N)}{|J(z_1, z_2, \ldots, z_N)|} \tag{2.37}$$

where Jacobian transformation $J(z_1, z_2, \ldots, z_N) = \begin{vmatrix} \frac{\partial \Psi_1}{\partial z_1} & \frac{\partial \Psi_1}{\partial z_2} & \cdots & \frac{\partial \Psi_1}{\partial z_N} \\ \frac{\partial \Psi_2}{\partial z_1} & \frac{\partial \Psi_2}{\partial z_2} & \cdots & \frac{\partial \Psi_N}{\partial z_N} \\ \cdots & \cdots & \cdots & \cdots \\ \frac{\partial \Psi_N}{\partial z_1} & \frac{\partial \Psi_N}{\partial z_2} & \cdots & \frac{\partial \Psi_N}{\partial z_N} \end{vmatrix}$.

2.5. IMAGE FORMATION

In general, image formation is a neighborhood process (7). One can assume that a radiant energy, such as a light source to illuminate an object, is represented by the function $f(\alpha, \beta, \gamma)$. For example, in case of photographic imaging, the object function $f(\alpha, \beta, \gamma)$ may be a distribution of the light reflected by the object. An image represented by the function $g(x, y, z)$ is obtained through an image formation system that transports the radiant energy from the object to the image plane (7–13). If the image plane is 2-D, such as in photographic imaging using a film camera, the projection of the 3-D object is acquired on a 2-D plane. If the image formation system is 3-D, a 3-D image is acquired and then can be manipulated to obtain 2-D views. For example, in X-ray transmission-based CT, a 3-D image can be reconstructed and used to compute any cross-sectional view as shown in Figure 2.5.

The image formation process can be similarly defined for other forms of imaging such as emission imaging, as shown in Figure 2.6. The only difference is that the object itself radiates the energy in emission imaging and therefore does not require any external radiation energy source. Although the imaging formation process can be described in a similar way, the radiant energy distribution has to be modeled differently in emission imaging.

2.5. IMAGE FORMATION

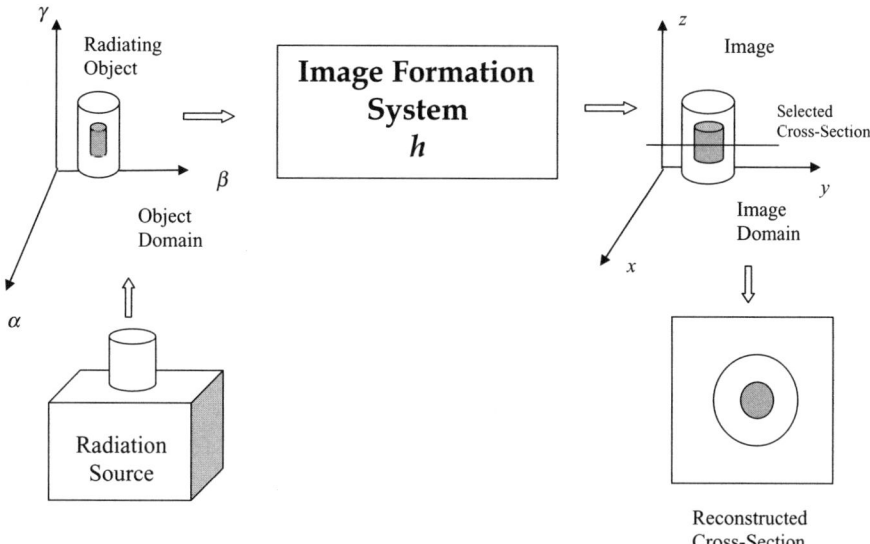

Figure 2.5 A schematic block diagram of a general 3-D image formation system requiring an external radiation source (such as light) for photographic imaging, or X ray for transmission imaging.

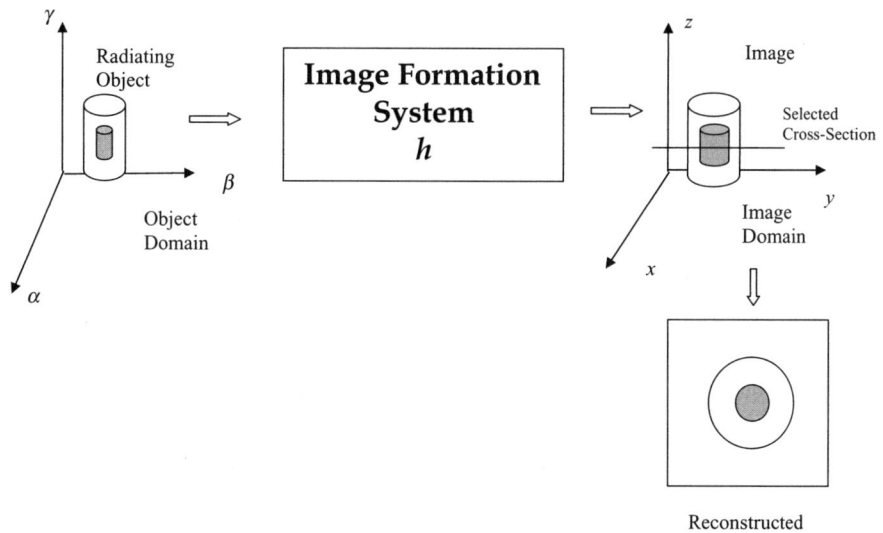

Figure 2.6 A schematic block diagram of an emission-based image formation system commonly used for fluorescence or nuclear medicine imaging modalities.

Whether the imaging process is 2- or 3-D, the image is formed through integration of a function of radiation energy distribution over the entire spatial extent from both object and image coordinates. This function is known as the response function of the image formation system. The parameters describing the response function could be very different and can be modeled differently across imaging systems. For example, X-ray and PET imaging modalities are characterized by different response functions involving different parameters. Diagnostic X rays attenuate while passing through the body because of the absorption properties of the medium within the body. On the other hand, PET imaging is influenced by absorption as well as scattering coefficients of the object being imaged.

Let us represent a generalized response function of an image formation system as h. A general image formation process follows the principles of non-negativity and superposition. Thus,

$$f(\alpha, \beta, \gamma) \geq 0$$
$$g(x, y, z) \geq 0. \quad (2.38)$$

Considering two spatial points $f_1(\alpha, \beta, \gamma)$ and $f_2(\alpha, \beta, \gamma)$ in the object domain and $g_1(x, y, z)$ and $g_2(x, y, z)$ in the image domain, the superposition principle follows as

$$g_1(x, y, z) + g_2(x, y, z) = h(x, y, z, \alpha, \beta, \gamma, f_1(\alpha, \beta, \gamma)) + h(x, y, z, \alpha, \beta, \gamma, f_2(\alpha, \beta, \gamma)). \quad (2.39)$$

where $h(x, y, z, \alpha, \beta, \gamma, f_i(\alpha, \beta, \gamma))$ for $i = 1, 2$ is the general response function that depends on the object and image coordinates and the spatial point $f_i(\alpha, \beta, \gamma)$ of the object distribution function.

If the image formation system is considered to be linear, the response function does not depend on the object distribution and hence

$$h(x, y, z, \alpha, \beta, \gamma, f(\alpha, \beta, \gamma)) = h(x, y, z, \alpha, \beta, \gamma) f(\alpha, \beta, \gamma). \quad (2.40)$$

Using the additive property of radiating energy distribution to form an image, one can write

$$g(x, y, z) = \int_{-\infty}^{+\infty} \int_{-\infty}^{+\infty} \int_{-\infty}^{+\infty} h(x, y, z, \alpha, \beta, \gamma, f(\alpha, \beta, \gamma)) \, d\alpha \, d\beta \, d\gamma. \quad (2.41)$$

If the image formation system is assumed to be linear, the image expression becomes

$$g(x, y, z) = \int_{-\infty}^{+\infty} \int_{-\infty}^{+\infty} \int_{-\infty}^{+\infty} h(x, y, z, \alpha, \beta, \gamma) f(\alpha, \beta, \gamma) \, d\alpha \, d\beta \, d\gamma. \quad (2.42)$$

As described above, the response function $h(x, y, z, \alpha, \beta, \gamma)$ is called the point spread function of the image formation system. The PSF depends on the spatial extent of the object and image coordinate systems. The expression $h(x, y, z, \alpha, \beta, \gamma)$ is the generalized version of the PSF described for the linear image formation system that can be further characterized as a spatially invariant (SI) or spatially variant (SV) system. If a linear image formation system is such that the PSF is uniform across the entire spatial extent of the object and image coordinates, the system is called a linear spatially invariant (LSI) system. In such a case, the image formation can be expressed as

$$g(x, y, z) = \int_{-\infty}^{+\infty} \int_{-\infty}^{+\infty} \int_{-\infty}^{+\infty} h(x - \alpha, y - \beta, z - \gamma) f(\alpha, \beta, \gamma) \, d\alpha \, d\beta \, d\gamma. \quad (2.43)$$

In other words, for an LSI image formation system, the image is represented as the convolution of the object is radiant energy distribution and the PSF of the image formation system. It should be noted that the PSF is basically a degrading function that causes a blur in the image and can be compared to the unit impulse response, a common term used in signal processing.

A 3-D LSI imaging system is very difficult to implement in real practice. Consider a photographic camera with a lens that has a fixed focal length. Such a camera will only focus on object points in a selected x–y plane in the object domain on a fixed x–y plane in the image domain. Depending on the depth of focus of the lens, all points out of the focused object plane (with different z-values in Fig. 2.1) will have different PSF and magnification to cause different amounts of blur in the 2-D image plane. Furthermore, the curvature of the lens will cause spatially variant PSF even within the focused object plane because of spherical aberrations. However, the spherical aberrations can be removed or minimized if high-quality lenses with appropriate aperture setting are used in the camera. Thus, a high-quality photographic camera can produce a sharp, spatially invariant image of the focused object plane. In this case, the above convolution equation for a fixed z value can be expressed as

$$g(x, y) = \int_{-\infty}^{+\infty} \int_{-\infty}^{+\infty} h(x-\alpha, y-\beta) f(\alpha, \beta) \, d\alpha \, d\beta \tag{2.44}$$

or

$$g = h \otimes f.$$

where $\otimes$ denotes a convolution operator.

As shown above, an image can be expressed as the convolution of the object distribution with the PSF for an LSI imaging system without any noise consideration. The noise in the detection instrumentation and data acquisition system can be modeled as additive and signal independent. This is a simplification but true for electronic instrumentation for linear imaging system. With additive noise assumption, the image formation process can be expressed as

$$g(x, y) = f(x, y) \otimes h(x, y) + n(x, y). \tag{2.45}$$

In most medical imaging systems, the instrumentation is designed in such a way so as to provide maximum linearity and spatially invariant properties of image formation. The advantage is rather obvious. Since it is easier to experimentally evaluate the PSF of an imaging system, the acquired image $g(x, y, z)$ can be updated or restored through image processing methods. General causes of blurry PSF include the finite size of the source, parallax and geometrical effects, radiation scatter, and nonlinear responses of the detector systems. The quality of medical images can be improved through image restoration and enhancement methods such as inverse filtering and Weiner deconvolution. These methods use the knowledge of the PSF of the imaging scanner in frequency filtering techniques that are described in Chapter 6.

2.5.1 PSF and Spatial Resolution

The PSF of an imaging system can be obtained experimentally by imaging a point source (defined above) and measuring the blur or spread of the point source. Usually, the PSF as the image of a point source (Fig. 2.7) is well approximated by a Gaussian

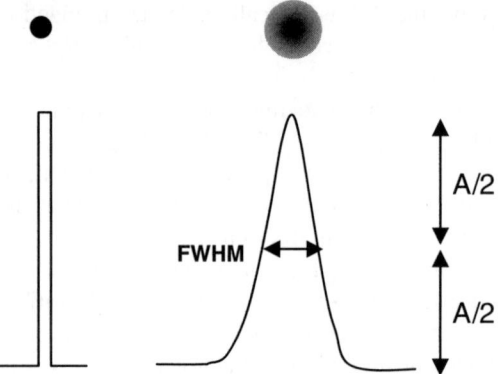

Figure 2.7 A point source (top left) and its point spread function (PSF) for an imaging system (top right); their one-dimensional intensity profiles are respectively shown in the second row.

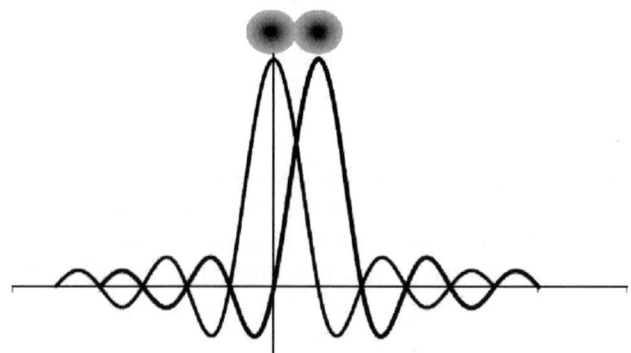

Figure 2.8 Two imaging point sources resolved through Rayleigh criterion applied to the respective sinc-based PSFs.

function as shown by the one-dimensional (1-D) intensity profile at the bottom right of Figure 2.7. If the PSF is arbitrarily approximated as a Gaussian function, the resolution of the image is described through full width at half maximum (FWHM) parameter of the Gaussian distribution. For example, in 1-D, the Gaussian distribution for PSF with mean μ and standard deviation σ can be represented as

$$h(x) = \frac{1}{\sqrt{2\pi\sigma^2}} e^{-\frac{(x-\mu)^2}{\sigma^2}}. \quad (2.46)$$

The FWHM in the above case is expressed as

$$\text{FWHM} = 2\sqrt{2\ln 2}\sigma \cong 2.36\sigma. \quad (2.47)$$

With an FWHM-based resolution criterion, two point sources are said to be resolved if they are separated by a distance greater than the FWHM. In case the PSF is described as a sinc function (see Fig. 2.8), a Rayleigh criterion can be used that

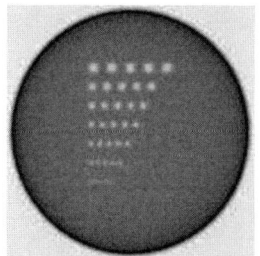

Figure 2.9 An X-ray imaging phantom with holes of different sizes.

requires the peak intensity of one PSF to at least coincide or be farther away from the first zero-crossing point of the second PSF in order to resolve two point sources.

For testing the spatial resolution performance of a medical imaging system, a physical phantom is used with a number of tubes of different diameters embedded in a cylindrical enclosure. For example, Figure 2.9 shows a spatial resolution phantom made out of aluminum with holes of different diameters. Such a phantom with holes acting as point sources can be used for X-ray imaging systems. There are varieties of phantoms that are used to meet specific needs of testing spatial resolution performance of a given imaging modality. Some phantoms are made out of an enclosure with circular tubes and hollow objects of different shapes and diameters. Based on imaging modality such as SPECT, PET, and MRI, the phantom is filled with a specific material (e.g., radioactive material for SPECT imaging system) for testing spatial resolution capabilities as well as contrast performance.

In addition to PSF, other measures are also often used in characterizing the spatial resolution performance of the imaging system. Such measures include line spread function (LSF) and modulation transfer function (MTF). The LSF is often used in X-ray imaging that is evaluated experimentally using a phantom with a grid of thin lead bars, and also defined as

$$LSF(y) = \int_{-\infty}^{\infty} PSF(x, y)\, dx. \qquad (2.48)$$

An MTF can be defined in the frequency domain that is characterized by the frequency response of the PSF as

$$MTF(\omega_x, \omega_y, \omega_z) = \iiint PSF(x, y, z) e^{-j2\pi\omega_x x} e^{-j2\pi\omega_x y} e^{-j2\pi\omega_x z}\, dx\, dy\, dz \qquad (2.49)$$

where $\omega_x, \omega_y, \omega_z$ are respectively spatial frequencies along x-, y-, and z-directions in the frequency domain (see Section 2.7 for Fourier transform).

2.5.2 Signal-to-Noise Ratio

The signal-to-noise ratio (SNR) is defined as the power ratio of original signal to noise. While the original signal can be regarded as useful information that is represented by the mean or expected value of the signal, noise can be considered variations in the background represented as standard deviation. Let us represent power of signal and noise as P_{signal} and P_{noise} respectively with A_{signal} and A_{noise} as amplitudes. SNR is then expressed as

$$\text{SNR} = \frac{P_{signal}}{P_{noise}} = \left(\frac{A_{signal}}{A_{noise}}\right)^2$$

$$\text{SNR(dB)} = 10\log\frac{P_{signal}}{P_{noise}} = 20\log\left(\frac{A_{signal}}{A_{noise}}\right). \quad (2.50)$$

For an image about which we have no other knowledge about the noise in its formation, the SNR can be represented by the ratio of mean and standard deviation or root-mean-square of all gray-level values of all pixels as

$$\text{SNR} = \frac{\bar{g}}{\sqrt{\frac{1}{MN}\sum_{x=1}^{M}\sum_{y=1}^{N}[g(x,y)-\bar{g}]^2}} \quad (2.51)$$

where $\bar{g} = \frac{1}{MN}\sum_{x=1}^{M}\sum_{y=1}^{N}g(x,y)$.

With additive noise assumption as used in Equation 2.45, image formation equation for an LSI imaging system can be expressed in frequency domain as

$$G(u,v) = F(u,v)H(u,v) + N(u,v) \quad (2.52)$$

where $G(u,v)$, $F(u,v)$ and $H(u,v)$ are, respectively, Fourier transform of acquired image, original object distribution, and PSF with u and v as spatial frequencies and $N(u,v)$ is the noise spectrum.

Considering that the acquired image represents the signal, and the noise spectrum can be estimated, the SNR can be computed through the ratio of signal and noise power spectra as

$$\text{SNR} = \frac{\sum_{u=0}^{P-1}\sum_{v=0}^{Q-1}|G(u,v)|^2}{\sum_{u=0}^{P-1}\sum_{v=0}^{Q-1}|N(u,v)|^2}. \quad (2.53)$$

Alternatively, with the knowledge of $f(x,y)$ (as is the case when a phantom is used for imaging), noise can be considered as the difference between the acquired image $g(x,y)$ and $f(x,y)$. The SNR then can be computed as

$$\text{SNR} = \frac{\sum_{x=1}^{M}\sum_{y=1}^{N}[g(x,y)]^2}{\sum_{x=1}^{M}\sum_{y=1}^{N}[f(x,y)-g(x,y)]^2}$$

$$= \frac{\sum_{x=1}^{M}\sum_{y=1}^{N}[g(x,y)]^2}{\sum_{x=1}^{M}\sum_{y=1}^{N}[n(x,y)]^2}. \quad (2.54)$$

2.5.3 Contrast-to-Noise Ratio

Medical images are often characterized by contrast-to-noise ratio (CNR) as a measure of image quality to discriminate an object of interest from its surrounding. In the context of medical imaging, CNR provides a measure of the capability to visualize physiological structures, lesions, or abnormalities in the image.

Contrast is a localized feature in the image that is described by the difference between the gray-level value of an object and its background. While there are several ways to define contrast feature, it is usually normalized in the 0–1 range as

$$C(x, y) = \frac{|f_{obj} - f_{back}|}{f_{obj} + f_{back}}$$

or

$$C(x, y) = \frac{|f_{obj} - f_{back}|}{\max\{f_{obj}, f_{back}\}}$$

or

$$C(x, y) = \frac{|f_{obj} - f_{back}|}{f_{ref}}. \tag{2.55}$$

where f_{obj} and f_{back} are, respectively, the average gray-level values or signal intensities in the object and background, and f_{ref} is a predetermined gray-level value or signal intensity in the image.

As described in the SNR section above, noise can be defined in different ways to determine CNR. Considering the image formation as expressed in Equation 2.52, the CNR can be expressed as

$$CNR = \frac{|f_{obj} - f_{back}|}{\sigma(x, y)}$$

or

$$CNR = \frac{\sum_{\text{for all objects}} |f_{obj} - f_{back}|^2}{[\sigma(x, y)]^2}. \tag{2.56}$$

where $\sigma(x, y)$ is the standard deviation of the noise in the image $f(x, y)$.

2.6. PIN-HOLE IMAGING

A pin-hole imaging method was originally developed for general-purpose photography. It is the simplest form of a camera for taking pictures on film or an array of sensors placed in the image plane. The pin-hole imaging method is used in many biomedical imaging systems including the nuclear medicine imaging modalities: SPECT and PET. The radiation from the object plane enters into the image plane through a pin hole. The plane containing the pin hole is called the focal plane. Figure 2.10 shows a schematic diagram of a pin-hole imaging system.

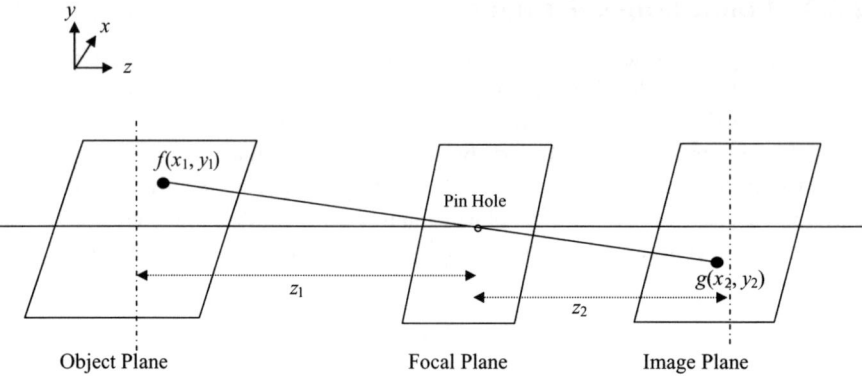

Figure 2.10 A schematic diagram of a pin-hole imaging camera.

If a point in the object plane is considered to have $(x_1, y_1, -z_1)$ coordinates mapped into the image plane as (x_2, y_2, z_2) coordinates, then

$$x_2 = -\frac{z_2 x_1}{z_1} \quad \text{and} \quad y_2 = -\frac{z_2 y_1}{z_1}. \tag{2.57}$$

It can be noted that such a pin-hole imaging system is inherently spatially variant providing a magnification factor, $M = -\frac{z_2}{z_1}$. However, if the collection efficiency of the radiant energy in the image plane is considered to be a constant throughout the image plane independent of the location of the source of the radiant energy point in the object plane, the imaging can be considered an LSI process. Generalizing the object plane with the 2-D coordinate system (α, β) and the corresponding image plane with the coordinate system (x, y), the general response function can include the magnification factor M so that the image formation equation can be expressed as

$$h(x, y; \alpha, \beta) = h(x - M\alpha, y - M\beta)$$

and

$$g(x, y) = \int_{-\infty}^{+\infty} \int_{-\infty}^{+\infty} h(x - M\alpha, y - M\beta) f(\alpha, \beta)\, d\alpha\, d\beta. \tag{2.58}$$

2.7. FOURIER TRANSFORM

The Fourier transform plays a very significant role in medical imaging and image analysis. The Fourier transform is a linear transform that provides information about the frequency spectrum of the signal, and is used in image processing for image enhancement, restoration, filtering, and feature extraction to help image interpretation and characterization. It is also used in image reconstruction methods for medical imaging systems. For example, the Fourier transform is used in image reconstruction in MRI. The Fourier transform can be applied to a signal to obtain frequency information if the function representing the signal is absolutely integrable over the entire domain and has only a finite number of discontinuities and a finite number of maxima and minima in any finite region. In addition, the function must not have any infinite discontinuities.

A 2-D Fourier transform, FT, of an image $g(x, y)$ is defined as*

$$G(u, v) = FT\{g(x, y)\} = \int_{-\infty}^{\infty} \int_{-\infty}^{\infty} g(x, y) e^{-j2\pi(ux+vy)} \, dx \, dy \qquad (2.59)$$

where u and v are the spatial frequencies in the x- and y-dimensions.

Once an image is transformed into the frequency domain, the degradation related to the noise and undesired frequencies can be filtered out. The filtered frequency information can then be used to recover the restored image through an inverse Fourier transform. Since the Fourier transform is a linear transform, the inverse transform can be used to obtain the original image from spatial frequency information if no filtering is performed in the frequency domain. A 2-D inverse Fourier transform is defined as

$$g(x, y) = FT^{-1}\{G(u, v)\} = \int_{-\infty}^{\infty} \int_{-\infty}^{\infty} G(u, v) e^{j2\pi(ux+vy)} \, du \, dv. \qquad (2.60)$$

The Fourier transform provides a number of useful properties for signal and image processing applications. Some of the important properties are briefly described below.

1. Linearity: Fourier transform, FT, is a linear transform.

$$FT\{ag(x, y) + bh(x, y)\} = aFT\{g(x, y)\} + bFT\{h(x, y)\} \qquad (2.61)$$

2. Scaling: It provides proportional scaling.

$$FT\{g(ax, by)\} = \frac{1}{ab} G\left(\frac{u}{a}, \frac{v}{b}\right) \qquad (2.62)$$

3. Translation: Translation of a function in the spatial domain introduces a linear phase shift in the frequency domain.

$$FT\{g(x-a, y-b)\} = G(u, v) e^{-j2\pi(ua+vb)} \qquad (2.63)$$

4. Convolution: The convolution of two functions in spatial domain is represented by multiplication of their respective spectra in the frequency domain.

$$FT\left\{\int_{-\infty}^{\infty} \int_{-\infty}^{\infty} g(\alpha, \beta) h(x-\alpha, y-\beta) \, d\alpha \, d\beta\right\} = G(u, v) H(u, v). \qquad (2.64)$$

5. Cross-correlation: The cross-correlation operation of two functions in the spatial domain is represented by the multiplication of the conjugate of one spectrum with another spectrum in the frequency domain.

---

*Using general notation, lowercase functions such as $g(x, y)$ are represented in the spatial domain with the spatial coordinate system (x, y) while upper case functions such as $G(u, v)$ are represented in the Fourier or frequency domain with the frequency coordinate system (u, v). Also, a and b have been used to represent constants for scaling, translation, and shifting operations.

$$FT\left\{\int_{-\infty}^{\infty}\int_{-\infty}^{\infty} g^*(\alpha,\beta)h(x+\alpha, y+\beta)\,d\alpha\,d\beta\right\} = G^*(u,v)H(u,v). \quad (2.65)$$

6. Auto-correlation: The Fourier transform of the auto-correlation of a function (such as a stochastic random signal) in the spatial domain is equal to the square of the absolute value of its Fourier transform, which is called the power spectrum.

$$FT\left\{\int_{-\infty}^{\infty}\int_{-\infty}^{\infty} g^*(\alpha,\beta)g(x+\alpha, y+\beta)\,d\alpha\,d\beta\right\} = G^*(u,v)G(u,v) = |G(u,v)|^2 \quad (2.66)$$

7. Parseval's theorem: The total energy is conserved in both spatial and frequency domains such that

$$\int_{-\infty}^{\infty}\int_{-\infty}^{\infty} g(x,y)g^*(x,y)\,dx\,dy = \int_{-\infty}^{\infty}\int_{-\infty}^{\infty} G(u,v)G^*(u,v)\,du\,dv. \quad (2.67)$$

8. Separability: If $g(x, y)$ is separable in x- and y-dimensions, the Fourier transform of $g(x, y)$ will also be separable.

$$g(x, y) = g_x(x)g_y(y).$$

then

$$FT\{g(x, y)\} = FT_x\{g_x(x)\}FT_y\{g_y(y)\}. \quad (2.68)$$

Figure 2.11a shows a vertical stripe image of 128 × 128 pixels generated from a sinusoid signal with a time period of 8 pixels. The image of the Fourier transform of the vertical stripe image is shown in Figure 2.11b. Two impulses corresponding to the frequency of the sinusoidal stripe signal can be seen in the Fourier transform image. Also, the vertical orientation of the stripes in the spatial domain and the horizontal orientation of the impulses in the Fourier domain should be noted. The effect of rotation in the spatial and frequency domains can be seen in Figure 2.12.

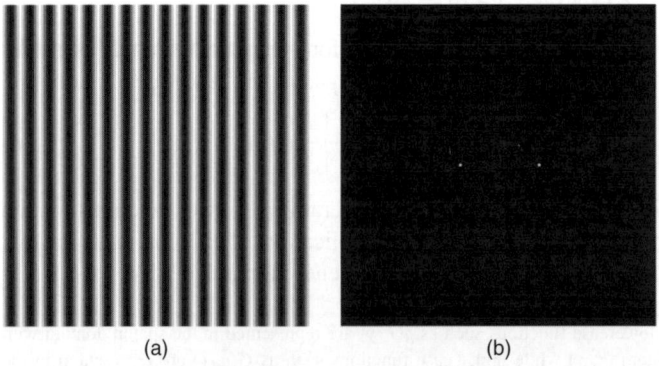

Figure 2.11 (a) A vertical stripe image generated from a sinusoidal waveform of a period of 8 pixels and (b) the magnitude image of its Fourier transform.

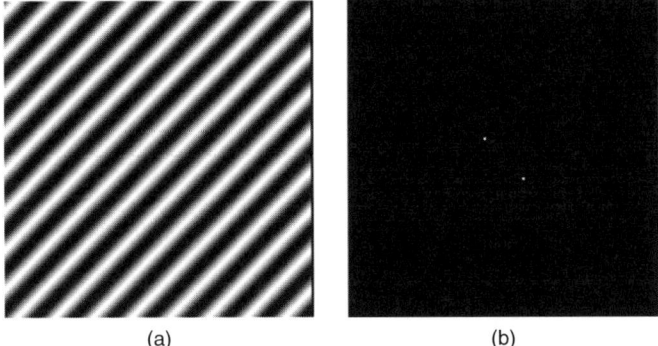

Figure 2.12 (a) A rotated stripe image and (b) magnitude image of its Fourier transform.

2.7.1 Sinc Function

The Fourier transform of a rectangular function is a sinc function. This has a specific significance in image processing because many image processing operations involve rectangular functions directly or indirectly. For example, a sampling period may be characterized by a rectangular window function, signal averaging is done over a rectangular window, and finite bandwidth is a specific case of the spectrum limited by a rectangular window function. Furthermore, a pixel in a digital image has a square shape, a specific instance of a rectangular function. For simplicity, let us consider a rectangular function in one dimension as

$$f(x) = \begin{cases} A & \text{for } |x| \leq \dfrac{w}{2} \\ 0 & \text{otherwise} \end{cases}. \quad (2.69)$$

Let $F(\omega)$ be the Fourier transform of $f(x)$ with ω as spatial frequency:

$$\begin{aligned} F(\omega) &= \int_{-\infty}^{\infty} f(x) e^{-j2\pi\omega x}\, dx = \int_{-w/2}^{w/2} A e^{-j2\pi\omega x}\, dx \\ &= \frac{-A}{j2\pi\omega}\left[e^{-j2\pi\omega x} \right]_{-w/2}^{w/2} \\ &= \frac{A}{j2\pi\omega}\left[e^{j\pi\omega w} - e^{-j\pi\omega w} \right] \\ &= Aw\frac{\sin(\pi\omega w)}{(\pi\omega w)} \\ &= Aw\operatorname{sinc}(z) \end{aligned} \quad (2.70)$$

where $\operatorname{sinc}(z) = \dfrac{\sin(\pi z)}{(\pi z)}$ and $z = \omega w$.

As shown in Figure 2.13, the $\operatorname{sinc}(z)$ function has high dc value with the oscillating lobes that go down in amplitude as frequency increases. The oscillatory

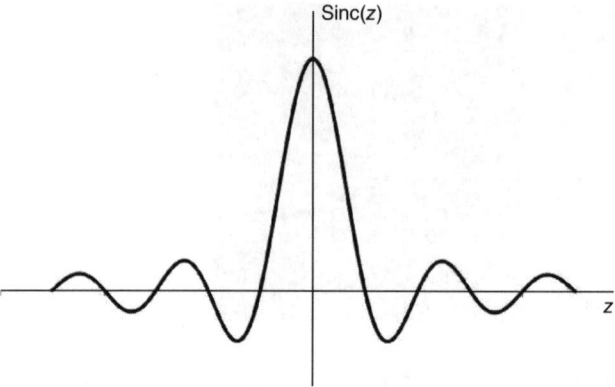

Figure 2.13 A sinc function: Fourier transform of a rectangular function.

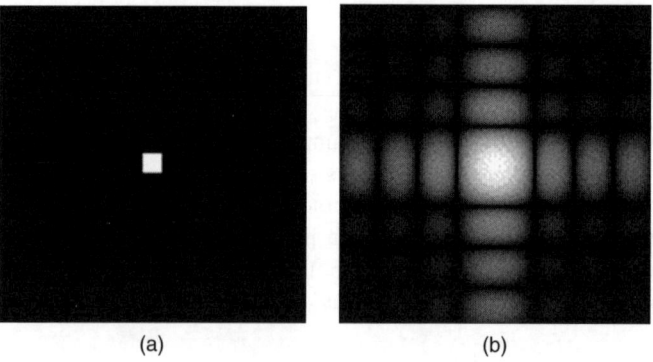

Figure 2.14 (a) An image with a square region at the center and (b) the logarithmic magnitude image of its Fourier transform.

nature of the sinc function creates dramatic effects in image reconstruction and processing. Figure 2.14 shows an image of a square region and its Fourier transform. The sinc-based oscillation pattern along both horizontal and vertical axes in the Fourier domain can be seen in Figure 2.14.

2.8. RADON TRANSFORM

The Radon transform defines projections of an object mapping the spatial domain of the object to its projection space. For example, the 2-D Radon transform of a 2-D object defines 1-D line integrals in the projection space, which is also called the Radon domain (14–17). In his paper published in 1917 (14), Radon provided a mathematical proof that an object can be reconstructed uniquely from its infinite continuous projections. In the early 1970s, Hounsfield and Cormack independently used the mathematical foundation established by Radon for reconstructing images of a human organ from its projections (15, 16). The projections were acquired through an X-ray CT imaging scanner (15).

2.8. RADON TRANSFORM

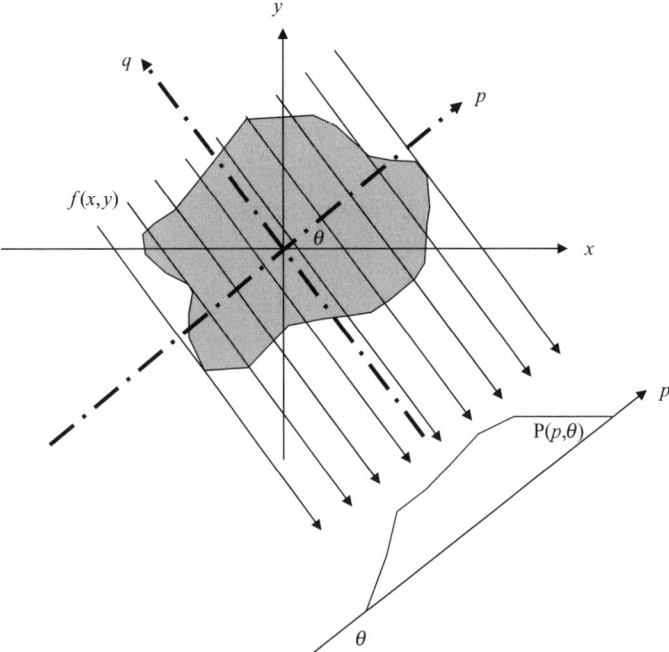

Figure 2.15 Line integral projection $P(p,\theta)$ of the two-dimensional Radon transform.

Let us define a 2-D object function $f(x, y)$ and its Radon transform by $\mathbf{R}\{f(x, y)\}$. Let us use the rectangular coordinate system (x, y) in the spatial domain. The Radon transform is defined by the projection $P(p, \theta)$ in the polar coordinate system as

$$P(p, \theta) = \mathbf{R}\{f(x, y)\} = \int_L f(x, y)\, dl$$

where the line integral $\int_L$ is defined along the path L such that

$$x\cos\theta + y\sin\theta = p. \tag{2.71}$$

Figure 2.15 shows a line integral that is computed along the parallel arrow lines that are sampled along the p axis and are defined by the angle θ. A set of line integrals or projections can be obtained for different θ angles.

The polar coordinate system (p,θ) can be converted into rectangular coordinates in the Radon domain by using a rotated coordinate system (p, q) as

$$x\cos\theta + y\sin\theta = p$$
$$-x\sin\theta + y\cos\theta = q. \tag{2.72}$$

The above implies

$$\mathbf{R}\{f(x, y)\} = \int_{-\infty}^{\infty} f(p\cos\theta - q\sin\theta,\, p\sin\theta + q\cos\theta)\, dq. \tag{2.73}$$

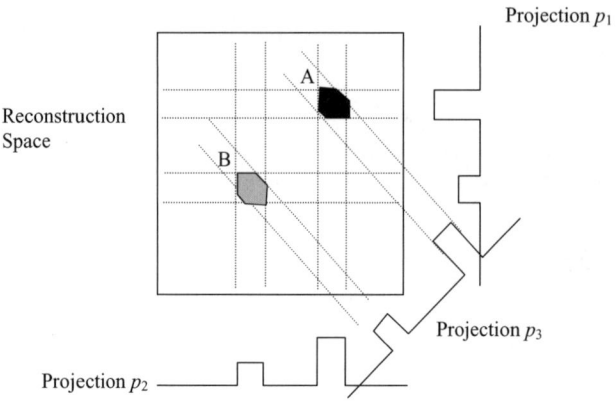

Figure 2.16 A schematic diagram for reconstructing images from projections. Three projections are back-projected to reconstruct objects A and B.

A higher-dimensional Radon transform can be defined in a similar way. For example, the projection space for a 3-D Radon transform would be defined by 2-D planes instead of lines.

The significance of using the Radon transform for computing projections in medical imaging is that an image of a human organ can be reconstructed by backprojecting the projections acquired through the imaging scanner. Figure 2.16 shows a schematic diagram of an image reconstruction process, called the backprojection method. Three simulated projections of two objects A and B are back-projected into the reconstruction space. Each projection has two segments of values corresponding to the objects A and B. When the projections are back-projected, the areas of higher values represent two reconstructed objects yielded by the intersection of back-projected data. It should be noted that the reconstructed objects may have geometrical or aliasing artifacts because of the limited number of projections used in the imaging and reconstruction processes. To improve the geometrical shape and accuracy of the reconstructed objects, a large number of projections should be used. The use of the Radon transform in image reconstruction from projection for applications in CT is described in Chapter 8.

2.9. SAMPLING

Computerized image processing and analysis requires that the image information be in a digital format. For example, a 2-D image $f_d[x, y]$ may be represented by a 2-D matrix of discrete numbers denoting the brightness levels placed uniformly in two dimensions. A picture element with a brightness level is called a pixel. The pixels are positioned in the image space based on the spatial sampling rate. Let us assume that a 2-D image signal $f_a(x, y)$ exists in the analog domain. This signal needs to sampled or discretized in order to create a digital image. One simple example is a digital camera with a charge-coupled device (CCD) array that provides a digital image through a 2-D array of light detectors. The physical size of each detector and its position provides the sampling of data points in the digital image. Thus, for a given object size and the discrete number of detectors, a sampling spatial frequency in the object space can be determined. The important question is whether the spatial sampling frequency is adequate to capture the fine details of the object. The sampling theorem provides the mathematical foundation of the Nyquist criterion to determine the optimal sampling rate for discretization of an analog signal without the loss of any frequency information. The Nyquist criterion states that to avoid any loss of information or aliasing artifact, an analog signal must be sampled with a sampling frequency that is at least twice the maximum frequency present in the original signal.

The sampling function is basically a series of delta functions represented in the same dimensions as of the signal. For example, when sampling a 1-D signal, a sampling function is defined as a series of 1-D delta functions. For a 2-D image, a 2-D distribution of delta functions is defined as

$$s(x, y) = \text{comb}(x, y) = \sum_{j_1=-\infty}^{\infty} \sum_{j_2=-\infty}^{\infty} \delta(x - j_1\Delta x, y - j_2\Delta y) \qquad (2.74)$$

where Δx and Δy are, respectively, the spacing of data points to be sampled in x- and y-directions.

Figure 2.17 shows an image of a 2-D distribution of Gaussian impulses (or comb function) and its Fourier transform.

The sampled version of the image $f_d[x, y]$ is given by

$$f_d[x, y] = f_a(x, y)s(x, y) = \sum_{j_1=-\infty}^{\infty} \sum_{j_2=-\infty}^{\infty} f_a(j_1\Delta x, j_2\Delta y)\delta(x - j_1\Delta x, y - j_2\Delta y). \qquad (2.75)$$

Let us consider, ω_x and ω_y to be the spatial frequencies in x- and y-directions, respectively, and $F_s(\omega_x, \omega_y)$ to be the Fourier transform of the sampled image $f_d[x, y]$.

Using the convolution theorem, it can be shown that

$$F_s(\omega_x, \omega_y) = \frac{1}{\Delta x \Delta y} \sum_{j_1=-\infty}^{\infty} \sum_{j_2=-\infty}^{\infty} F_a(\omega_x - j_1\omega_{xs}, \omega_y - j_2\omega_{ys}) \qquad (2.76)$$

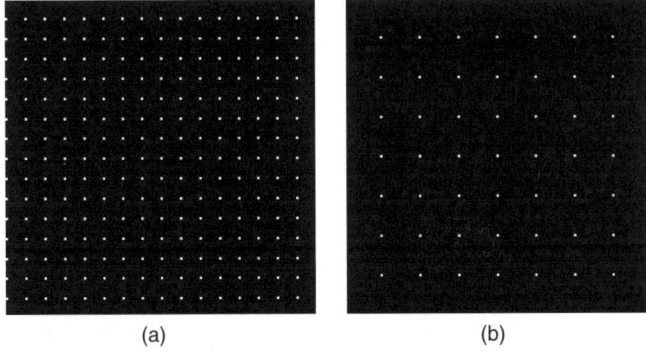

(a) (b)

Figure 2.17 (a) A 2-D distribution of Gaussian impulses (or comb function) in the spatial domain and (b) its representation in the Fourier domain.

where $F_a(\omega_x, \omega_y)$ is the Fourier transform of the analog image $f_a(x, y)$ and ω_{xs} and ω_{ys} represent the Fourier domain sampling spatial frequencies such that

$$\omega_{xs} = 2\pi/\Delta x \quad \text{and} \quad \omega_{ys} = 2\pi/\Delta y. \tag{2.77}$$

For a good discrete representation, the analog signal should be sampled in such a way that the information from the sampled signal can be recovered without any loss or artifact. In other words, the sampling process must not cause any loss of frequency information.

It can be easily shown that the multiplication operation of $f_a(x, y)$ with the sampling signal $s(x, y)$ would create a convolution operation in the Fourier domain resulting in multiple copies of the sampled image spectrum with the $2\pi/\Delta x$ and $2\pi/\Delta y$ spacing in ω_x and ω_y directions, respectively.

Let us assume that the image as the 2-D signal in the spatial domain is bandlimited, for example, the Fourier spectrum $F_a(\omega_x, \omega_y)$ is zero outside the maximum frequency components ω_{xmax} and ω_{ymax} in x- and y-directions as shown in Figure 2.18a.

To recover the signal without any loss, the multiple copies of the image spectrum must not overlap. If this condition is not met, the overlapped region of image spectrum will create aliasing and the original signal or image cannot be recovered by any filtering operation. Thus, to avoid overlapping of image spectra, it is necessary that

$$\omega_{xs} \geq \omega_{xmax} = 2\pi f_{xmax}$$
$$\omega_{ys} \geq \omega_{ymax} = 2\pi f_{ymax} \tag{2.78}$$

where f_{xmax} and f_{ymax} are the maximum spatial frequencies available in the image in x- and y-directions, respectively.

Figure 2.18b shows a good sampling of the bandlimited image signal shown in Figure 2.18a. Since the sampling frequency is higher than the Nyquist rate, multiple copies of the sampled spectrum do not overlap. Such a sampling does not cause any loss of information.

If the above condition is not satisfied, the undersampling will cause the overlapping of the high-frequency regions of the copies of image spectrum in the frequency domain. Such a sampled image will show an aliasing artifact, making it difficult to visualize the high-frequency information such as edges. Figure 2.18c shows undersampling of the bandlimited image signal shown in Figure 2.18a. Since the sampling frequency is lower than the Nyquist rate, multiple copies of the sampled spectrum overlap, causing the loss of high-frequency information in the overlapped regions. Due to the loss of information, the overlapping of high-frequency regions results in aliasing artifacts in the image.

To remove the aliasing artifact, a low-pass filter is required in the Fourier domain, prior to sampling, to remove the potential overlapped region of image spectra. After filtering the high-frequency information from the analog image, an inverse Fourier transform can recover the image in the spatial domain, but the recovered image will suffer from the lack of high-frequency information. Therefore, it is important to sample the image acquisition space adequately (preferably at a higher rate than the Nyquist rate) in medical imaging by placing an appropriate array

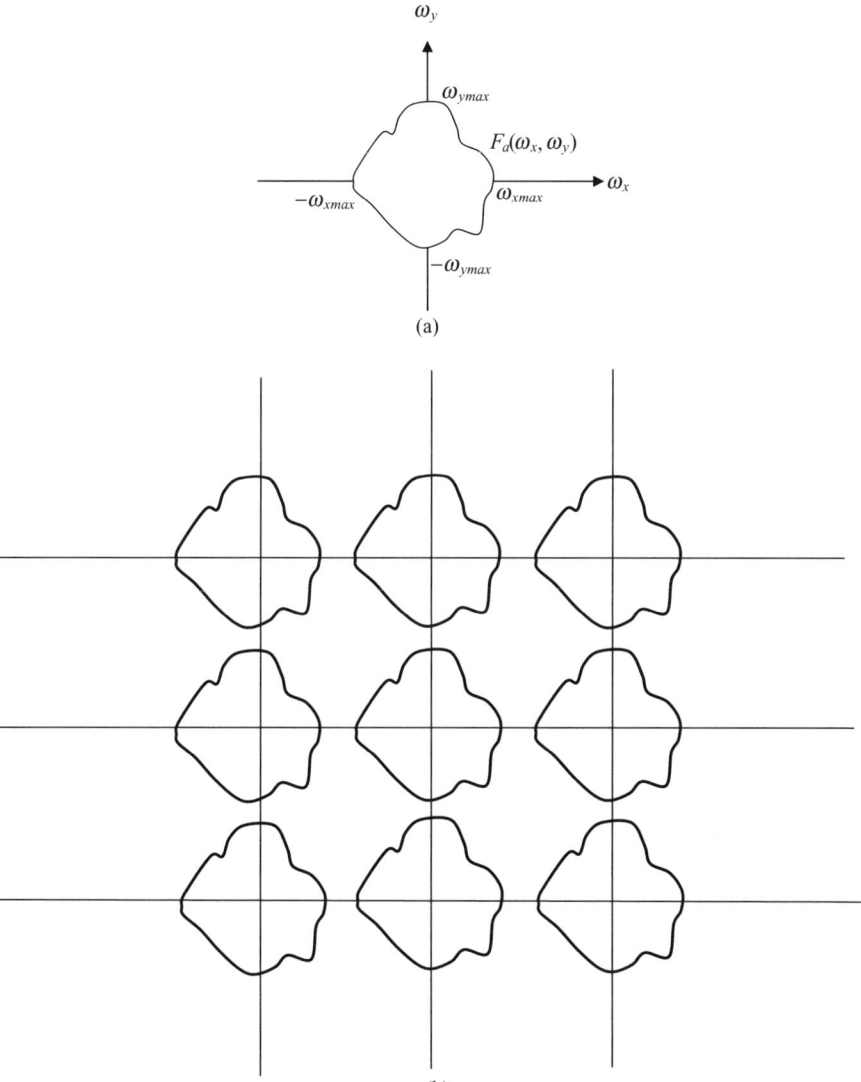

Figure 2.18 (a) The Fourier spectrum of a bandlimited two-dimensional signal; (b) sampling of the bandlimited signal with a sampling frequency higher than the Nyquist rate; (c) undersampling of the bandlimited signal with a sampling frequency lower than the Nyquist rate.

of detectors so that the acquired images do not suffer from aliasing artifacts. Figure 2.19 shows the effect of aliasing. An aliasing sinusoidal signal of a period of 1.8 pixels is shown in Figure 2.19a. The logarithmic magnitude of the Fourier transform of the aliasing signal shown in Figure 2.19a is shown in Figure 2.19b. Figure 2.19c shows the central cross section of the logarithmic magnitude of the Fourier transform, along the horizontal direction, of the image shown in Figure 2.11a, which is

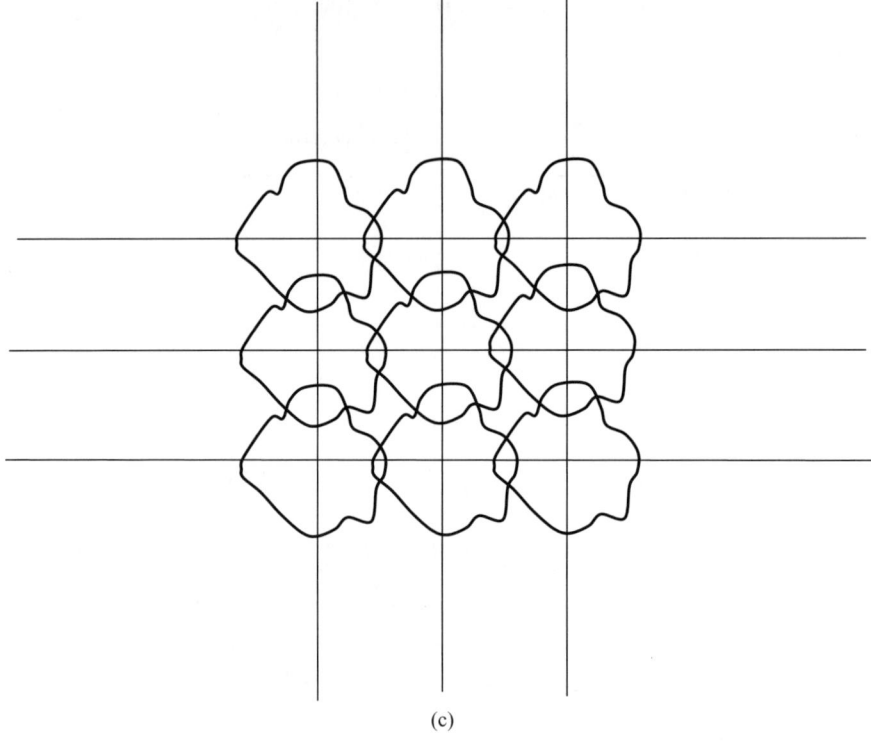

(c)

Figure 2.18 *Continued*

sampled satisfying the Nyquist criterion. The two peaks of the Fourier transform can be seen without any distortion in Figure 2.19c. Figure 2.19d shows the central cross-section along the horizontal direction of the logarithmic magnitude of the Fourier transform of the aliasing pattern shown in Figure 2.19a showing the distortion of the Fourier spectrum.

2.10. DISCRETE FOURIER TRANSFORM

The discrete Fourier transform (DFT), $F(u, v)$ of an image $f(x, y)$ is defined as

$$F(u, v) = \frac{1}{MN} \sum_{x=0}^{M-1} \sum_{y=0}^{N-1} f(x, y) e^{-j2\pi\left(\frac{xu}{M} + \frac{yv}{N}\right)} \qquad (2.79)$$

where u and v are frequency coordinates in the Fourier domain such that $u = 0, 1,..., M - 1$ and $v = 0, 1,..., N - 1$.

The inverse DFT in two dimensions can be defined as

$$f(x, y) = \frac{1}{MN} \sum_{u=0}^{M-1} \sum_{v=0}^{N-1} F(u, v) e^{j2\pi\left(\frac{xu}{M} + \frac{yv}{N}\right)}. \qquad (2.80)$$

2.10. DISCRETE FOURIER TRANSFORM 51

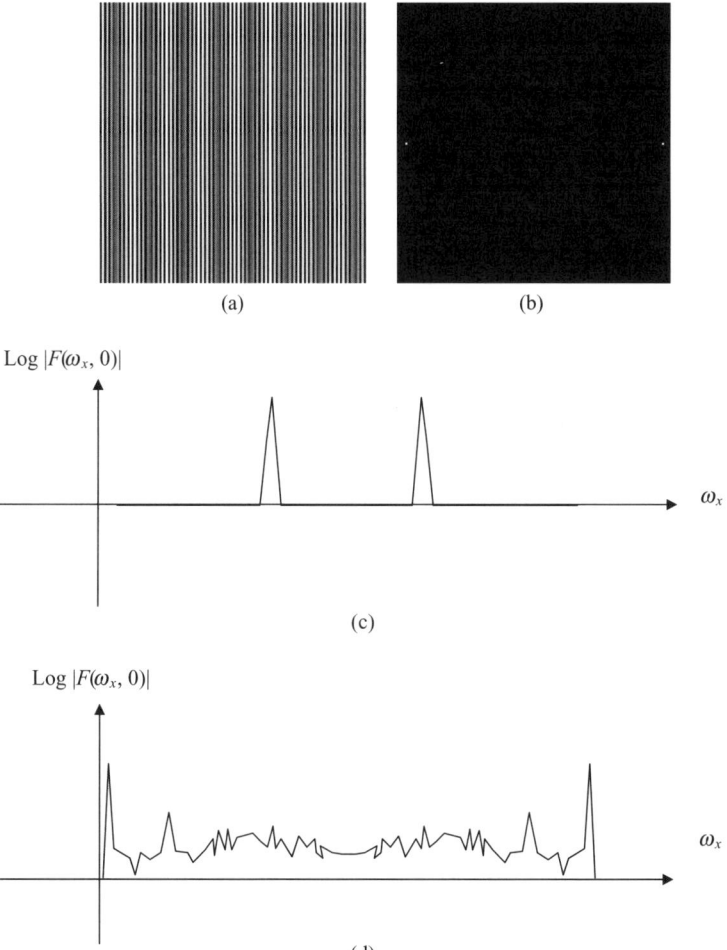

Figure 2.19 (a) A vertical stripe image generated from a sinusoidal waveform of a period of 1.8 pixels; (b) the logarithmic magnitude image of its Fourier transform; (c) the central cross-section of the logarithmic magnitude of the Fourier transform, along the horizontal direction, of the signal shown in Figure 2.8a, which is sampled, satisfying the Nyquist criterion; and (d) the central cross-section along the horizontal direction of the logarithmic magnitude of the Fourier transform of the aliasing pattern shown in Figure 2.15a.

The properties of the Fourier transform as described above are valid for the DFT as well. However, the numerical implementation of the DFT and fast Fourier transform (FFT) may make some approximations and finite computations. The errors in computations and approximations may cause artifacts in the image spectrum and may not allow an implementation of Fourier transform to be exactly reversible.

2.11. WAVELET TRANSFORM

The wavelet transform is a method for the complete frequency localization of a signal. The Fourier transform provides information about the frequency components present in the signal. However, Fourier analysis suffers from the drawback of the loss of localization or time information when transforming information from the time domain to the frequency domain. When the frequency representation of a signal is analyzed, it is impossible to tell when a particular frequency event took place. If the signal properties do not change much over time, this drawback may be ignored. However, signals change with interesting properties over time or space. An electrocardiogram signal changes over the time marker with respect to heartbeat events. Similarly, in the context of 2- and 3-D images, a signal or a property represented by the image (such as blood flow) may change over the sampled data points in space. Thus, Fourier analysis, in general, does not provide a specific event (frequency) localized information with respect to time (in time series signals) or space (in images). This drawback of Fourier transfer can be somewhat addressed with the use of short-time Fourier Transform (STFT) (19–22). This technique computes the Fourier transform to analyze only a small section of the signal at a time. As a matter of fact, STFT maps a signal into separate functions of time and frequency. The STFT provides some information about frequency localization with respect to a selected window. However, this information is obtained with limited precision determined by the size of the window. A major shortcoming of STFT is that the window size is fixed for all frequencies, once a particular size for the time window is chosen. In real applications, signals may require a variable window size in order to accurately determine event localization with respect to frequency and time or space.

Wavelet transform may use long sampling intervals where low-frequency information is needed, and shorter sampling intervals where high-frequency information is available. The major advantage of wavelet transform is its ability to perform multiresolution analysis for event localization with respect to all frequency components in data over time or space. Thus, wavelet analysis is capable of revealing aspects of data that other signal analysis techniques miss, such as breakdown points, and discontinuities in higher derivatives (19–22).

Wavelet transform theory uses two major concepts: scaling and shifting. Scaling, through dilation or compression, provides the capability to analyze a signal over different windows (sampling periods) in the data, while shifting, through delay or advancement, provides translation of the wavelet kernel over the entire signal. Daubechies wavelets (20) are compactly orthonormal wavelets that make discrete wavelet analysis practicable. Wavelet analysis has been used in numerous applications in statistics, time series analysis, and image processing (21–25).

The wavelet transform is based on the principle of linear series expansion of a signal using a set of orthonormal basis function. Through linear series expansion, a signal $f(t)$ can be uniquely decomposed as a weighted combination of orthonormal basis functions as

$$f(t) = \sum_n a_n \varphi_n(t) \quad (2.81)$$

where n is an integer index with $n \in Z$ (Z is a set of all integers), a_k are weights, and $\varphi_n(t)$ are orthonormal basis functions.

It follows that $f(t) \in V$ as the closed span of the expansion set $\{\varphi_n(t)\}$ denoted by V and expressed as

$$V = \overline{\underset{n}{Span}\{\varphi_n(t)\}}. \tag{2.82}$$

The weights or coefficients of expansions can then be expressed as

$$a_n = \langle \tilde{\varphi}_n(t), f(t) \rangle \tag{2.83}$$

where $\{\tilde{\varphi}_n(t)\}$ is set of dual basis function, and $\langle \rangle$ represents the inner product.

Using the orthonormality condition of the set of basis functions, Equation 9.46 can be expressed as

$$a_n = \langle \varphi_n(t), f(t) \rangle$$

$$\text{with } \langle \varphi_j(t), \varphi_k(t) \rangle = \delta_{jk} = \begin{cases} 0 & j \neq k \\ 1 & j = k \end{cases}. \tag{2.84}$$

The wavelet transform utilizes the series expansion of a signal using a set of orthonormal basis functions that are generated by scaling and translation of the mother wavelet $\psi(t)$ and the scaling function $\phi(t)$. The wavelet transform decomposes the signal as a linear combination of weighted basis functions to provide frequency localization with respect to the sampling parameter such as time or space. The multiresolution approach of the wavelet transform establishes a basic framework of the localization and representation of different frequencies at different scales.

If the sampling parameter is assumed to be time, a scaling function $\phi(t)$ in time t can be defined as

$$\phi_{j,k}(t) = 2^{j/2} \phi(2^j t - k) \tag{2.85}$$

where j is a scaling parameter, and k is a translation parameter, and $j, k \in Z$, set of all integers, and $\{\phi_{j,k}(t)\}$ spans over the subspace $V_j \in L^2(\mathbf{R})$ where $\mathbf{R}$ is the space of all real numbers.

The scaling and translation generates a family of functions using the following "dilation" equations:

$$\phi(t) = \sqrt{2} \sum_{n \in Z} h_\phi(n) \phi(2t - n) \tag{2.86}$$

where $h_\phi(n)$ is a set of filter (generally called as low-pass filter) coefficients.

To induce a multiresolution analysis in $L^2(\mathbf{R})$, it is necessary to have a nested chain of closed subspaces defined as

$$\cdots \subset V_{-1} \subset V_0 \subset V_1 \subset V_2 \subset \cdots \subset L^2(\mathbf{R}). \tag{2.87}$$

Let us define a function $\psi(t)$ as the "mother wavelet" such that its translated and dilated versions form an orthonormal basis of $L^2(\mathbf{R})$ to be expressed as

$$\psi_{j,k}(t) = 2^{j/2} \psi(2^j t - k). \tag{2.88}$$

The wavelet basis induces an orthogonal decomposition of $L^2(R)$, that is, one can write

$$\cdots \subset W_{-1} \subset W_0 \subset W_1 \subset W_2 \subset \cdots \subset L^2(R) \qquad (2.89)$$

where W_j is a subspace spanned by $\psi(2^j t - k)$ for all integers $j, k \in Z$.

This basic requirement of a multiresolution analysis is satisfied by the nesting of the spanned subspaces similar to scaling functions, that is, $\psi(t)$ can be expressed as a weighted sum of the shifted $\psi(2t-n)$ as

$$\psi(t) = \sqrt{2} \sum_{n \in Z} h_\psi(n) \psi(2t - n) \qquad (2.90)$$

where $h_\psi(n)$ is a set of filter (generally called high-pass filter) coefficients.

The wavelet-spanned multiresolution subspace satisfies the relation

$$V_{j+1} = V_j \oplus W_j$$
$$= V_{j-1} \oplus W_{j-1} \oplus W_j$$
$$= V_{j-2} \oplus W_{j-2} \oplus W_{j-1} \oplus W_j$$

where $\oplus$ denotes the union operation of subspaces, and

$$L^2(R) = \cdots \oplus W_{-2} \oplus W_{-1} \oplus W_0 \oplus W_1 \oplus W_2 \oplus \cdots \qquad (2.91)$$

Figure 2.20 shows the wavelet multiresolution space showing the distribution of the original $L^2(R)$ space into subspaces through wavelet decomposition. Three levels of decomposition are shown. In the first level of decomposition, the original space V_{j+1} is divided into V_j and W_j spectral subspaces as the output of the low-pass and high-pass filters, respectively. These subspaces are then further decomposed into smaller spectral bands. It can be seen from the hatched spaces that for a complete spectral representation of the original signal in V_{j+1} space, it is sufficient to include the last low-pass filter space V_{j-2} and all high-pass filter spaces W_{j-2}, W_{j-1} and W_j. However, other combinations involving different spectral bands are possible.

Wavelet functions span the orthogonal complement spaces. The orthogonality requires the scaling and wavelet filter coefficients to be related through the following:

$$h_\psi(n) = (-1)^n h_\phi(1-n). \qquad (2.92)$$

Let $x[n]$ be an arbitrary square summable sequence representing a signal in the time or space domain such that

$$x[n] \in L^2(R). \qquad (2.93)$$

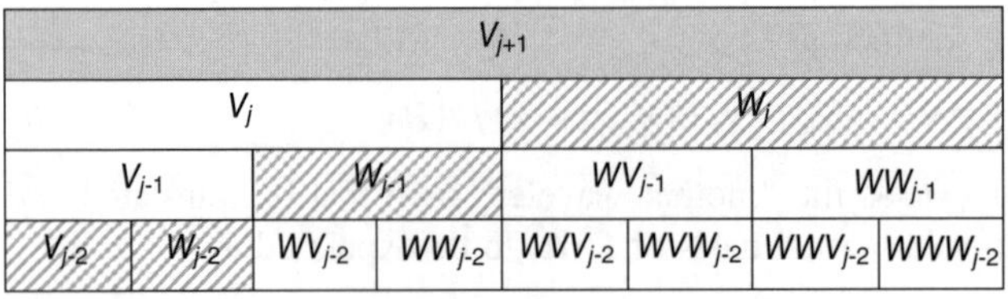

Figure 2.20 The wavelet multiresolution space with three levels of decomposition.

The series expansion of a discrete signal $x[n]$ using a set of orthonormal basis functions $\phi_k(n)$ is given by

$$x[n] = \sum_{k \in Z} \langle \phi_k[l], x[l] \rangle \phi_k[n] = \sum_{k \in Z} X[k]\varphi_k[n] \qquad (2.94)$$

where $X[k] = \langle \phi_k[l], x[l] \rangle = \sum_l \phi_k^*(l)x[l]$.

where $X[k]$ is the transform of $x[n]$. All basis functions must satisfy the orthonormality condition, that is,

$$\langle \phi_k[n], \phi_l[n] \rangle = \delta[k-l]$$

with

$$\|x\|^2 = \|X\|^2. \qquad (2.95)$$

The series expansion is considered complete if every signal can be expressed using the expression in Equation 2.95. Similarly, using a set of bi-orthogonal basis functions, the series expansion of the signal $x[n]$ can be expressed as

$$x[n] = \sum_{k \in Z} \langle \phi_k[l], x[l] \rangle \tilde{\phi}_k[n] = \sum_{k \in Z} \tilde{X}[k]\tilde{\varphi}_k[n]$$

$$= \sum_{k \in Z} \langle \tilde{\phi}_k[l], x(l) \rangle \phi_k[n] = \sum_{k \in Z} X[k]\phi_k[n] \qquad (2.96)$$

where $\tilde{X}[k] = \langle \phi_k[l], x[l] \rangle$ and $X[k] = \langle \tilde{\phi}_k[l], x[l] \rangle$ and $\langle \phi_k[n], \tilde{\phi}_l[n] \rangle = \delta[k-l]$.

Using the quadrature-mirror filter theory, the orthonormal bases $\phi_k[n]$ can be expressed as low-pass and high-pass filters for decomposition and reconstruction of a signal. It can be shown that a discrete signal $x[n]$ can be decomposed into $X[k]$ as

$$x[n] = \sum_{k \in Z} \rangle \varphi_k[l]x[l]\langle \varphi_k[n] = \sum_{k \in Z} X[k]\varphi_k[n]$$

where

$$\varphi_{2k}[n] = h_0[2k-n] = g_0[n-2k]$$
$$\varphi_{2k+1}[n] = h_1[2k-n] = g_1[n-2k]$$

and

$$X[2k] = \langle h_0[2k-l], x[l] \rangle$$
$$X[2k+1] = \langle h_1[2k-l], x[l] \rangle. \qquad (2.97)$$

In Equation 2.97, h_0 and h_1 are, respectively, the low-pass and high-pass filters for signal decomposition or analysis, and g_0 and g_1 are, respectively, the low-pass and high-pass filters for signal reconstruction or synthesis. A perfect reconstruction of the signal can be obtained if the orthonormal bases are used in decomposition and reconstruction stages as

$$x[n] = \sum_{k \in Z} X[2k]\phi_{2k}[n] + \sum_{k \in Z} X[2k+1]\phi_{2k+1}[n]$$

$$= \sum_{k \in Z} X[2k]g_0[n-2k] + \sum_{k \in Z} X[2k+1]g_1[n-2k]. \qquad (2.98)$$

As described above, the scaling function provides low-pass filter coefficients and the wavelet function provides the high-pass filter coefficients. A multiresolution signal representation can be constructed based on the differences of information available at two successive resolutions 2^j and 2^{j-1}. Such a representation can be computed by decomposing a signal using the wavelet transform. First, the signal is filtered using the scaling function, a low-pass filter. The filtered signal is then subsampled by keeping one out of every two samples. The result of low-pass filtering and subsampling is called the scale ransformation. If the signal has the resolution 2^j, the scale transformation provides the reduced resolution 2^{j-1}. The difference of information between resolutions 2^j and 2^{j-1} is called the "detail" signal at resolution 2^j. The detail signal is obtained by filtering the signal with the wavelet, a high-pass filter, and subsampling by a factor of two. Thus, wavelet-based decomposition of a signal $x[n]$ is obtained using a low-pass filter $h_0[k]$ (obtained from the scaling function) and a high-pass filter $h_1[k]$ (obtained from the wavelet function). The signal decomposition at the jth stage can thus be generalized as

$$X^{(j)}[2k] = \langle h_0^{(j)}[2^j k - l], x[l] \rangle$$
$$X^{(j)}[2k+1] = \langle h_1^{(j)}[2^j k - l], x[l] \rangle. \quad (2.99)$$

The signal can be reconstructed back from the decomposed coefficients using the reconstruction filters as

$$x[n] = \sum_{j=1}^{J} \sum_{k \in z} X^{(j)}[2k+1] g_1^{(j)}[n - 2^j k] + \sum_{k \in z} X^{(j)}[2k] g_0^{(j)}[n - 2^j k]. \quad (2.100)$$

The signal decomposition and reconstruction stages implementing Equations 2.99 and 2.100 are schematically shown in Figure 2.21, where H_0 and H_1 are shown,

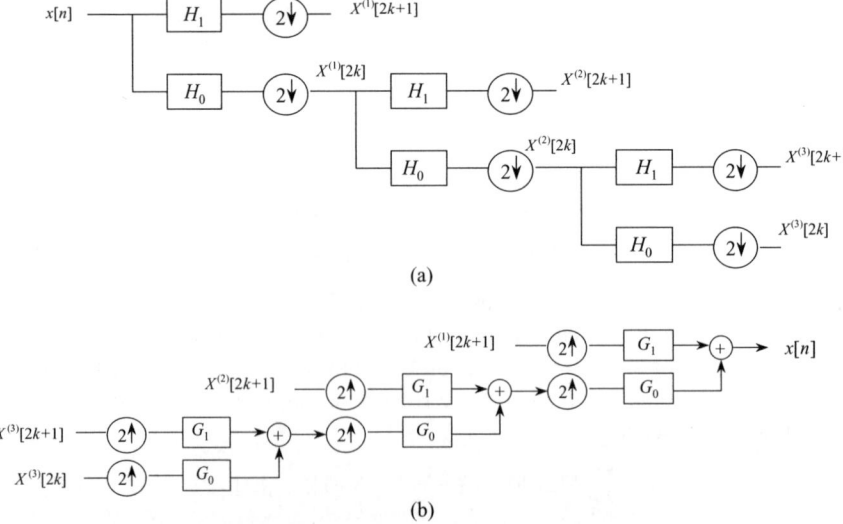

Figure 2.21 (a) A multiresolution signal decomposition using wavelet transform and (b) the reconstruction of the signal from wavelet transform coefficients.

respectively, as low-pass and high-pass filters for signal decomposition, and G_0 and G_1 are shown, respectively, as low-pass and high-pass filters for signal reconstruction.

In order to apply wavelet transform for image processing, the above method for 1-D wavelet transform for signal decomposition is applied to two individual 1-D vectors extracted from the 2-D image: the first vector reading pixels along the rows of the image (horizontal sampling), and the second vector reading pixels along the columns of the image (vertical sampling). The image (say at resolution 2^{j+1}) is first low-pass and high-pass filtered along the rows (Fig. 2.22). The result of each filtering process is subsampled. Next, the subsampled results are low-pass and high-pass filtered along each column. The results of these filtering processes are again subsampled. The combination of filtering and subsampling processes essentially provides the band-pass information. The frequency band denoted by A_j in Figure 2.22 is referred to as the low-low-frequency band. It contains the scaled low-frequency information. The frequency bands labeled D_j^1, D_j^2, and D_j^3 denote the detail information. They are referred to as low-high, high-low, and high-high-frequency bands, respectively. Thus, an image is decomposed into four quadrants: low-low, low-high, high-low, and high-high-frequency bands. This scheme can be iteratively applied to an image for further decomposition into narrower frequency bands; that is, each frequency band can be further decomposed into four narrower bands. However, for wavelet decomposition as shown in Figure 2.20, only low-low band is further decomposed into four quadrants of the next lower resolution. A two-level wavelet decomposition-based quadrant structure is shown in Figure 2.21b. Since each level of decomposition reduces the resolution by a factor of two, the length of the filter limits the number of levels of decomposition.

Several wavelets satisfying the mathematical constraints of providing orthonormal bases for signal decomposition have been developed by Daubechies (20). Least asymmetric wavelets computed with different support widths have been designed for signal and image processing applications (20–22). Figure 2.23 shows the scaling and wavelet functions with the corresponding decomposition and reconstruction low-pass and high-pass filters for Daubechies's db4 wavelet. Each filter is limited to eight coefficients in length. Figure 2.24 shows an X-ray mammographic image and its complete three-level decomposition using the db4 wavelet-based low-pass and high-pass decomposition filters shown in Figure 2.23. Figure 2.25 shows a denoised image of the X-ray mammogram shown in Figure 2.23 after soft thresholding the coefficients in the wavelet decomposition domain and then reconstructing the image using the reconstruction filters (shown in Figure 2.23). The wavelet description and operations can be found in the MATLAB wavelet toolbox. Image processing operations using wavelets are further described in Chapter 9.

Wavelet transform has been widely used in signal and image processing applications as well as in data mining and information processing applications. Wavelet transform provides many favorable properties, such as hierarchical and multiresolution decomposition structure, linear time and space relationships, and a wide variety of basis functions to extract specific spectral features for analysis (20–27).

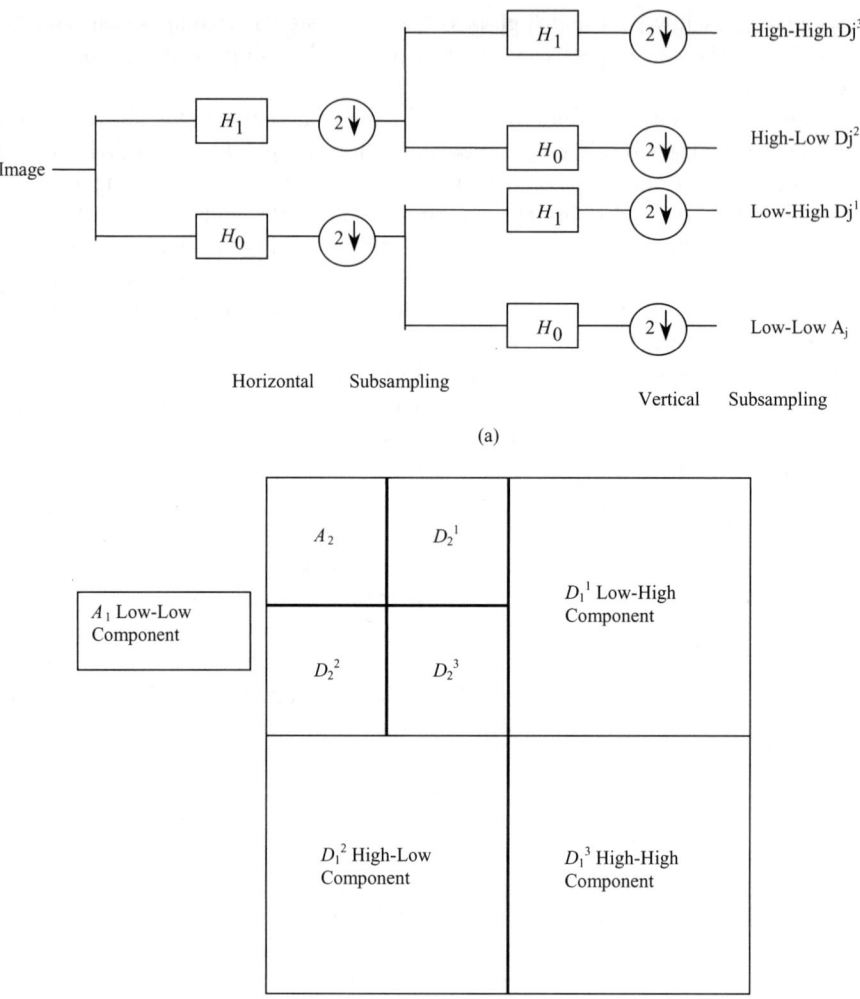

Figure 2.22 (a) Multiresolution decomposition of an image using the wavelet transform. (b) Wavelet transform-based image decomposition: the original resolution image ($N \times N$) is decomposed into four low-low A_1, low-high D_1^1, high-low D_1^2, and high-high D_1^3 images, each of which is subsampled to resolution $\left(\dfrac{N}{2} \times \dfrac{N}{2}\right)$. The low-low mage is further decomposed into four images of $\left(\dfrac{N}{4} \times \dfrac{N}{4}\right)$ resolution each in the second level of decomposition. For a full decomposition, each of the "Detail" component can also be decomposed into four sub-images with $\left(\dfrac{N}{4} \times \dfrac{N}{4}\right)$ resolution each.

2.11. WAVELET TRANSFORM   59

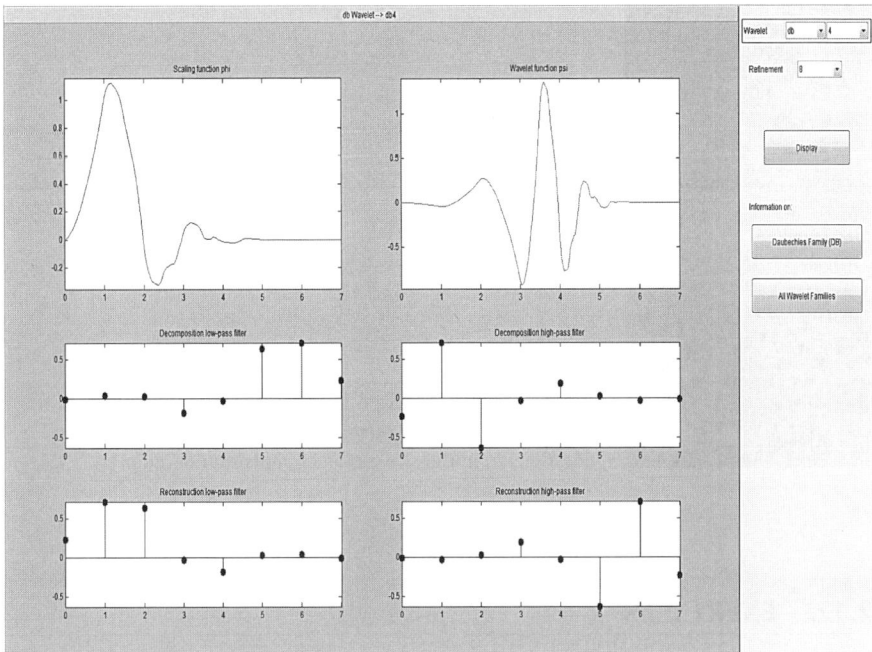

Figure 2.23   Scaling and wavelet functions with corresponding decomposition and reconstruction low-pass and high-pass filters for Daubechies's db4 wavelet. The image is produced using the MATLAB wavelet toolbox GUI.

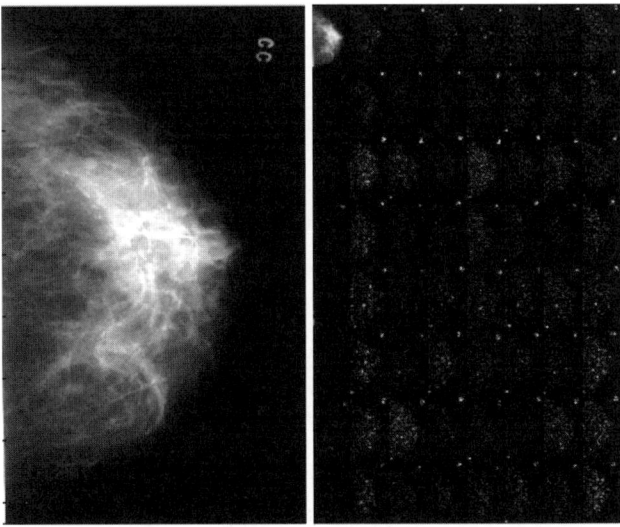

Figure 2.24   An image of X-ray mammogram (left) and its complete decomposition using Daubechies's db4 wavelet.

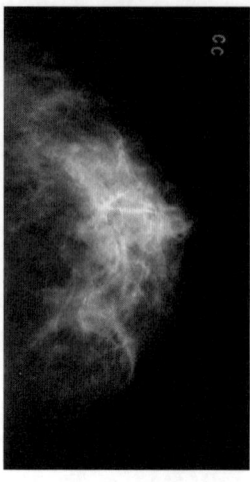

Figure 2.25 A denoised image of the X-ray mammogram (shown in Fig. 2.23) reconstructed after soft thresholding coefficients in the wavelet decomposition domain.

2.12. EXERCISES

2.1. What is the difference between a linear and a nonlinear imaging system? What problems would you expect if an imaging system is nonlinear and spatially variant?

2.2. Why it is important to design instrumentation in medical imaging that can provide spatially invariant point spread function (PSF)? What is the main advantage in dealing with linear spatially invariant medical imaging systems?

2.3. Prove Parseval's theorem in two dimensions.

2.4. Extend the Radon transform to three dimensions. Develop the mathematical expressions defining the projection domain.

2.5. Prove and explain the convolution and correlation properties of two-dimensional discrete Fourier transform (DFT).

2.6. Show that the frequency spectrum of a circularly symmetric function is also circularly symmetric.

2.7. Show that the Fourier transform of a unit impulse function located at the origin is a constant.

2.8. Show that the Fourier transform of a spatially distributed impulse function as $comb(x, y)$ is a $comb(u, v)$ function in the frequency domain.

2.9. Show that Fourier transform of a sampled function is an infinite periodic sequence of copies of Fourier transform of the original continuous function.

2.10. For the image formation as represented by Equation 2.44, show that $S_{gg}(u, v) = S_{ff}(u, v)|H(u, v)|^2$ where $S_{ff}(u, v)$ and $S_{gg}(u, v)$ are, respectively, the spectral densities of the random fields represented by $f(x, y)$ and $g(x, y)$; and $H(u, v)$ is the Fourier transform of point spread function, $h(x, y)$.

2.11. Show that the Fourier transform of 1-D rectangular function of amplitude A and duration t is a sinc function given by $\left(At\dfrac{\sin(\pi ut)}{\pi ut}\right)$.

2.12. Define the Nyquist criterion for sampling a 2-D signal. What should be the maximum sampling period to avoid aliasing if the highest frequency in the signal is 27 KHz?

2.13. A medical imaging scanner has a detector system that cannot acquire the data faster than 1.0 KHz with a spatial resolution of 1 mm × 1 mm. Let us assume that the object is dynamically changing its contrast with a period 0.1 ms and needs to see pathology with circular dimension of about 1 mm diameter on average. Can this imaging system provide sufficient information through its images? Explain your answer.

2.14. Display an image in MATLAB. Mark five landmarks in the image and note their positions. Create a rotation transform to rotate the image by 30 degrees along the horizontal axis and 45 degrees along the vertical axis. Implement the transformation in MATLAB. Find the landmarks and note their positions. Are all landmarks rotated by exactly the same vector? If not, why not?

2.15. Apply the reverse rotation transformation to the rotated image in Problem 2.3. Subtract this image from the original image in the MATLAB environment. Does the resulting image contain all zeros? If not, explain the reason.

2.16. Write a program in MATLAB to implement and display 2-D Radon transform. Obtain eight projections of a chest radiograph covering the angular span of 180 degrees around the image. Display the line-integral projections.

2.17. Create a phantom image by assigning 255 gray-level value to the 2 × 2 pixel area in the center of a 256 × 256 pixel image. All other pixels are assigned zero value. Use 2-D FFT routine in MATLAB and display the Fourier spectrum image.

2.18. Use the chest radiograph image and apply the 2-D FFT routine in MATLAB. Display the Fourier spectrum image. Now take 2-D inverse Fourier transform of the spectrum image to recover the spatial domain image. Subtract this image from the original image. Does the image contain all zero values?

2.19. Can Fourier transform provide localization of spatial frequencies in an image? Elaborate your answer with an example.

2.20. Explain the wavelet transform with respect to scaling and wavelet functions.

2.21. How is the wavelet transform different from the short-time Fourier transform?

2.22. Why must the bases in wavelet decomposition-based series expansion satisfy the condition of orthonormality?

2.23. Describe a three-level wavelet processing with decomposition filters. Using the output of the decomposition filters, describe a method for loss-less perfect reconstruction.

2.24. Use a brain image for wavelet-based three-level decomposition using the following wavelets in the MATLAB environment:

  a. HAAR
  b. db2
  c. db4
  d. db8

2.25. Use the denoised operation on the brain image used in Exercise 2.24 with db6 (level 3) wavelet in the MATLAB wavelet graphical user interface (GUI). Use three sets of different soft thresholds at each level with the fixed thresholding method to obtain three denoised images. Compare these images and explain the variations in the denoised images with respect to the threshold values. (You may add Gaussian noise in the original image and then repeat the denoised operations to observe performance variations better.)

2.13. REFERENCES

1. J.C. Russ, *The Image Processing Handbook*, 2nd Edition, CRC Press, Boca Raton, FL, 1995.
2. B. Jahne, *Practical Handbook on Image Processing for Scientific Applications*, CRC Press, Boca Raton, FL, 1997.
3. R.C. Gonzalez and R.E. Woods, *Digital Image Processing*, 2nd Edition, Prentice Hall, Englewood Cliffs, NJ, 2002.
4. A.P. Dhawan and A. Sicsu, "Segmentation of images of skin-lesions using color and surface pigmentation," *Comput. Med. Imaging Graph.*, Vol. 16, pp. 163–177, 1992.
5. L.K. Arata, A.P. Dhawan, A.V. Levy, J. Broderick, and M. Gaskil, "Three-dimensional anatomical model based segmentation of MR brain images through principal axes registration," *IEEE Trans. Biomed. Eng.*, Vol. 42, pp. 1069–1078, 1995.
6. A.P. Dhawan, L.K. Arata, A.V. Levy, and J. Mantil, "Iterative principal axes registration method for analysis of MR-PET brain images," *IEEE Trans. Biomed. Eng.*, Vol. 42, pp. 1079–1087, 1995.
7. H.C. Andrews and B.R. Hunt, *Digital Image Restoration*, Prentice Hall, Englewood Cliffs, NJ, 1977.
8. H. Barrett and W. Swindell, *Radiological Imaging: The Theory of Image Formation, Detection and Processing, Volumes 1–2*, Academic Press, New York, 1981.
9. R.N. Bracewell, *Two-Dimensional Imaging*, Prentice Hall, Englewood Cliffs, NJ, 1995.
10. Z.H. Cho, J.P. Jones, and M. Singh, *Fundamentals of Medical Imaging*, John Wiley & Sons, New York, 1993.
11. M.P. Ekstrom, *Digital Image Processing Techniques*, Academic Press, Inc, New York, 1984.
12. P. Stucki, *Advances in Digital Image Processing*, Plenum Press, New York, 1979.
13. A. Rosenfield and A.C. Kak, *Digital Picture Processing*, 2nd Edition, Volumes 1 and 2, Academic Press, Englewood Cliffs, NJ, 1982.
14. J. Radon, "Uber die Bestimmung von Funktionen durch ihre Integralwerte langs gewisser Mannigfaltigkeiten," *Ber. Verb. Saechs. AKAD. Wiss., Leipzig, Match Phys.*, Kl 69, pp. 262–277, 1917.
15. G.N. Hounsfield, "A method and apparatus for examination of a body by radiation such as X or gamma radiation," Patent 1283915, The Patent Office, London, 1972.
16. A.M. Cormack, "Representation of a function by its line integrals with some radiological applications," *J. Appl. Phys.*, Vol. 34, pp. 2722–2727, 1963.
17. G.T. Herman, *Image Reconstruction from Projections*, Academic Press, New York, 1980.
18. A. Papoulis and S.U. Pillai, *Probability, Random Variables and Stochastic Processes*, McGraw-Hill, New York, 2001.

19. S. Mallat, "A theory for multiresolution signal decomposition: the wavelet representation," *IEEE Trans. Pattern Anal. Mach. Intell.*, Vol. 11, No. 7, pp. 674–693, 1989.
20. I. Daubechies, *Ten Lectures on Wavelets*, Society for Applied Mathematics, Philadelphia, PA, 1992.
21. S. Mallat, "Wavelets for a vision," *Proc. IEEE*, Vol. 84, No. 4, pp. 604–614, 1996.
22. M. Vetterli and J. Kovacevic, *Wavelets and Subband Coding*, Prentice Hall, Englewood Cliffs, 1995.
23. A. Raheja and A.P. Dhawan, "Wavelet based multiresolution expectation maximization reconstruction algorithm for emission tomography," *Comput. Med. Imaging Graph.*, Vol. 24, No. 6, pp. 359–376, 2000.
24. J.B. Weaver, X. Yansun, D.M. Healy Jr., and L.D. Cromwell, "Filtering noise from images with wavelet transforms," *Magn. Reson. Med.*, Vol. 21, No. 2, pp. 288–295, 1991.
25. S. Patwardhan, A.P. Dhawan, and P. Relue, "Classification of melanoma using tree-structured wavelet transform," *Comput. Methods Programs Biomed.*, Vol. 72, No. 3, pp. 223–239, 2003.
26. A. Laine, "Wavelets in spatial processing of biomedical images," *Annu. Rev. Biomed. Eng.*, Vol. 2, pp. 511–550, 2000.
27. M. Unser, A. Aldroubi, and A. Laine, "IEEE transactions on medical imaging," Special Issue on Wavelets in Medical Imaging, 2003.

CHAPTER 3

INTERACTION OF ELECTROMAGNETIC RADIATION WITH MATTER IN MEDICAL IMAGING

Historically, the foundation of medical imaging was laid when Wilhelm Conrad Roentgen invented X rays and described their diagnostic capabilities in 1895 (1). Roentgen received the first Nobel Prize for his discovery of X rays in 1901. X rays were first used in three-dimensional (3-D) medical imaging using computed tomography (CT) methods in 1972, independently by Godfrey Hounsfield and Allen Cormack, who shared the Nobel Prize for medicine in 1979 (2–4). Today, X rays are the primary and most widely used radiation source for radiological imaging in X-ray radiography, X-ray mammography, and X-ray CT. After the discovery of natural radioactivity by Antonio Henri Becquerel in 1896, the first use of radioactive tracers in medical imaging through a rectilinear scanner was reported by Cassen et al. in 1951 (5). This was followed by the development of a gamma-ray pinhole camera for in vivo studies by Anger in 1952 (6). The clinical use of positron emission tomography (PET) was demonstrated by G. Brownell in 1953 (7). Later, visual light-based imaging methods including fluoroscopy and endoscopy became useful in biomedical and clinical sciences (8, 9). All of these modalities deal with the radiation emerging from the electromagnetic (EM) spectrum as discussed in Chapter 1. Recently, other modalities including magnetic resonance imaging (MRI) and ultrasound have been applied to many medical applications (10–14). It is apparent that medical imaging modalities dealing with radiation sources related to the EM spectrum are most widely used in diagnostic and therapeutic radiological imaging. In this chapter, the basic principles of interaction of EM with matter are briefly discussed.

3.1. ELECTROMAGNETIC RADIATION

In general, radiation is a form of energy that can be propagated through space or matter. It travels in vacuum with a speed of 2.998×10^8 m/s. In other media, the propagation of EM radiation would depend on the transport characteristics of the

---

Medical Image Analysis, Second Edition, by Atam P. Dhawan
Copyright © 2011 by the Institute of Electrical and Electronics Engineers, Inc.

matter. The behavior of EM radiation can be described by a wave or by particle-like bundles of energy called quanta or photons. The wave nature of EM radiation explains reflection, refraction, diffraction, and polarization. However, the physics of EM radiation is often better understood in terms of particles. Short EM waves, such as X rays, may react with matter as if they were treated as particles rather than waves.

EM radiation can be broken down into two mutually dependent perpendicular components. The first carries the electrical properties and is therefore called the electrical field. The other component exhibits the magnetic properties of the radiation and is therefore known as the magnetic field. Both fields propagate in space with the same frequency, speed, and phase. Thus, the combination of the two fields justifies the name "electromagnetic" radiation. The EM radiation wave is characterized by its wavelength λ, frequency ν, and speed c, which is a constant. This provides an inverse relationship between the wavelength and frequency with the following equation:

$$c = \lambda \nu. \tag{3.1}$$

The particle-like quantum or photon is described by a specific amount of energy in EM radiation. The energy, E, of a quantum or photon is proportional to the frequency and is given by

$$E = h\nu \tag{3.2}$$

where h is Planck's constant (6.62×10^{-34} J/s or 4.13×10^{-18} keV/s).

It is apparent from above that the energy of a photon can also be given by

$$E = hc/\lambda = 1.24/\lambda \text{ keV} \tag{3.3}$$

where c (3×10^8 m/s) is the velocity of light by which a photon can travel in space, and λ is in nanometer (nm).

The particle nature of EM radiation, particularly at short wavelengths, is important in diagnostic radiology. EM radiation usually travels in a straight line within a medium but sometimes can change direction due to scattering events. With respect to energy, the interaction of a photon with matter may lead to penetration, scattering, or photoelectric absorption. While the scattering causes a partial loss of energy and a change of the direction, the photoelectric absorption leads to a complete loss of energy and removal of the photon from the radiation beam.

3.2. ELECTROMAGNETIC RADIATION FOR IMAGE FORMATION

The interaction of photons with matter leads to the formation of an image that carries the information about the absorption properties of the medium. The human body has several types of matter such as bone, soft tissue, and fluid. When a beam of short-wavelength EM radiation such as X ray is transmitted through the body, the X-ray photons usually travel in a straight line and are attenuated depending on the density and atomic properties of the matter in the medium. Thus, the X rays when passed through the body carry the attenuation information that is used to form an image. Since different body matters have different absorption coefficients, an X-ray image reflects an anatomical map of the spatial distribution of the absorption coefficients of the various body matters.

Another form of EM radiation commonly used in nuclear medicine is gamma-ray emission obtained through the radioactive decay of a nucleus. Through a selective administration of radioactive pharmaceuticals, the body matter becomes a source of radioactive decay with emission of gamma rays or other particles such as positrons that eventually lead to the emission of gamma rays. A gamma-ray image shows a spatial distribution of the activity of the source emission. Since body matters, depending on the metabolism, absorb different quantities of radioactive material, the gamma-ray image shows a metabolic or functional map along with some information about anatomical regions.

Since the purpose of gamma-ray imaging is to provide a distribution of the radioactive tracer in the object, the attenuation caused by the object medium is undesirable. In X-ray imaging, the attenuation caused by the object medium is the imaging parameter. Another major difference in these two imaging modalities is radiation dose. The amount and duration of radioactivity caused by the administration of radioactive pharmaceuticals in the body needs to be kept at low levels for the safety of the patient. This is another reason why attenuation and scattering cause a significant problem in nuclear medicine imaging. The gamma-ray photons are approximately in the same energy range as X-ray photons, yet low energy photons are not desirable because they are more likely to be absorbed within the body. Any gamma-ray photon absorbed in the body causes a loss of signal and therefore reduces the signal-to-noise ratio in the image, leading to a poor image quality. Also, any scattering event within the body will degrade the localization of the signal and therefore will cause a poor image with unreliable information.

Due to these differences in imaging, the image reconstruction, processing, and interpretation require different strategies for X-ray and nuclear medicine imaging modalities. These issues are discussed in the subsequent chapters.

3.3. RADIATION INTERACTION WITH MATTER

The photons that are transmitted through a medium either penetrate, scatter, or are removed from the beam due to complete loss of energy. The removal of photons from the radiation beam is called absorption. If a photon is not absorbed, it may continue traveling in the same direction or be scattered in another direction with or without any loss of energy. An X-ray radiation beam for body imaging is selected with an appropriate energy level to provide a reasonable absorption and negligible or very low scattering.

With EM radiation, there are four different types of interaction of photons with matter: (1) coherent or Rayleigh scattering, (2) photoelectric absorption, (3) Compton scattering, and (4) pair production.

3.3.1 Coherent or Rayleigh Scattering

This is an elastic collision of the photon with the matter that causes a slight change in the direction of the photon travel with no loss of energy. This type of elastic scattering occurs with the low-energy photons in the range of a few kilo-electron-volts (keV). It is not a major form of interaction in diagnostic radiology, as photons with energy levels of 20 keV or higher are used, but is often used in X-ray diffraction studies.

3.3.2 Photoelectric Absorption

At lower energy levels, the photon interaction with matter is dominated by photoelectric absorption, which is a major factor in attenuation. The amount of attenuation is described by the attenuation coefficient. In a general model of an atom, electrons are organized in shells or orbits around the nucleus based on their energy levels. During photoelectric absorption, a photon loses its energy by interacting with a tightly bound electron in the body matter, which is subsequently ejected from the atom due to the increased kinetic energy. The ejected electron is dissipated in the matter, leaving a vacancy that is filled by another electron falling from the next shell. The energy dissipation associated with this event is accompanied by the emission of a fluorescent radiation. The photoelectric absorption increases significantly with the increase in atomic number, in other words, the density of the material. It should be noted that low-energy photons are usually absorbed by M and L shells of the atomic structure, while the high-energy photons are absorbed in the inner K-shell. The increase in the energy level associated with the K-shell is characterized by the K absorption edge. Figure 3.1 shows the component of mass attenuation coefficients of water and lead.

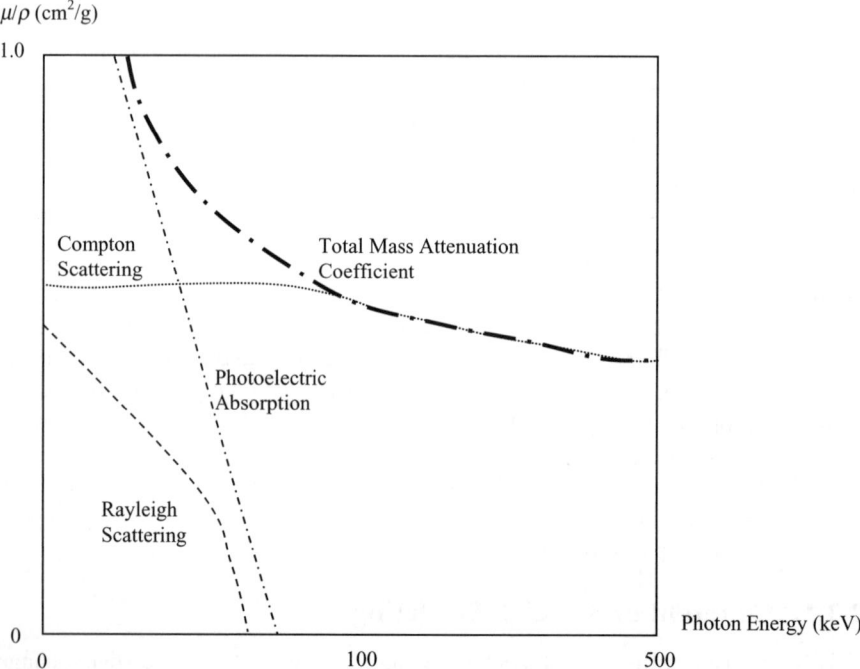

Figure 3.1 The mass attenuation coefficients of water under the 511 keV energy range.

3.3.3 Compton Scattering

Compton scattering is caused by an inelastic collision of a photon with an outer-shell electron with a negligible binding energy. After the collision, the photon with reduced energy is deflected, while the electron with an increased energy is ejected from the atom. With the conservation of energy, the loss of photon energy is equal to the gain in energy for the electron. While the photoelectric effect dominates in materials with high atomic numbers, Compton scattering is more significant in materials with lower atomic numbers. Also, Compton scattering dominates with high-energy photons. Since the higher energy photons would cause a larger deflection angle, a higher energy radiation is not desirable in radiological imaging. In diagnostic radiology and nuclear medicine, Compton scattering is the most problematic interaction of photons with the body matter. The deflections in scattering events cause uncertainties in photon localization as it becomes difficult to keep the desired radiation transmission path. The scattering events not only cause degrading image artifacts such as blur but also lead to a lower signal-to-noise ratio.

3.3.4 Pair Production

Pair production occurs when a high-energy photon on the order of 1 MeV interacts near the nucleus of an atom in a manner similar to the positron emission in a radioactive decay. The transfer of high energy from a photon to the nucleus causes ionization of the atom with a negatron (negatively charged) and a positron (positively charged) electron, each of 511 keV. The positron after coming to rest can interact with an electron, resulting in an annihilation creating two photons of 511 keV, each moving in the opposite direction. Since the high-energy photons are not used in diagnostic radiology, pair production does not play a significant role in radiological imaging.

In diagnostic radiology, the total attenuation coefficient, μ, is the sum of attenuation coefficients caused by Ralyeigh scattering, photoelectric absorption, and Compton scattering. Since Rayleigh scattering is negligible in diagnostic radiological imaging with X rays at energy levels of 20 keV or higher, the effective attenuation coefficient is the sum of photoelectric absorption and Compton scattering.

$$\mu = \mu_{Rayl} + \mu_{Photo} + \mu_{Comp}$$
$$\mu_{Rayl} = \rho Z^2 E^{-1}$$
$$\mu_{Photo} = \rho Z^3 E^{-3}$$
$$\mu_{Comp} = \rho \left(\frac{N_{av} Z}{A_m} \right) E^{-1} \tag{3.4}$$

where μ_{Ray}, μ_{Photo}, and μ_{Com} are, respectively, the attenuation coefficients caused by Rayleigh scattering, photoelectric absorption, and Compton scattering and ρ, Z, E, N_{av}, and A_m are, respectively, the density, atomic number of the material, energy of the photon, Avogadro's number (6.023×10^{23}), and atomic mass.

3.4. LINEAR ATTENUATION COEFFICIENT

Due to absorption, a radiation beam experiences attenuation when transmitted through a medium. A linear attenuation coefficient, μ, of a medium can be represented as

$$N_o = N_{in} e^{-\mu t} \tag{3.5}$$

where N_{in} is the total number of photons entering into the medium of thickness t with a linear attenuation coefficient μ, and N_o is the total number of photons that come out of the medium.

Let us consider $I_{in}(E)$ to be the intensity of input radiation of energy, E, and $I_d(x, y)$ to be the intensity of the beam detected at a plane perpendicular to the direction of the input beam. Considering no loss of photons due to the detector, $I_d(x, y)$ can be represented by

$$I_d(x, y) = \int I_{in}(x, y, E) e^{-\int \mu(x,y,z,E) dz} d(E) \tag{3.6}$$

where $\mu(x, y, z, E)$ is the linear attenuation coefficient at each region of the object in the field of view of radiation.

If we assume that the medium is homogeneous with a uniform linear attenuation coefficient μ_0 throughout the volume of thickness, t, and the radiation beam is obtained from a monochromatic energy source, $I_d(x, y)$ can be represented by

$$I_d(x, y) = I_{in}(x, y) e^{-\mu_0 t}. \tag{3.7}$$

The linear attenuation coefficient of a material is dependent on the energy of the photon and the atomic number of the elements in the material. Due to the dependency on the mass of the material, often a mass attenuation coefficient (μ/ρ) of a material is considered more useful and is defined by a ratio of the linear attenuation coefficient (μ) and the density (ρ) of the material. Figure 3.2 shows X-ray mass attenuation coefficients for compact bone and fat found in human body.

3.5. RADIATION DETECTION

Spectrometric detectors are used for detection of EM radiation, particularly for X-ray and gamma-ray imaging modalities. There are two basic principles used in spectrometric detectors: ionization and scintillation. Ionization-based detectors create a specific number of ion pairs depending on the energy of the EM radiation. In scintillation detectors, charged particles interact with the scintillation material to emit optical photons. Photomultiplier tubes (PMTs) are used to amplify the light intensity and to convert the optical photons into voltage proportional to the energy of charged particles. Semiconductor detectors have been developed for improving the detection performance of small sized detectors with minimal power requirements.

3.5.1 Ionized Chambers and Proportional Counters

The family of ionized detectors includes ionization chambers and proportional counters. The quantum or photon particle interacts with the sensitive volume of the

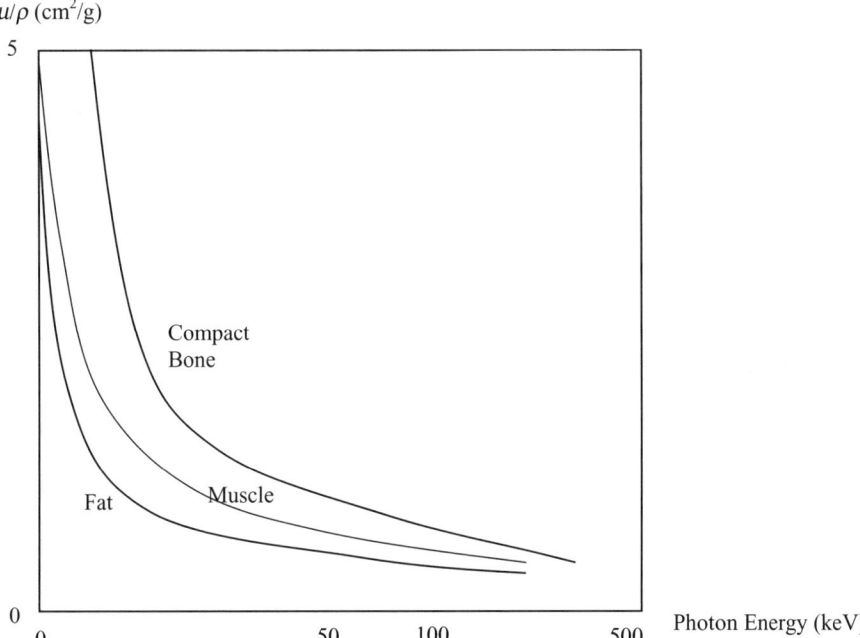

Figure 3.2 The mass attenuation coefficients of compact bone, muscle, and fat.

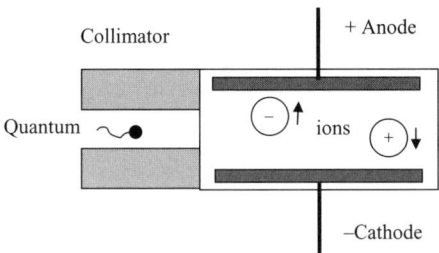

Figure 3.3 A schematic diagram of an ionization chamber-based detector.

detector material and produces a specific number of ion pairs, which is proportional to the energy of the quantum.

An ionized chamber-based detector is comprised of a hermetically sealed vessel filled with gas such as N_2 or Ar_2. A high electric field is used across the electrodes in the presence of a stimulating gas to improve ionization performance. An incoming quantum causes ionization in the gas medium (Fig. 3.3). The positive ions are collected at the cathode and negative ions are collected at the anode to charge an interelectrode capacitance to produce voltage proportional to the energy of the quantum. The electrodes in the ionization chambers are designed in different shapes to maximize the probability of uniform distribution of ions along the surface of the electrodes. Grids are used to improve the movements of charged particles for better efficiency. Since the origin or the traveling path of a scattered quantum from source to the detector cannot be determined with accuracy, the scattered radiations create error in image reconstruction and subsequent quantitative analysis. To avoid the errors in measurements due to scattered events that lower the signal-to-noise ratio, these scattered events must be rejected by the detector. One efficient way of achieving this is to use a collimator with a high density material such as lead. Lead absorbs the scattered quantum that approaches the detector area at an angle.

Let us assume that a quantum of energy, E, produces N number of ions. Let us also assume q to be the charge of an ion. The ionization would ideally lead to a voltage V such that

$$V = Nq/C \qquad (3.8)$$

where C is the interelectrode capacitance.

If e_{ion} is the net energy required to create an ion, then

$$N = E/e_{ion}. \qquad (3.9)$$

In proportional counters, additional grids are used with an increased voltage on the electrode in the ionization chamber. The proportional counters are usually of cylindrical form because such a shape permits a high potential gradient near the collecting electrode that is placed at the center. This creates a region of impact ionization of gas molecules. The impact ionization improves the process of ionization and increases the number of electrons reaching the collecting electrode. As a result, the proportional counters have a gas multiplication factor to produce better voltage transformation. However, linearity of proportional counters may be affected in the presence of impurities. In practice, gas multiplication factors can provide a gain up to 10,000. Thus, they are more efficient than simple pulse ionization chambers.

3.5.2 Semiconductor Detectors

Recently, emphasis has been given to semiconductor detectors because of their compactness, low power requirements, and potential for high sensitivity and specificity. In ionized detectors, an electric field is established with the help of electrodes. In semiconductor detectors, the particle energy is transformed into electric pulses at the junction region of the semiconductor material. On the surface of the detector a thin layer of p-type material is created over the n-type of material that serves as the base. With a p-n junction, the holes in p-type of material diffuse into n-type material and electrons in n-type material diffuse into p-type material to create a barrier potential across the junction to stop any further movement. The depletion layer across which the barrier potential exists can be modified by applying an external voltage to the p and n regions. The thickness of the depletion layer and, hence, the barrier voltage can be increased by applying positive voltage to the n region and negative voltage to the p region. This creates a high potential gradient in the depletion layer, which serves as an ionization chamber. A quantum interacting with the surface of the detector will create electron-hole pairs in the depletion layer, resulting in the movement of electrons toward positive electrodes and holes toward the negative electrodes to produce a voltage. The voltage that is produced through charging a capacitor is proportional to the energy of the input quantum. The thickness of the depletion layer is analogous to the diameter of an ionization chamber. The voltage produced in the semiconductor detectors can be modeled in terms of number of electron-hole pairs generated, the mobility of the holes, and depletion layer field. Let us assume that there are N numbers of electron-hole pairs generated by a quantum when the voltage across the p-n junction is $V_{p\text{-}n}$, and the mobility of holes in the depletion layer is μ_p. The voltage produced by an incoming quantum of energy E can then be modeled as:

$$v(t) = \frac{Nq}{C}(1 - e^{-t/t_0})e^{-t/\tau}$$

$$\text{with } t_0 = \frac{w^2}{4\mu_p V_{p\text{-}n}}. \tag{3.10}$$

where C is the capacitance across the p-n junction with τ time constant, q is the charge of a hole, and w is the width of depletion layer.

3.5.3 Advantages of Semiconductor Detectors

It should be noted that for accurate measurement, the thickness of the depletion layer must be much larger than the range of measured particles. This can create a problem in fabricating semiconductor detectors for specific energy ranges. Nevertheless, there are several advantages for using semiconductor detectors. These are listed below.

1. Semiconductor detectors can be fabricated with smaller e (minimum energy needed to create an electron-hole pair), which is ~3.6 eV for silicon. This leads to better detector resolution.
2. Due to the strong electric potential gradient across the depletion layer, the e value becomes independent of the mass and charge of the particle.
3. Semiconductor detectors provide a small charge collection time (<10 ns).
4. Semiconductor detectors cause very small recombination losses due to fast charge collection.

3.5.4 Scintillation Detectors

Scintillation detectors use a scintillation phosphor and a PMT coupled together through an optical contact. The charged particles interact with the scintillation material to excite molecules. The excited molecules emit optical photons during the relaxation process to return to the ground state. The intensity of each scintillation event (amount of light) is proportional to the energy lost by the charged particle or quantum in the phosphor. Thus, scintillation absorbs the energy of ionized radiation quantum and converts it into small flash of light usually in the visible spectrum. Scintillation materials are also called phosphors, or fluorescent materials. For medical imaging applications, a good scintillation material should have a high efficiency of conversion of incident radiation energy into scintillation photons with a linear response over the required energy range, high-energy resolution, good spectral response to match with spectral sensitivity of the connected PMT, a short rise time for fast timing applications, and a fast decay time to reduce detector dead time for faster sampling of dynamic events. While efficiency is defined as the percentage of incident particles that are detected by the detector, energy resolution is measured as the ratio of the full width at half maximum (FWHM) of a given energy peak to the peak position. A good scintillation detector must have a strong stopping power over the required energy range. Stopping power, based on the absorption length, is the ability to stop the quantum in as little material as possible to keep the overall size of the scintillation detector as small as possible. The density of the material is also an important factor in determining the size of the detector to meet spatial resolution requirements of the imaging application.

There are several types of scintillation materials including organic crystals, organic liquids, inorganic crystals, plastics, gaseous scintillators, and glasses. Organic crystals for scintillation, such as anthracene ($C_{14}H_{14}$), stibene ($C_{14}H_{14}$), and naphthalene ($C_{14}H_{14}$), have the advantage of very fast decay time but suffer from anisotropic response, resulting in poor energy resolution. They are hard to develop in the shape and sizes required for medical imaging applications. Organic liquids are also not very practical to use in medical imaging applications, as they provide low efficiency and require sealed chambers. Plastic scintillation materials such as polyvinyltoluene and polystyrene provide high light output and can be molded into any desirable shape. However, they have not been used in the clinical environment because of their low density (approximately 1.1 to 1.2 g/cm^3). Because of their low density, plastic scintillators have poor stopping power and are therefore not used for medical imaging applications. Inorganic crystal materials such as sodium iodide doped with thallium (Na(TI)) are most commonly used because of their high luminescence efficiency, excellent spectral response, and economic price. Other inorganic alkali halide crystals suitable for medical imaging applications include bismuth germanate (BGO), cesium iodide activated by thallium (CsI(TI)), lutetium oxyorthosilicate (LSO), and yttrium oxyorthosilicate activated by cerium (YSO(Ce)). Table 3.1 provides the decay time and light yield for popular scintillation materials used in producing detectors in medical imaging.

PMTs are used to amplify the optical photon intensity or light produced by scintillation materials to provide measurable electric voltage proportional to the energy of the incident quantum. A typical PMT consists of a photocathode, focusing

TABLE 3.1 Characteristic Properties of Commonly Used Scintillation Materials

Material	Density g/cm^3	Refraction index	Decay time ns	Emission wavelength nm	Light yield quanta/keV
NaI(TI)	3.67	1.85	230	410	38
BGO	7.13	2.15	300	480	8.2
LSO	7.44	1.82	40	420	15–27
YSO(Ce)	4.54	1.8	35	420	10–24
CsI(TI)	4.51	1.79	1100	540	38

electrodes, a number of dynodes that work as electron multiplier, and an anode (electron collector electrode) sealed in a vacuum tube. The light photons that are emitted by absorption of an incident quantum in the scintillation material now strike the photocathode of the PMT. As these light photons strike the photocathode, photoelectrons are emitted. The number of photoelectrons emitted by the photocathode, N_c, can be given as

$$N_c = kg_0 w E / E_{ph} \tag{3.11}$$

where g_0 is the coefficient to account for losses at the photocathode, w is quantum efficiency, and E_{ph} is the average energy of photon.

The primary emission of photoelectrons from the photocathode is focused on a series of dynodes with increasing higher voltage levels that stimulate a secondary emission due to a high potential gradient, working as positive feedback to provide a multiplication factor to N_c. The multiple dynodes with increasing voltage levels also accelerate the movement of electrons to provide an amplification factor for the transformation of voltage. Thus, the repetition of secondary emission through multiple dynodes creates electronic multiplication such that photoelectrons are increased up to one million times or more with 10–12 dynodes, making the PMT the most sensitive to the energy of the incident quantum.

In a scintillation detector system, a quantum of energy E produces a time-dependent process of photon emission that decays in a manner similar to an exponential radioactive decay with a time constant t_0. Let us assume that N_0 is the number of photons at time $t = 0$, the total number of photons N generated by a quantum can be expressed as

$$N = N_0 e^{-t/t_0}. \tag{3.12}$$

The decay of photons emission, dN/dt, can then be expressed as

$$\frac{dN}{dt} = \frac{N_0}{t_0} e^{-t/t_0}. \tag{3.13}$$

Although the PMT provides a multiplication factor through secondary emission, the voltage produced by the PMT is a time-dependent function due to the photon emission decay process. A voltage pulse $v(t)$ yielded by the PMT can be modeled as

$$v(t) = k \frac{N_0 q}{C} (1 - e^{-t/t_0}) e^{-t/\tau} \tag{3.14}$$

where C is the interelectrode capacitance of the PMT with a time constant τ, k is the multiplication factor, and it is assumed that $\tau \gg t_0$.

Photomultiplier tubes provide excellent amplification factor with low noise as the signal is amplified within the vacuum tube. Figure 3.4 shows a schematic diagram of a scintillation detector showing a collimator to reject scattering events, scintillation phosphor or crystal area, and PMT with multiple dynodes. The spectral response of the scintillation material must be matched with spectral sensitivity of the PMT to provide maximum possible efficiency. Figure 3.5 shows typical quantum efficiency with respect to spectral sensitivity of PMTs manufactured by Hamamatsu. It can be noted that the typical quantum efficiency of PMT is usually within the

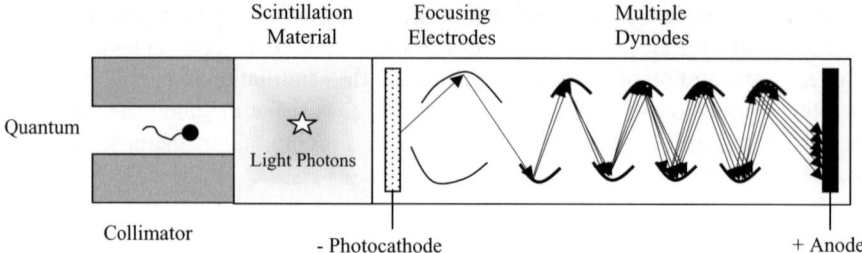

Figure 3.4 A schematic diagram of photomultiplier tube.

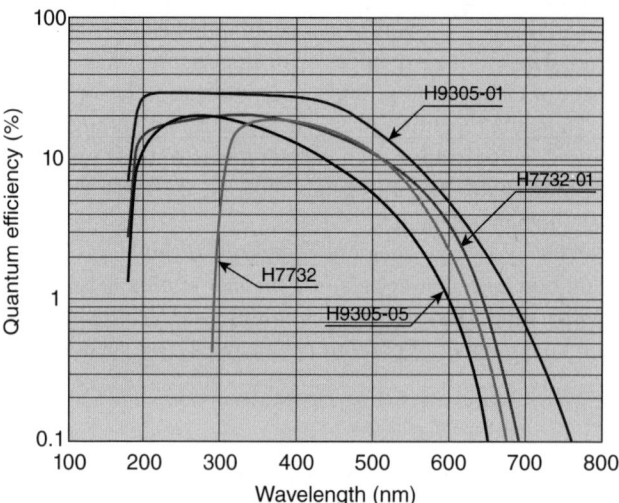

Figure 3.5 Typical spectral sensitivity and quantum efficiency of some of the Hamamatsu photomultiplier tubes (from http://sales.hamamatsu.com).

20–30% range. There are multianode position-sensitive enclosures that are available today in a square-shaped configuration of 8×8 PMTs. These position-sensitive PMT blocks are used in modern nuclear medicine as well as CT single photon emission computed tomography (SPECT) and CT–PET dual modality imaging cameras.

3.6. DETECTOR SUBSYSTEM OUTPUT VOLTAGE PULSE

As described above, the primary detector, such as a scintillation phosphor, crystal, or semiconductor material, is interfaced to a PMT and/or gain amplifier that provides a multiplication factor and produces a voltage pulse in an electronic circuit. The design of the electronic circuit may vary but it usually carries an output circuit

3.6. DETECTOR SUBSYSTEM OUTPUT VOLTAGE PULSE

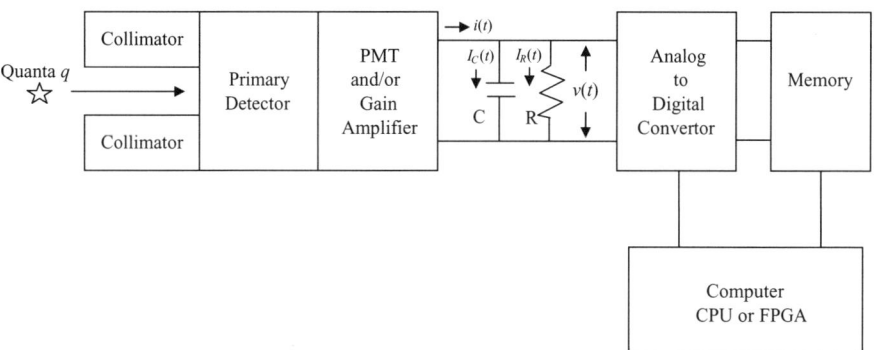

Figure 3.6 A schematic diagram of detector subsystem with output pulse shaping and storage.

segment with a capacitor connected with a load resistor in parallel to shape the output voltage pulse as shown in Figure 3.6. The output voltage pulse is then sampled by an analog-to-digital convertor and the values can be stored in a memory unit using a computer or field programmable gate arrays (FPGA) board.

As shown in Figure 3.6, the current $i(t)$ from the PMT or gain amplifier circuit is split into a capacitor current $i_C(t)$ and a load resistor current $i_R(t)$, producing an output voltage pulse $v(t)$. The output voltage pulse can be shaped using a proper time constant τ, determined by the values of capacitor C and load resistance R. It can be seen from Figure 3.6 that

$$i(t) = i_R(t) + i_C(t)$$

and

$$i_R(t)R = \frac{1}{C}\int i_C(t)dt \qquad (3.15)$$

$$i_C(t) = RC\frac{di_R(t)}{dt}.$$

The relationship between the capacitor and resistor currents is given by

$$\frac{di_R(t)}{dt} + \frac{i_R(t)}{RC} = \frac{i(t)}{RC}$$

with $i_R(t) = \frac{1}{\tau}e^{-t/\tau}\int_0^t i(t')e^{-t'/\tau}dt'$ and $\tau = RC$. \qquad (3.16)

The output voltage pulse $v(t)$ can then be expressed as

$$v(t) = i_R(t)R = \frac{1}{C}e^{-t/\tau}\int_0^t i(t')e^{-t'/\tau}dt'. \qquad (3.17)$$

It should be noted that the final shape of the output voltage pulse also depends on the detector, PMT, and gain amplifier responses with their respective time decay constants, as they are critical in shaping the current pulse $i(t)$.

3.7. EXERCISES

3.1. Find the wavelength of a quantum with 511 keV.

3.2. What is the linear attenuation coefficient? Why is it important in medical imaging?

3.3. What is Rayleigh scattering? What is its significance in medical imaging?

3.4. Define Compton scattering and photoelectric absorption and describe their differences.

3.5. What happens when photons higher than 1 MeV interact with matter? Describe how this process is different from Compton scattering.

3.6. Why is a monochromatic energy source preferred in medical imaging? Explain your answer.

3.7. Describe the operation of semiconductor detectors and their advantages over the ionized chambers.

3.8. Describe the gain function of a photomultiplier tube on the secondary emission.

3.9. Does a PMT provide better signal-to-noise ratio than a semiconductor amplifier? Explain your answer.

3.10. Why are the photomultiplier tubes extensively used in nuclear medicine imaging?

3.11. Why is it important to have a short decay time for a detector?

3.8. REFERENCES

1. W.K. Roentgen (translation by A. Stanton), "On a new kind of rays," *Nature*, Vol. 53, pp. 274–276, 1896.
2. G.N. Hounsfield, "A method and apparatus for examination of a body by radiation such as X or gamma radiation," Patent 1283915, The Patent Office, London, 1972.
3. G.N. Hounsfield, "Computerized transverse axial scanning tomography: Part-1, description of the system," *Br.J. Radiol.*, Vol. 46, pp. 1016–1022, 1973.
4. A.M. Cormack, "Representation of a function by its line integrals with some radiological applications," *J. Appl. Phys.*, Vol. 34, pp. 2722–2727, 1963.
5. B. Cassen, L. Curtis, C. Reed, and R. Libby, "Instrumentation for ^{131}I used in medical studies," *Nucleonics*, Vol. 9, pp. 46–48, 1951.
6. H. Anger, "Use of gamma-ray pinhole camera for in-vivo studies," *Nature*, Vol. 170, pp. 200–204, 1952.
7. G. Brownell and H.W. Sweet, "Localization of brain tumors," *Nucleonics*, Vol. 11, pp. 40–45, 1953.
8. H. Barrett and W. Swindell, *Radiological Imaging: The Theory of Image Formation, Detection and Processing*, Volumes 1–2, Academic Press, New York, 1981.
9. J.T. Bushberg, J.A. Seibert, E.M. Leidholdt, and J.M. Boone, *The Essentials of Medical Imaging*, Williams & Wilkins, Philadelphia, 1994.
10. Z.H. Cho, J.P. Jones, and M. Singh, *Fundamentals of Medical Imaging*, John Wiley & Sons, New York, 1993.
11. A. Macovski, *Medical Imaging Systems*, Prentice Hall, Englewood Cliffs, NJ, 1983.
12. K.K. Shung, M.B. Smith, and B. Tsui, *Principles of Medical Imaging*, Academic Press, San Diego, CA, 1992.
13. Z. Liang and P.C. Lauterbur, *Prinicples of Magnetic Resonance Imaging*, IEEE Press, Piscataway, NJ, 2000.
14. F.W. Kremkau, *Diagnostic Ultrasound Principles and Instrumentation*, Saunders, Philadelphia, 1995.

CHAPTER 4

MEDICAL IMAGING MODALITIES: X-RAY IMAGING

As introduced in Chapter 1, medical imaging is an essential aspect of radiological sciences for visualization of anatomical structures and metabolic information of the human body. Structural and functional imaging of a human body is important for understanding human anatomy, function of organs, and associated physiological processes. Imaging also becomes a critical source of information to study the physiological behavior of an organ or tissue under a treatment. Thus, imaging is an essential tool for diagnosis as well as evaluation of the treatment of an illness.

Medical imaging modalities can be broadly classified into two classes: (1) anatomical or structural and (2) functional or metabolic (1–4). The characterization of a specific anatomical imaging modality depends on its ability to discriminate different constituents of the body such as water, bone, soft tissue, and other biochemical fluids. Examples of major anatomical imaging modalities include X-ray imaging (X-ray radiography, X-ray mammography, X-ray computer tomography [CT]), ultrasound, and magnetic resonance imaging (MRI). The characterization of a specific functional imaging modality depends on its ability to discriminate different levels of metabolism caused by specific biochemical activity that may be generated by the uptake of a radiopharmaceutical substance. The biochemical activity describing the functional behavior of the tissue or organ can be caused by any internal or external stimulation. Major functional imaging modalities include functional MRI (fMRI), single photon emission computed tomography (SPECT), positron emission tomography (PET), and fluorescence imaging. For example, fMRI methods can be used to measure the blood flow or oxygenation level in brain tissue. The changes in blood flow or oxygen level in the tissue reflect neural activity in the brain caused by stimulation such as sound or light. In nuclear medicine imaging modalities, blood flow in the tissue or an organ can be measured through an emission process of a radioactive tracer that is administered in the blood. For example, a PET image obtained through the administration of flurodeoxyglucose (FDG) may show blood flow and glucose metabolism in the tissue that may be affected by a disease such as a tumor or epilepsy (1–8).

Medical Image Analysis, Second Edition, by Atam P. Dhawan
Copyright © 2011 by the Institute of Electrical and Electronics Engineers, Inc.

4.1. X-RAY IMAGING

X rays were discovered in 1895 by Conrad Roentgen, who described them as a new kind of ray that could penetrate almost anything. He described the diagnostic capabilities of X rays for imaging human body and received the Nobel Prize in 1901. X-ray radiography is the simplest form of medical imaging with the transmission of X rays through the body, which are then collected on a film or an array of detectors. The attenuation or absorption of X rays is described by the photoelectric and Compton effects, with more attenuation through bones than soft tissues or air (1–5).

X rays are a part of the electromagnetic spectrum with smaller wavelengths than the ultraviolet or visible light spectrum. Because of their smaller wavelength, X rays have high energy providing excellent capability of straight penetration and transmission in human body. Soft X rays are identified as having wavelengths from 10 nm to 0.10 nm (or 100 Å to 1 Å), corresponding to 120 eV to 12.3 keV or 3×10^{16} Hz to 3×10^{18}, respectively. Wavelengths shorter than 0.1 nm (1 Å) up to 0.001 nm (0.01 Å) are considered hard X rays. For medical applications, it is important to select X rays with wavelengths that provide linear attenuation coefficients for human body. X-ray radiation photons can be used for both diagnostic and therapeutic applications. Lower energy X rays are used for diagnostic imaging, while higher energy photons are utilized in radiation therapeutic applications. Usually, X rays between 0.1 nm and 0.01 nm (1 Å to 0.1 Å, with corresponding 12.3 keV to 123 keV energy range) are used for diagnostic purposes. In this range the attenuation is quite reasonable to discriminate bones, soft tissue, and air. In addition, the wavelength is short enough for providing excellent resolution of images, even with submillimeter accuracy. Wavelengths shorter than those used for diagnosis provide much higher photon energy and therefore less attenuation. Increasing photon energy makes the human body transparent for the loss of any contrast in the image. The diagnostic X-ray wavelength range provides sufficient energy per photon with a refractive index of unity for almost all materials in the body. This guarantees that the diffraction will not distort the image and rays will travel in straight lines (1–8).

For medical imaging applications, an X-ray imaging tube is used as an external ionized radiation source to generate an X-ray radiation beam that is transmitted through human body in a scanning mode. As the radiation beam passes through a specific location, X rays undergo absorption and scattering as described in Chapter 3. In other words, the radiation beam is attenuated due to the mass attenuation coefficients of physiological structures in the body. The attenuation of radiation intensity is determined at each scan location by measuring the difference of intensity between the source and detector. A two-dimensional (2-D) attenuation map, as obtained through scanning the object in the respective geometry, can be recorded on a radiographic film for an X-ray (film) radiograph. Alternatively, the attenuation map can be stored digitally using X-ray detectors and electronic instrumentation to display a digital X-ray radiograph. Furthermore, the attenuation measurements can be obtained through a three dimensional (3-D) scanning geometry to define projections all around the object. Attenuation projection data are then used in image reconstruction algorithm (described in Chapter 8) to reconstruct and display 3-D CT images. More details are provided later in this chapter.

4.2. X-RAY GENERATION

X rays are generated as the result of interactions of high-speed electrons with heavy target atoms such as tungsten or molybdenum. In principle, an accelerated electron loses energy in interaction with an atom and the loss of energy emits X-ray photons in a scattered direction. The basic principle is explained in detail below.

An atom is comprised of a nucleus and electrons that revolve around the nucleus in orbits called shells. In a nucleus, protons carry positive charge while neutrons possess no charge. Protons and neutrons basically provide mass to an atom, while the number of electrons defines the atomic number. As an atom is neutral in charge, the number of protons is equal to the number of electrons. Each electron shell has a characteristic energy level that represents the binding energy of the electron to the corresponding shell. Also each shell has a maximum energy level depending on its position from the nucleus for the stability of the atom. The K-shell that is closest to the nucleus has greater binding energy than the next L-shell. An electron can be ejected or transferred to another shell from its original place depending on the energy exchange that is caused by an interaction of the atom with a quantum. In each interaction, the total energy is preserved according to the principle of energy preservation. The energy lost by an electron due to change in path is emitted in the form of X-ray photon. For example, if an incident electron with energy greater than the binding energy of K-shell interacts with an atom, the K-shell electron is ejected, leaving an ionized atom with a vacancy in the K-shell. This vacancy is filled by an electron from the outer L-shell. Because the total energy has to be preserved, the difference between the binding energies of K- and L-shells causes the release of a characteristic X-ray photon as a result of the transition of the electron from the L- to K-shell.

Since each element has its own shell-binding energy levels that are specific to its atomic structure, the energy of the X-ray photon emitted in the interaction process is a characteristic feature of that element. For example, in the case of tungsten, a commonly used element for X-ray generation, the specific K- and L-shell binding energy levels are, respectively, 69.5 and 10.2 keV. Thus, an interaction of incident electron of energy greater than 69.5 keV with an atom of tungsten yields an emission of X-ray photon of 59.3 keV (Fig. 4.1). In the case of tungsten, an incident electron, also called an accelerating electron, must have energy greater than 69.5 keV. It is apparent that in such interactions, electrons striking the target material can go through interactions with several nuclei before they are stopped, resulting in electrons with different energy levels. Therefore, emitted X-ray photons also produce a distribution of energy called white radiation or Bremsstrahlung radiation spectrum. Along with the white radiation, characteristic emissions occur due to specific transitions of electrons from different shells such as L to K, M to K, or N to K, as shown in Figure 4.2. The energy of X-ray photons emitted from transitions of electrons to regions other than the K-shell are not used in diagnostic radiology because they are usually of low energy that can be easily absorbed in the medium.

In an X-ray generation tube electrons are released by the source cathode and are accelerated toward the target anode in a vacuum under the potential difference ranging from 20,000 to 150,000 V. Depending on the radiological application,

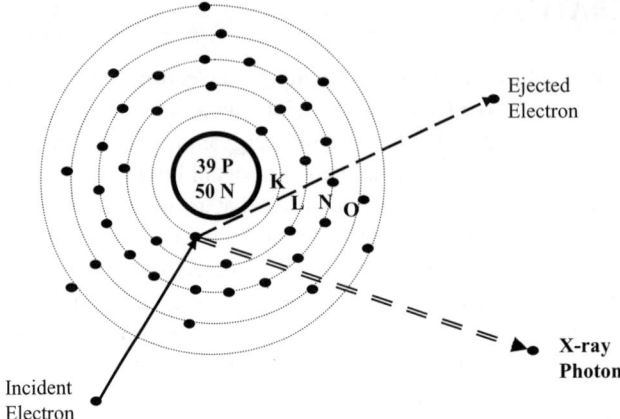

Figure 4.1 Atomic structure of a tungsten atom. An incident electron with energy greater than K-shell binding energy is shown striking a K-shell electron for the emission of an X-ray photon.

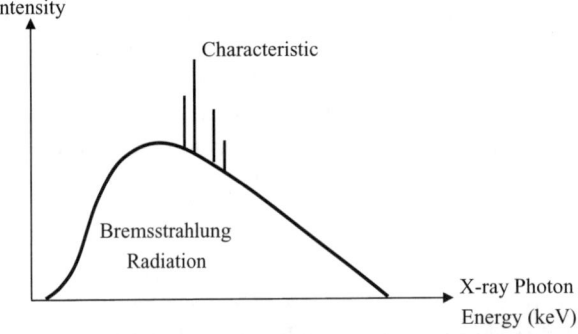

Figure 4.2 A typical X-ray radiation distribution spectrum with characteristic radiations.

specific element materials are used in the X-ray tubes for building the source cathode and target anode in a suitable configuration to maximize X-ray emission. The desired energy level of X-ray photons as a focused monochromatic beam is achieved through appropriate filtration using attenuation mediums absorbing the undesired low-energy emissions. Lead-based collimators are used to define an adequate field dimension of the radiation beam suitable for the specific area of the patient to be radiated for imaging.

Important parameters for selection of X-ray tube for diagnostic imaging include the size of the focal spot, spectrum of X-ray energies, and the X-ray intensity. It is obvious that the focal spot size defines the potential spatial resolution in the X-ray imaging system such as digital radiography, mammography, and CT. Since the attenuation coefficients of X rays and their penetration capabilities in human tissue are wavelength-dependent, it is important that the X-ray source system provides a monochromatic or short band spectrum of appropriate energy at the suitable intensity level. The X-ray intensity level directly defines the signal-to-noise ratio

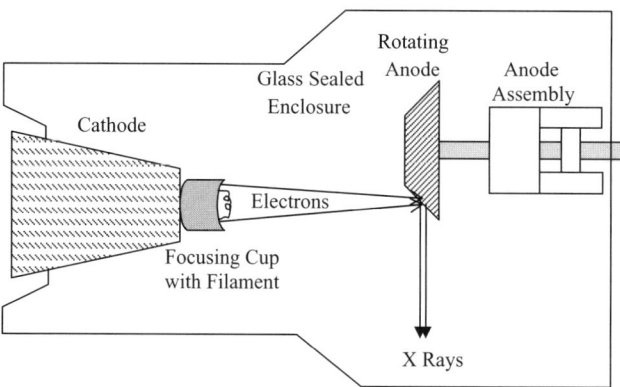

Figure 4.3 A simplified schematic diagram of an X-ray generation tube with rotating anode.

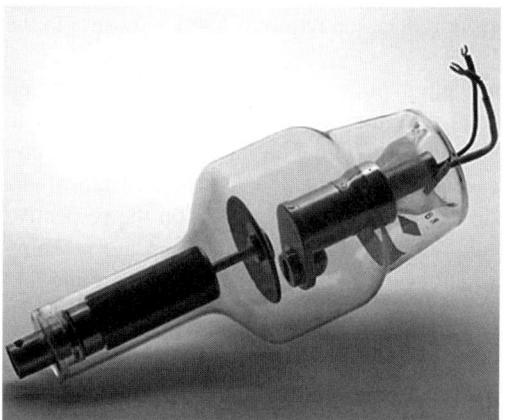

Figure 4.4 A picture of rotating anode X-ray tube.

(SNR) of the imaging system. Higher intensity levels provide more reliable counts at the detector.

An X-ray tube has a cathode block with a focusing cup and a hot filament that determines the focal spot size. Often a dual filament assembly is used to provide two focal spot sizes. X-ray CT systems typically utilize spot sizes ranging from 0.5 to 2 mm. The higher the spot size, the larger the power requirement. For example, a spot size of 1.8 mm may require a 2000 W power load, versus a spot size of 0.8 mm for which a power load of 500 W may be sufficient. Figure 4.3 shows a simplified schematic diagram of an X-ray generation tube; an actual tube is shown in Figure 4.4. As shown in Figure 4.1, the accelerated electrons bombard the target atoms available at the stationary or rotating anode where X rays are generated in a scattered direction through an exit window of a sealed glass enclosure. The rotating anode with an annular target close to the edge (Fig. 4.4) is very efficient in X-ray production and quite commonly used in X-ray tubes. Because the focal spot can become very hot, the anode is made out of material that can withstand high temperatures (in the range of 2000–3000°C). High-performance digital radiography and CT systems utilize X-ray tubes of less than 1 mm focal spot size and a power rating up to 100 kW.

4.3. X-RAY 2-D PROJECTION IMAGING

Two-dimensional projection radiography is the oldest medical imaging modality and is still one of the most widely used imaging methods in diagnostic radiology (1, 2). Conventional film radiography uses an X-ray tube to focus a beam on the imaging area of a patient's body to record an image on a film. The image recorded on the film is a 2-D projection of the three-dimensional (3-D) anatomical structure of the human body. The image is thus obtained through transmission of X rays through the body. The film is developed to show the image that represents the localized sum of attenuation coefficients of material (such as air, blood, tissue, or bone) present in the body along the X-ray path. X-ray screens are used to improve the sensitivity of X-ray detection on the film and therefore reduce the required X-ray exposure to the patient (1, 2).

Scattering can create a major problem in projection radiography. The scattered photons can create artifacts and artificial structures in the image that can lead to an incorrect interpretation or at least create a difficult situation for diagnosis. Projection imaging assumes that all photons travel in a straight line so that the sum of the attenuation coefficients along the path can be recorded correctly on the respective location in the image. If there are additional scattered photons that are reaching the same location, the exposure recorded at the location would be inaccurate and may cause a spurious structure in the image that is actually not present in the patient's body. Also, the scattered photon leads to an incorrect exposure and therefore may cause loss of diagnostic information. For example, in X-ray mammography, scattered radiation can mislead a radiologist in the identification of microcalcifications. In quantitative imaging and analysis applications, such as digital subtraction angiography (DSA), scattered radiation can introduce major errors. In film-screen radiography, the scattered radiation also reduces the overall contrast in the image (2, 3, 8).

Antiscatter grids and collimators are used to reduce the number of scattered radiation reaching at the detector or film (see Fig. 4.2). The grids provide tunnels for passing the radiation with no attenuation of the photons that are traveling parallel to the axis. The primary photons are thus unaffected as they are aligned with the axis. The bars are made of high-density material such as lead or tantalum, causing photoelectric absorption of the scattered X-ray photons. Scattered photons enter the tunnel at an angle and hit the lead walls for absorption (2).

X-ray intensifying screens, also called X-ray screens are used to improve the detection of X-ray photons to produce a better quality image on X-ray films. These screens are used along with an antiscatter grid as shown in Figure 4.5. A complete X-ray intensifying screen contains several layers including an outer plastic protective layer that is transparent to X rays (about 15–20 μm thick), a phosphor layer (100–500 μm thick), a light reflecting layer (20 μm thick), and a plastic base layer

4.3. X-RAY 2-D PROJECTION IMAGING

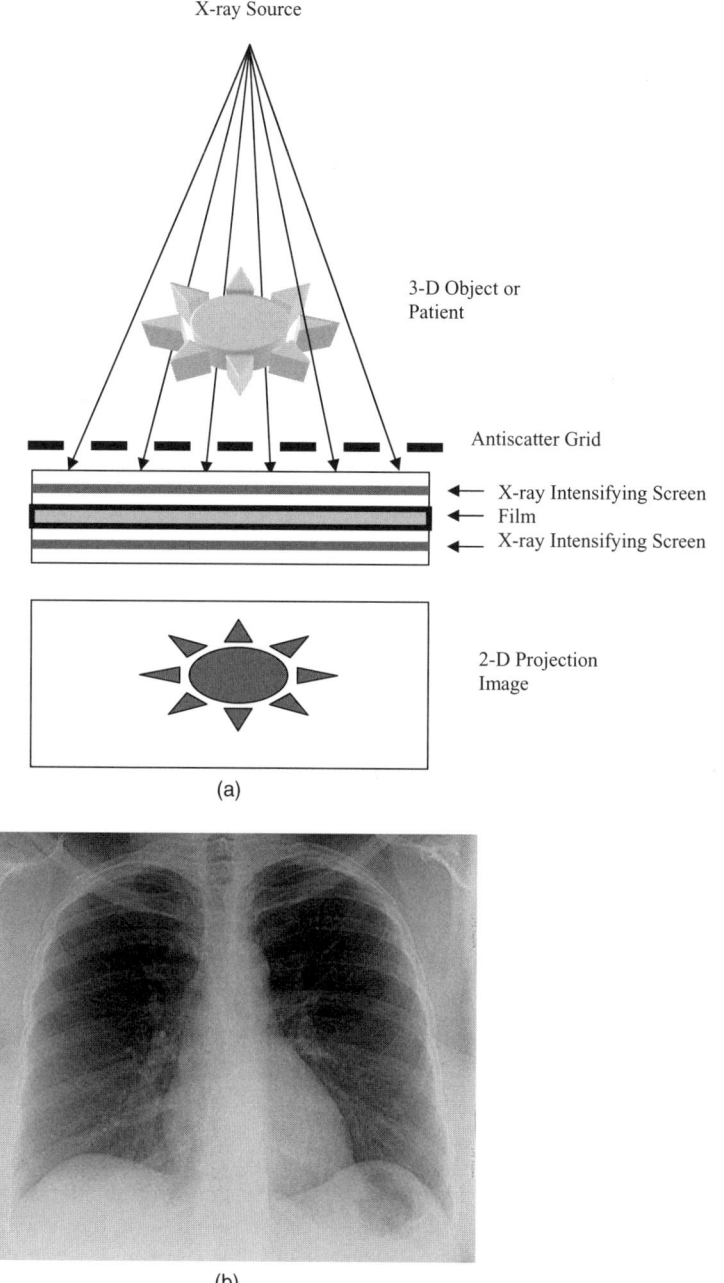

Figure 4.5 (a) A schematic diagram of a 2-D X-ray film-screen radiographic system. A 2-D projection image of the 3-D object is shown at the bottom. (b) X-ray radiographic image of a normal male chest.

(20 μm thick). The phosphor layer absorbs X-ray photons and produces light that is reflected toward the film for better exposure. The phosphor layer is formed from specific materials with high X-ray-to-light photon conversion efficiency such as terbium-doped gadolinium oxysulfide (Gd_2O_2S:Tb) or terbium-doped lanthanum oxybromide (LaOBr:Tb). The X-ray image intensifying screen improves SNR and image quality on X-ray film.

In case of digital radiography, the combination of intensifying screen and film is replaced by a phosphor layered screen coupled with a charge-coupled device (CCD)-based panel. A solid-state detector system in digital radiography and mammography may use a structured thallium-doped cesium iodide (CsI) scintillation material to convert X-ray photons into light photon, which are then converted into electrical signal by CCDs through a fiber optics coupling interface. Other scintillation material (discussed in Chapter 3) or phosphor screens along with thin CCD-based panels have also been investigated for specific digital radiographic applications.

Film-based radiography provides a very high-resolution image depending on the granular structure of the film emulsion. It may suffer from some artifacts such as uneven contrast due to inconsistencies in film processing and chemical effects in the film-developing process. Underexposed and overexposed films are usually of significant concern because they can contribute to incorrect interpretation or conjecture by the physician. On the other hand, brightness levels are much better controlled with digital detector systems instead of film-based systems. As described above, digital radiographic systems use scintillation crystals optically coupled with CCDs in which electrical output signal sensitivity can be controlled much more efficiently than in a film-based system. The digital detector system also provides excellent linearity and gain control, which directly affects the SNR of the acquired data. For this reason, a digital detection system provides a superior dynamic range compared with the film-based systems. However, the resolution of a digital image is limited by the detector size and data collection method (2).

4.4. X-RAY MAMMOGRAPHY

X-ray film-screen mammography is a specialized radiographic imaging method used for breast imaging for diagnosis of breast diseases. Detection of breast cancer in the early stages, an important clinical health care issue for women, imposes much more challenging requirements for imaging than conventional radiography. Breast tissue is quite vascular and soft with low X-ray attenuation coefficients as compared to other anatomical structures. Detection of architectural distortions, small lesions, and particularly microcalcifications require high spatial resolution on the order of 50–100 microns. The mammographic images are required to have high sensitivity and specificity for early detection of breast cancer, but at the same time, mammographic imaging techniques must minimize scattering radiation to provide accurate imaging of breast tissue with a relatively low radiation dose. Recent advanced X-ray film-screen imaging methods use specialized X-ray tubes, breast compression devices, antiscatter grids, and optimized detector systems to optimize diagnostic capabilities for the early detection of breast cancer (2, 3).

4.4. X-RAY MAMMOGRAPHY

X-ray tubes for mammography operate on a low operating voltage, typically less than 30 kV. X-ray tubes with X-ray energies between 17 and 25 keV are preferred for breast imaging. Typically, molybdenum or rhodium is used as a target material in X-ray mammography tubes to provide the characteristic X-ray radiation in the desired range. The K-, L-, and M-shell binding energies for molybdenum are 20, 2.8, and 0.5 keV, respectively. The shell-binding energy levels of molybdenum yield the characteristic X-ray radiation with energies around 17 keV. Rhodium can provide the characteristic X-ray radiation with energies around 20 keV as its K-, L-, and M-shell binding energies, respectively, are around 23, 3.4, and 0.6 keV. With a specific design of the cathode and anode, the X-ray tube used in mammography provides a small focal spot on the order of 0.1 mm required for high-resolution magnification imaging. Inherent filtration methods are used to make the X-ray tube monochromatic with the X-ray radiation beam tightly distributed around a single energy level. Antiscatter grids and compression devices are used to minimize the scattered radiation along with computer-controlled processing to compensate for breast thickness, breast density, and grid effects. Compression of the breast is critical in obtaining good mammographic images. An appropriate compression of the breast along with oscillations of the moving antiscatter grid provides a significant reduction in X-ray scatter and radiation dose. Magnification of the image is obtained by adjusting the distance between the X-ray source, compressed breast, and the film, as shown in Figure 4.6. However, the magnification factor is critically limited by the blurring effect caused by the size of the cathode focal spot and its distance from the breast tissue. In recent film-screen mammography scanners, a double screen with double film emulsions is used for breast imaging. However, digital X-ray mammographic

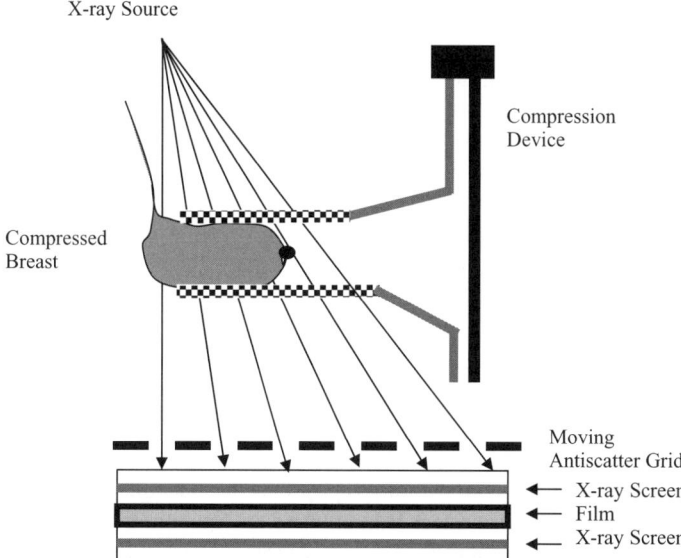

Figure 4.6 A film-screen X-ray mammography imaging system.

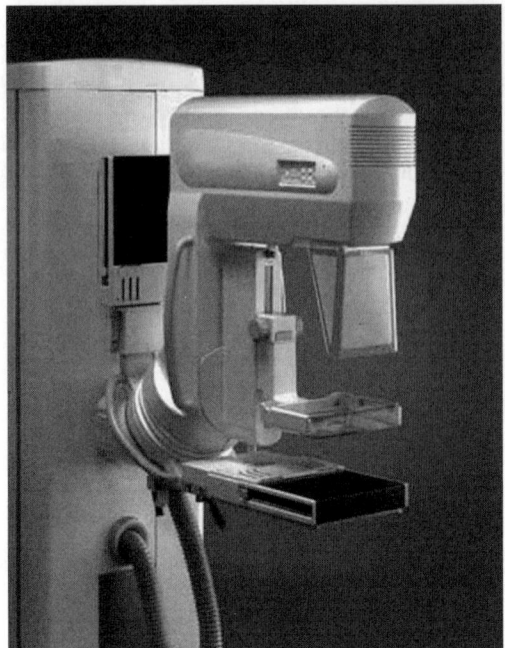

Figure 4.7 A digital X-ray mammography scanner.

scanners are also replacing film-screen with scintillation crystal- and semiconductor technology-based digital detector systems (2).

The low-dose X-ray mammographic imaging systems use a tungsten–rhenium target with a power load of about 8 kW to produce low-energy X-ray photons for breast imaging. Recently, digital mammographic systems have been developed with high sensitivity to low-dose mammograms and portability. They utilize a solid-state semiconductor technology-based detection system instead of vacuum tubes-based photomultiplier technology. The detector system in digital mammographic systems use a phosphor screen or scintillation material thallium-doped CsI layer optically coupled with CCDs. Some portable systems such as SenoScan® digital mammography systems can complete a scan in a few seconds with resolution as small as $0.027 \, mm^2$ pixel size. A digital X-ray mammographic scanner is shown in Figure 4.7, and a mammographic image of a female breast is shown in Figure 4.8.

4.5. X-RAY CT

X-ray conventional radiography creates a 2-D image of a 3-D object projected on the detector plane. While 2-D projection radiography may be adequate for many diagnostic applications, it does not provide 3-D qualitative and quantitative information about the anatomical structures and associated pathology necessary for diagnostics and treatment of a number of diseases or abnormalities. For example, a tumor

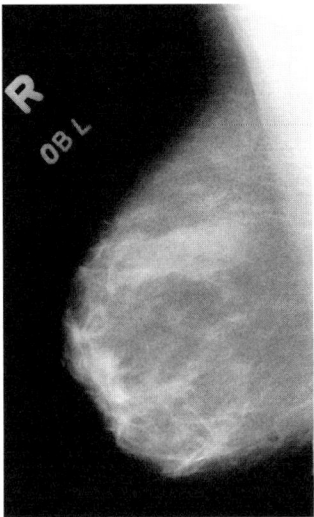

Figure 4.8 An X-ray film-screen mammographic image of a female breast.

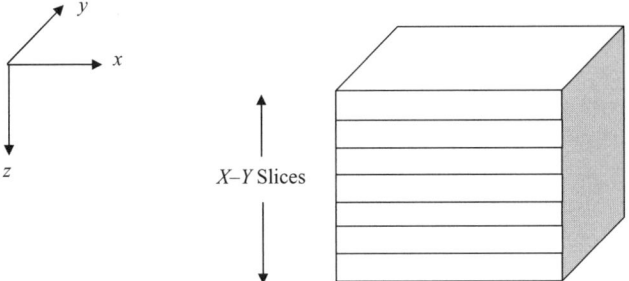

Figure 4.9 3-D object representation as a stack of 2-D x–y slices.

size and its 3-D shape are important features for diagnostic and therapeutic purposes. Also, a fracture in a bone may require 3-D information for better treatment. Other examples may include 3-D imaging of the heart and brain.

Combining 2-D projection radiography with 3-D scanning geometry and advances in image processing algorithms, 3-D CT provides a very useful and sophisticated imaging tool in diagnostic radiology and therapeutic intervention protocols. The basic principle of X-ray CT is the same as that of X-ray digital radiography. X rays are transmitted through the body and collected by an array of detectors to measure the total attenuation along the X-ray path.

Let us assume a 3-D object to be a stack of 2-D slices as shown in Figure 4.9. Let us consider a monochromatic X-ray radiation source aligned with a detector such that the source–detector pair translates to cover the entire 2-D slice for scanning (Fig 4.10). The output intensity of a radiation beam parallel to the x-direction for a specific y-coordinate location, $I_{out}(y; x, z)$ would be given by

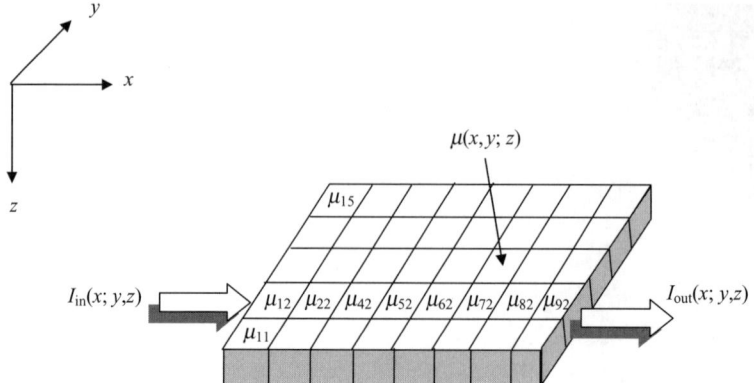

Figure 4.10 Source–detector pair-based translation method to scan a selected 2-D slice of a 3-D object to give a projection along the y-direction.

$$I_{out}(y; x, z) = I_{in}(y; x, z)e^{-\int \mu(x,y;z)dx}. \quad (4.1)$$

One simple way of performing a 3-D scan is to use a pair of point X-ray source and point detector aligned along the ray parallel to the x-axis (2, 8–10). For each position along the y-axis, the source–detector pair will provide one measurement for the y-direction projection of the selected slice. Now, if a projection along x-direction is to be obtained, the source and detector are aligned along the y-direction and then translated along the x-axis. To obtain a projection of the 2-D slice at a different angle, we need to translate the source–detector pair along the direction parallel to the viewing angle. Thus, the angular scan is obtained through the rotation of the source–detector assembly around the object. For a specific viewing angle, the 2-D scan is performed through a linear motion involving translation of the source and detector pair. Figure 4.11 shows a translate–rotate parallel-beam geometry for obtaining a set of projection around a selected 2-D slice of the 3-D object. Such a principle was used in first generation CT scanners. From 1-D projections obtained at different angles around the selected 2-D slice, a 2-D image is reconstructed on a computer using a reconstruction algorithm such as the filtered backprojection method (image reconstruction algorithms are presented in Chapter 8). Thus, a 3-D object can be scanned slice-by-slice along the z-axis as shown in the 3-D representation of stacked slices in Figure 4.9. Correspondingly, a 3-D reconstructed image can be displayed by stacking the reconstructed 2-D slice images. The 3-D reconstructed image is usually interpolated between the slices to obtain a smooth 3-D representation.

The scanner geometry for X-ray CT had several stages of development through four generations. As described above, the first-generation CT scanner utilized an X-ray source–detector pair that was translated in parallel-beam geometry to acquire projections related to a viewing angle. The source–detector pair geometry was then rotated to obtain additional views as shown in Figure 4.12. The second-generation X-ray CT scanners used a fan-beam geometry with a divergent X-ray source and a linear array of detectors. The scanning technique was still based on translation to

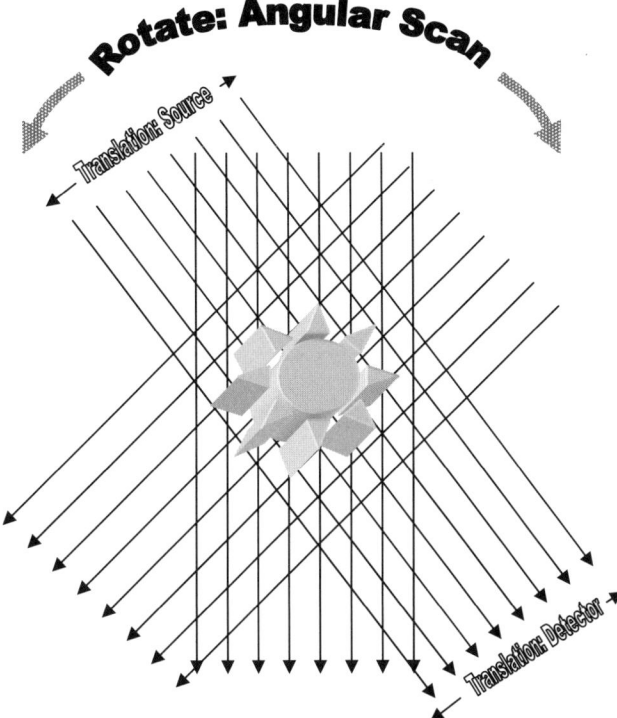

Figure 4.11 The translate–rotate parallel-beam geometry of first-generation CT scanners.

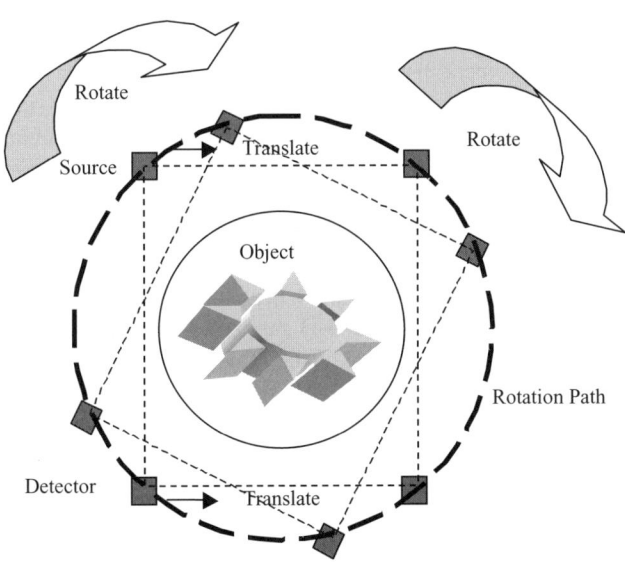

Figure 4.12 The first-generation X-ray CT scanner geometry.

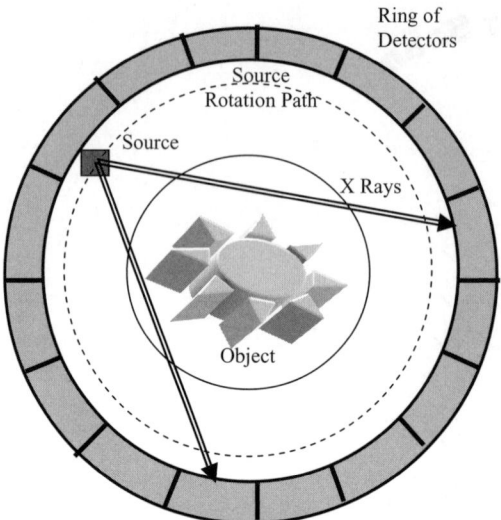

Figure 4.13 The fourth-generation X-ray CT scanner geometry.

cover the object and rotation to obtain additional views. The third-generation X-ray CT scanner used a fan-beam geometry with a divergent X-ray source and an arc of detectors. The divergence of the X-ray fan beam was designed to cover the object without any translation. Thus, the entire projection was obtained from a single position of the X-ray source. Additional views were obtained by simultaneous rotation of the X-ray source and detector assembly. This scanning geometry was called "rotate-only." The fourth-generation X-ray CT scanners use a detector ring around the object as shown in Figure 4.13. The X-ray source provides a divergent fan beam of radiation to cover the object for a single ring of detectors. Scanners with multiple rings of detectors utilize a cone beam to cover multiple slices (8–12). Recent fast spiral CT scanners use a spiral movement instead of parallel movement for selection of axial slices (see the next section). Fourth-generation scanners normally use a ring of 720 or more detectors that are equally spaced around the circumference of a circle. The detectors used in X-ray CT scanners are ionization chambers filled with xenon gas or scintillators with photomultiplier tubes. Recent hybrid X-ray CT scanners such as CT-PET or CT-SPECT also utilize scintillation detectors coupled with photomultiplier tubes or flat panel scintillation detectors coupled with solid-state CCDs.

A modern X-ray CT scanner is shown in Figure 4.14. Figure 4.15 shows a CT reconstructed image of a selected 2-D slice of the 3-D cardiac cavity of a cadaver. For comparison purposes, the pathological section of the selected slice is shown in Figure 4.16.

4.6. SPIRAL X-RAY CT

Certain applications such as brain imaging requires high-resolution imaging that is produced by collecting data for consecutive axial slices (with parallel sections) by

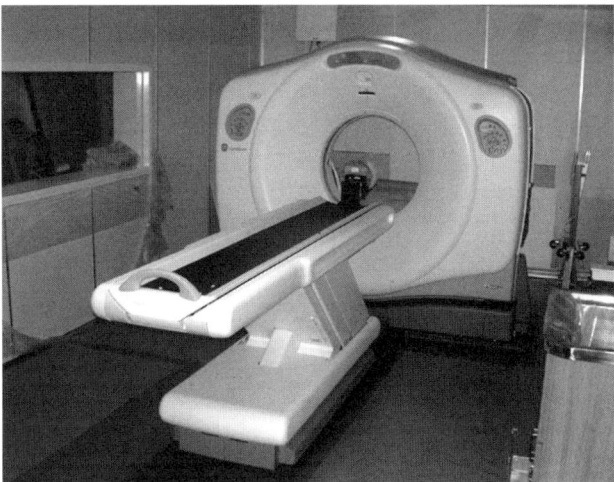

Figure 4.14 An X-ray CT scanner.

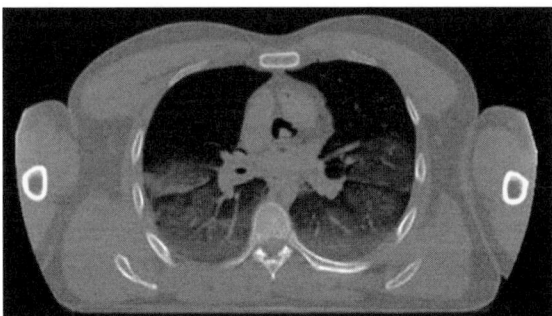

Figure 4.15 X-ray CT image of a selected slice of cardiac cavity of a cadaver.

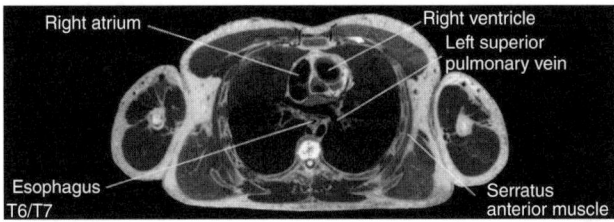

Figure 4.16 The pathological image of the selected slice shown with the X-ray CT image in Figure 4.15.

an X-ray CT scanner. This usually requires longer scan time. A faster scan at lower radiation dose can be obtained for other body imaging applications by spiral (helical) CT while slightly sacrificing image resolution and sharpness. Nevertheless, a faster spiral CT scan provides images with higher temporal resolution to allow investigation of the bolus of the contrast agent administered in the body. In full-resolution

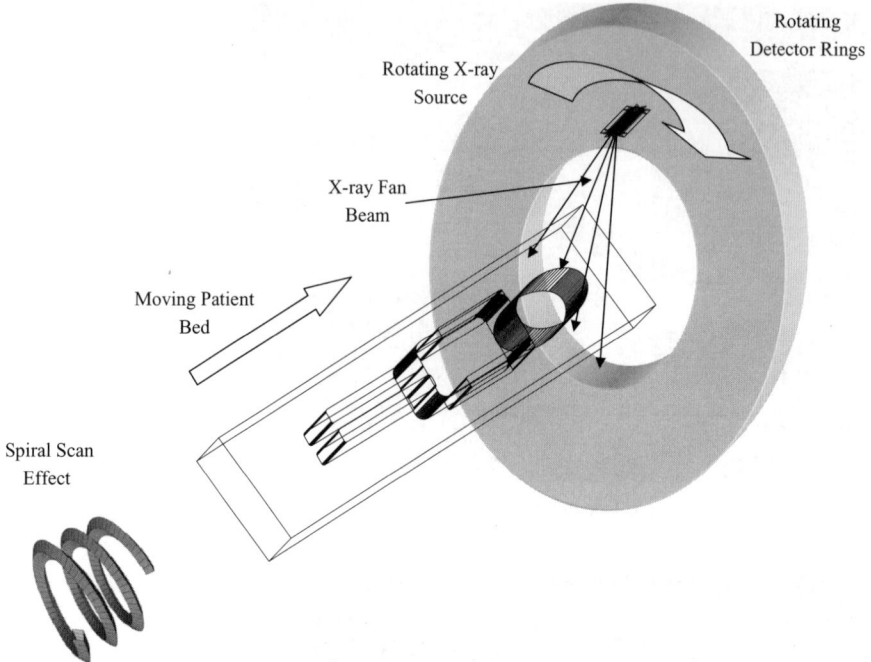

Figure 4.17 A schematic diagram of a spiral CT scanner with spiral effect caused by the movement of patient bed.

CT imaging the patient bed is kept stationary while the source–detector ring gantry is translated to select axial slices. In spiral CT, the patient bed is moved at a constant speed into the gantry space during imaging while the gantry is rotated within the circular opening. The forward movement of the patient bed enables the sampling points to provide the data along a spiral or helical path as shown in Figure 4.17. Due to the motion of patient bed, total scan time for collecting data for multiple sections is significantly reduced. For a single detector ring-based configuration, an X-ray source with a fan-shaped beam is used with width ranging from one to several millimeters. For multislice volume imaging, spiral CT scanners use multiple detector rings with an X-ray source that emits a cone-shaped beam to cover multiple sections at the same time. The spiral CT scans collect continuous data during the entire scan with the rotating gantry. Therefore, a spiral CT scanner requires an X-ray source with better cooling capabilities and detectors with better efficiency. The slip-ring configuration of a spiral CT scanner allows rotation of both X-ray source and detector ring for faster gantry rotation. The slip-ring gantry utilizes a set of rings with electrical components that can rotate and slide seamlessly to enable continuous scanning. During the scanning, slice thickness (t in mm) is determined by the pitch, which is defined by the movement of bed (d in mm) one complete rotation (360 degrees) of gantry as

$$p = \frac{d}{t}. \tag{4.2}$$

For example, a pitch of value "1" for a slice thickness of 2 mm would require the patient's bed to move 2 mm per second if the gantry is rotated 360 degrees per second. In this case, the total scan time of raw data collection will be 30 s to cover a 60 mm wide scanning volume with 2 mm thick contiguous slices. The raw data collected at sampling points distributed along the spiral (helix) is re-binned and interpolated (and even extrapolated as needed) to create projection data that is then used to reconstruct sectional images of desired slice thickness. By combining the detector outputs, images of different slice thickness can be easily reconstructed from the same data. Details about the projection data and reconstruction methods are discussed in Chapter 8.

Multislice spiral CT scanners are used for fast scanning (higher temporal resolution) in dynamic volume imaging in a number of clinical applications including trauma, cardiovascular, abdominal, skeletal, and pediatric imaging.

4.7. CONTRAST AGENT, SPATIAL RESOLUTION, AND SNR

To improve contrast of selected physiological structures in X-ray images, materials that increase the total attenuation coefficient of X rays are used orally or through an intravenous injection. For example, barium sulfate is administered orally to the patent to enhance contrast in upper gastrointestinal (GI) tract imaging, including the esophagus and stomach. Barium atom has a K-edge at 37.4 keV, which causes much higher attenuation of X rays. Thus, when barium sulfate is consumed through the GI tract, respective areas in the image are seen with higher contrast because of increased attenuation. Iodine also has a K-edge at 33.2 keV, causing greater attenuation of X rays. Iodine-based contrast agents are used through intravenous injection in angiography, urography, and intra-arterial DSA to improve visibility of arteries and blood vessels. In X-ray angiography, a series of images with and without contrast agent are compared to visualize the arteries and blood vessels. In DSA, digital images of the tissue before and after administering the contrast agent are taken and subtracted to enhance to contrast between the blood vessels and tissue. Iodine-based contrast agents can also be used in brain imaging for detection of tumors and metastases.

Spatial resolution in X-ray imaging modalities depends on the effective size of the focal spot of X-ray tube, and distance between the X-ray source and the patient due to magnification of the point spread function as discussed in Chapter 2. In addition, the thickness of the intensifying screen and the speed of X-ray film directly affect the spatial resolution in X-ray film-screen imaging. The size and shape of the collimators and detectors also impact considerably on the spatial resolution of X-ray images.

The signal-to-noise ratio of X-ray imaging modalities depends on the X-ray exposure, source and detector instrumentation, thickness and heterogeneity of the tissue, scattering, and contrast agents. The SNR of X-ray imaging is proportional to the square root of the product of the exposure time and X-ray tube current. X rays with higher monochromatic energy provide higher SNR. As X rays are attenuated in the body, they lose energy as they move forward in thicker tissue. Since the attenuation coefficients are energy-dependent (higher energy photons attenuate less), the X-ray beam does not provide same attenuation coefficients for the same type of tissue at the entrance and exit levels of a thick medium. This is called beam hardening, which causes errors and lower SNR in reconstructed images in CT. Specific estimation methods can be used to compensate for the beam-hardening effect based on the thickness of the medium (2, 9). In addition, nonuniform responses of the intensifying screen, phosphor, and scintillation detectors causes lower SNR in X-ray images. In X-ray CT, spatial resolution and SNR of reconstructed images are directly correlated with the number of projections (angular sampling) and number of detectors (projection sampling). For higher spatial resolution, data must be acquired with higher sampling rate in the projection space. However, in practice, the higher sampling rate is compromised by the limitations on scan time, method of data collection, and detector size and efficiency.

4.8. EXERCISES

4.1. Describe the major differences between the anatomical and functional imaging modalities. Identify at least two imaging modalities in each category.

4.2. What is the principle of X-ray computed tomography (CT)?

4.3. How are X rays generated? What is the range of diagnostic X rays? Justify the selection of this range.

4.4. What types of detectors are commonly used in X-ray CT?

4.5. How is the mammography imaging different from conventional X-ray chest radiography? What are the challenges in mammography imaging?

4.6. What is the detector system used in digital mammography systems?

4.7. What contrast agents can be used with X-ray imaging? Describe their significance.

4.8. What are the advantages of fourth-generation CT scanners over the second generation systems?

4.9. What is the difference between a fourth-generation X-ray CT and spiral CT imaging systems?

4.10. If the pitch of a spiral scan is changed from 1 to 2, what will be the effect on the radiation dose?

4.11. X rays of 25 keV are received with an X-ray intensifying screen that produces light photons at 425 nm. If the conversion efficiency of intensifying screen is 20%, calculate how many light photons will be generated by an X-ray photon.

4.12. What is an X-ray contrast agent and why is it used in imaging?

4.13. What consideration should be taken to improve the signal-to-noise ratio (SNR) of X-ray CT images? Describe if there is any harmful effect associated with them.

4.14. Display an axial brain image of a CT scan with brain hemorrhage in MATLAB. In another window, display axial MR brain images including proton density, T_1-, and T_2-weighted images of a stroke patient. Compare and comment on the contrast of the primary hemorrhage and soft tissue regions in the CT and MR images.

4.9. REFERENCES

1. H. Barrett and W. Swindell, *Radiological Imaging: The Theory of Image Formation, Detection and Processing*, Volumes 1–2, Academic Press, New York, 1981.
2. J.T. Bushberg, J.A. Seibert, E.M. Leidholdt, and J.M. Boone, *The Essentials of Medical Imaging*, Williams & Wilkins, Philadelphia, 1994.
3. Z.H. Cho, J.P. Jones, and M. Singh, *Fundamentals of Medical Imaging*, John Wiley & Sons, New York, 1993.
4. A.P. Dhawan, "A review on biomedical image processing and future trends," *Comput. Methods Programs Biomed.*, Vol. 31, No. 3–4, pp. 141–183, 1990.
5. K.K. Shung, M.B. Smith, and B. Tsui, *Principles of Medical Imaging*, Academic Press, San Diego, CA, 1992.
6. G.N. Hounsfield, "A method and apparatus for examination of a body by radiation such as X or gamma radiation," Patent 1283915, The Patent Office, London, 1972.
7. G.N. Hounsfield, "Computerized transverse axial scanning tomography: Part-1, description of the system," *Br.J. Radiol.*, Vol. 46, pp. 1016–1022, 1973.
8. A.M. Cormack, "Representation of a function by its line integrals with some radiological applications," *J. Appl. Phys.*, Vol. 34, pp. 2722–2727, 1963.
9. E. Seeram, *Computed Tomography: Physical Principles, Clinical Applications, and Quality Control*, Saunders, Philadelphia, 2001.
10. E.K. Fisherman and R.B. Jeffrey (Eds), *Spiral CT: Principles, Techniques and Applications*, Lippincott-Raven, Philadelphia, 1998.
11. T. Fuchs, M. Kachelriess, and W.A. Kalender, "Technical advances in multi-slice spiral CT," *Eur. J. Radiol.*, Vol. 36, pp. 69–73, 2000.
12. W.A. Kalender and M. Prokop, "3D CT angiography," *Crit. Rev. Diagn. Imaging*, Vol. 42, pp. 1–28, 2001.

CHAPTER 5

MEDICAL IMAGING MODALITIES: MAGNETIC RESONANCE IMAGING

Like X-ray computed tomography (CT), magnetic resonance imaging (MRI) is a tomographic imaging method that produces 3-D images of the human body, but it is not based on the transmission of external radiation for imaging. MRI uses the nuclear magnetic resonance (NMR) property of selected nuclei of the matter of the object. MRI provides high-resolution images with excellent soft-tissue contrast superior to X-ray CT because of the underlying physics of the imaging process. It is difficult to produce images with good soft-tissue contrast, and information about changes in physiological parameters (such as oxygenation level) and functions (such as diffusion and perfusion) through X-ray CT because X rays do not provide measurable differentiation (leading to contrast in the image) for them. MRI uses selected nuclei, such as hydrogen protons, available in the body for NMR, which produces an electromagnetic signal for imaging. Thus, differentiation (or contrast) in the MRI signal is based on the difference of hydrogen protons in the tissue and physiological structures. Hydrogen protons are readily available in water and other fluids in the body and vary in density within a tissue if its chemical composition changes, providing the basis for better imaging. MRI is a powerful modality for imaging anatomical structures as well as biochemical properties based on physiological function, including blood flow and oxygenation (1–3).

The principle of NMR was independently explained by Felix Bloch and Edward Purcell in 1946. Later, Paul Lauterbur used the NMR principle in MRI to obtain physical and chemical properties based images of an object (2, 3). Paul Lauterbur and Sir Peter Mansfield were jointly awarded Nobel Prize in Medicine in 2003 for their discoveries concerning MRI. Today, MRI techniques are used in multidimensional imaging of the human body, providing both structural and physiological information about internal organs and tissues (1–3).

Magnetic resonance imaging is a complex multidimensional imaging modality that produces extensive amounts of data. Imaging methods and techniques applied in signal acquisition allow reconstruction of images with multiple parameters that represent various physical and chemical properties of the matter of the object. Figure 5.1 shows three images of the same cross-section of a human brain with different

---

Medical Image Analysis, Second Edition, by Atam P. Dhawan
Copyright © 2011 by the Institute of Electrical and Electronics Engineers, Inc.

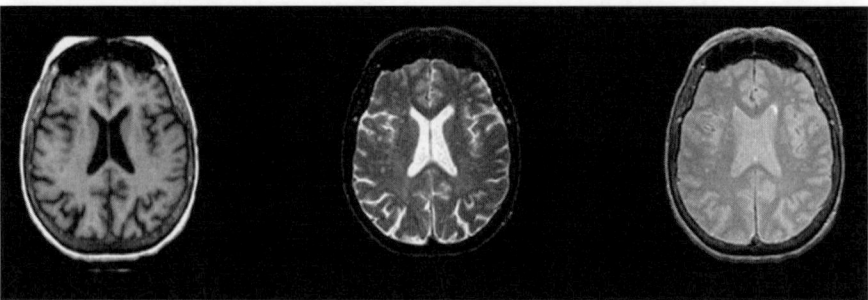

Figure 5.1 MR images of a selected cross-section that are obtained simultaneously using a specific imaging technique. The images show (from left to right), respectively, the T_1-weighted, T_2-weighted and the spin-density property of the hydrogen protons present in the brain.

parameters: T_1 weighted, T_2 weighted, and spin density (also called proton density). These images are reconstructed from the data generated through specialized imaging techniques called pulse sequences. MRI pulse sequences provide signal timing and spatial encoding of the object space for data acquisition. Recent advances in MRI include MR spectroscopy, functional (fMRI), and diffusion tensor imaging (DTI) modalities that have sophisticated means of obtaining localized characteristic information about the physiological behavior of the human organ or tissue. For example, a sequence of fMRI images of the brain can show the changes in blood flow or oxygenation levels in the auditory cortex when a signal for auditory stimulation is presented to a subject. A significant advantage of MRI is that it can create any directional cross-sectional images along with multidimensional image sequences without making any physical changes in the instrumentation during imaging. Another advantage of MRI is fast signal acquisition (of the order of a fraction of a second) with a very high spatial resolution in the range of a millimeter to one-hundredth of a millimeter. However, in practice, due to the limitations of instrumentation used in data acquisition methods, these parameters are realized with a lower range to maintain a reasonable signal-to-noise ratio (SNR) for acceptable image quality.

5.1. MRI PRINCIPLES

The basic objective of MR imaging is to map the spatial location and associated properties of specific nuclei or protons present in the object being imaged. The hydrogen proton is the most common form of nuclei used in MRI. Figure 5.1 shows three images displaying three properties of hydrogen nuclei (protons) mapping their spatial locations present in a selected cross-section of the brain. These properties are the spin–lattice relaxation time T_1, spin–spin relaxation time T_2, and the spin density ρ. These properties and their significance in diagnostic radiology are described later in this chapter. The high-resolution anatomical information can be seen with different contrast features in Figure 5.1.

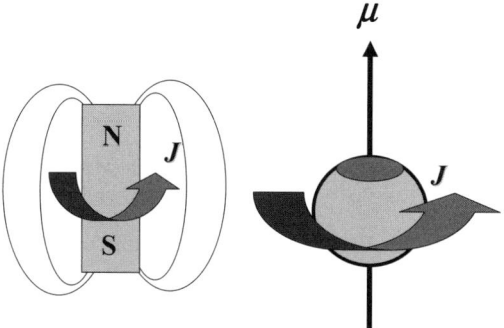

Figure 5.2 Left: A tiny magnet representation of a charged proton with angular moment, *J*. Right: A symbolic representation of a charged proton with angular moment, *J*, and a magnetic moment, μ.

The principle of NMR is based on the quantum properties of nuclei and protons. A fundamental property of nuclei with odd atomic weight and/or odd atomic numbers is the possession of angular moment, generally called spin. These protons carry an electric charge and spin around their axes (Fig. 5.2). Because of the spinning, the charged protons create a magnetic field around them and thus act like tiny magnets possessing both angular moment and magnetic moment. The magnetic moment is proportional to the spin angular moment and is related through a constant, called the gyromagnetic ratio, a quantum property of the proton. Thus, the relationship between the spin angular moment, $\vec{J}$, and the magnetic moment, $\vec{\mu}$, is described by

$$\vec{\mu} = \gamma \vec{J} \quad (5.1)$$

where γ is a gyromagnetic ratio defined in megahertz/Tesla.

A hydrogen atom, for example, has only one proton in its nucleus and thus exhibits the property of nuclear spin. Its gyromagnetic ratio is 42.58 MHz/T, providing a corresponding magnetic moment that is excellent for imaging the human body under an external magnetic field of 0.5 to 1.5 T. The hydrogen proton is also an important in NMR imaging of the human body because of its presence in water molecules, which are available in abundance in the body. However, other protons that exhibit the NMR phenomenon and are available in the body for MRI include ^{13}C, ^{19}F, and ^{31}P (1–5).

The spinning protons with both angular and magnetic moment possess a specific spin quantum number that characterizes their orientations and corresponding energy levels with or without the presence of an external magnetic field. In the absence of an external magnetic field, the direction of the magnetic moments of spinning protons or nuclei is completely random. In the presence of an external magnetic field, the magnetic moments of nuclei result in a nuclear paramagnetic polarization with specific orientations and energy levels as characterized by their spin quantum number. Also, the interaction between the magnetic moment of nuclei with the external magnetic field causes the spinning nuclei to precess, similar to the wobbling of a spinning top, under the gravitational field. The precession of a

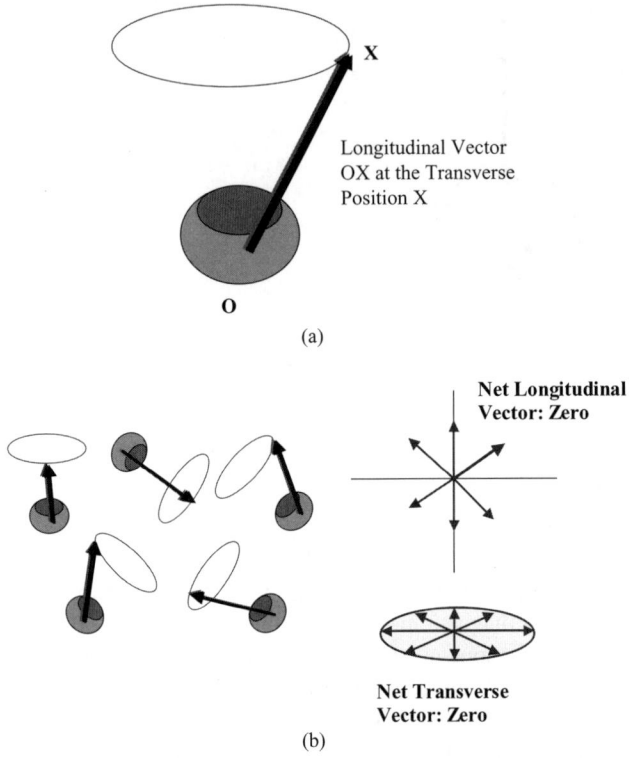

Figure 5.3 (a) A symbolic representation of a proton with precession that is experienced by the spinning proton when it is subjected to an external magnetic field. (b) The random orientation of protons in matter with the net zero vector in both longitudinal and transverse directions.

spinning proton (or nucleus) is shown in Figure 5.3. The spin quantum number of hydrogen proton (^{1}H) and other nuclei such as ^{13}C, ^{19}F, and ^{31}P is ½. When such nuclei are placed under an external magnetic field, they are aligned either along the external magnetic field or against the magnetic field. The energy level of nuclei aligning themselves along the external magnetic field is lower than the energy level of nuclei aligned against the external magnetic field. Upon establishing a thermal equilibrium in the presence of an external magnetic field, the total number of nuclei aligned along the external magnetic field is slightly larger than the number of nuclei aligned against the external magnetic field. This results in a net magnetization vector in the direction of the external magnetic field as shown in Figure 5.4. However, the precession phase is still random, providing a net zero vector in the transverse direction.

Using the principle of classical mechanics, the torque generated by the interaction of magnetic moment of a proton and the external magnetic field is equal to the rate of change of angular momentum and can be given by the equation of motion for isolated spin as (1–3)

5.1. MRI PRINCIPLES

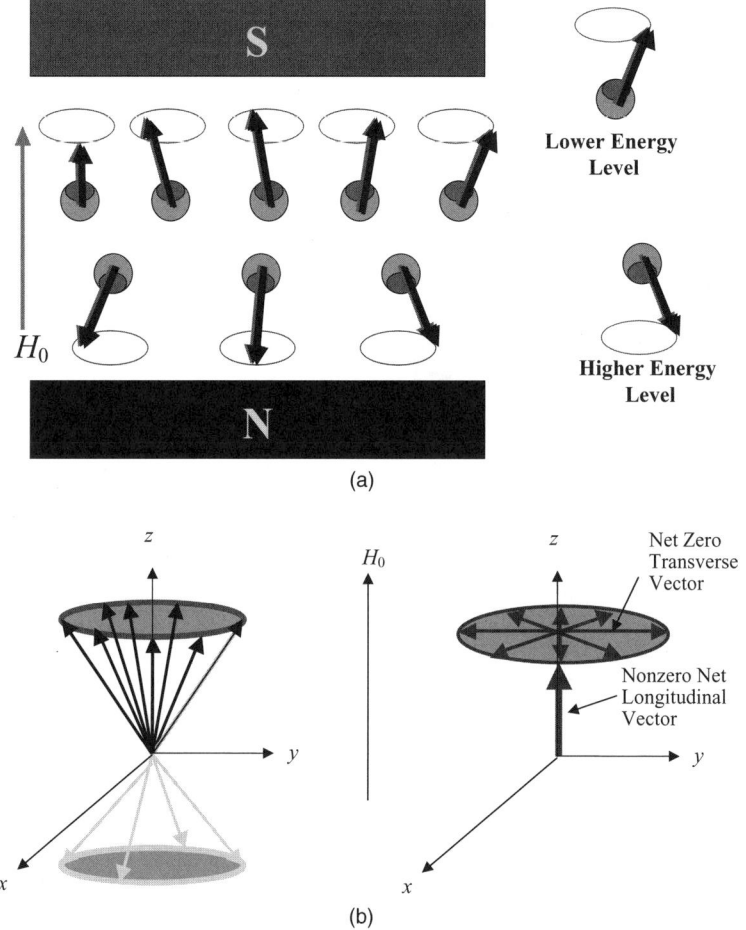

Figure 5.4 (a) Nuclei aligned under thermal equilibrium in the presence of an external magnetic field. (b) A nonzero net longitudinal vector and a zero transverse vector provided by the nuclei precessing in the presence of an external magnetic field.

$$\frac{d\vec{J}}{dt} = \vec{\mu} \times \vec{H}_0 = \vec{\mu} \times H_0 \vec{k}. \tag{5.2}$$

Since $\vec{\mu} = \gamma \vec{J}$, the derivative equation can be written as

$$\frac{d\vec{\mu}}{dt} = \gamma \, \vec{\mu} \times H_0 \vec{k} \tag{5.3}$$

where H_0 is the strength of the external magnetic field and $\vec{k}$ is the unit vector in z-direction with $\vec{H}_0 = H_0 \vec{k}$.

The solution of the above equation leads to an important relationship that provides the angular frequency, ω_0, of nuclear precession as

$$\omega_0 = \gamma H_0 \tag{5.4}$$

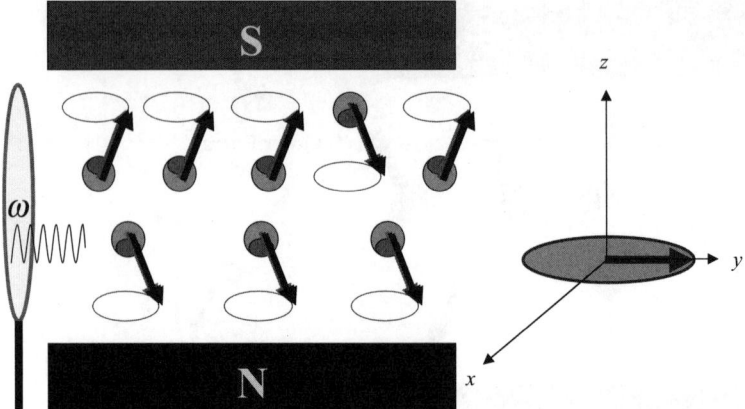

Figure 5.5 The 90-degree pulse causing nuclei to precess in phase with the longitudinal vector shifted clockwise by 90 degrees as a result of the absorption of RF energy at the Larmor frequency.

The above relationship in Equation 5.4 is also known as the Larmor equation. Thus, the precession frequency depends on the type of nuclei with a specific gyromagnetic ratio and the intensity of the external magnetic field. This is the frequency on which the nuclei can receive the radio frequency (RF) energy to change their states to exhibit NMR. The excited nuclei return to the thermal equilibrium through a process of relaxation, emitting energy at the same precession frequency, ω_0.

During NMR, the nuclei can receive energy to move from the lower-energy state to the higher energy state. In other words, upon receiving the RF energy at the Larmor frequency, the nuclei spinning with an orientation along the external magnetic field can flip to an orientation against the magnetic field. As a result of the change in the orientation of the excited nuclei, the net longitudinal vector is no longer in the direction of the external magnetic field (z-direction). It starts moving away from the z-direction. An RF energy pulse required to shift the longitudinal vector by 90 degrees is called the "90-degree pulse." Upon receiving energy at the Larmor frequency, the transverse vector also changes as nuclei start to precess in phase. After the completion of the 90-degree pulse, all of the nuclei precess in phase and therefore form a net nonzero transverse vector that rotates in the x-y plane perpendicular to the direction of the external magnetic field (see Fig. 5.5).

If enough energy is supplied, the longitudinal vector can be completely flipped over with a 180-degree clockwise shift in the direction against the external magnetic field. The RF energy pulse required to flip the net longitudinal magnetization vector over is called the "180-degree pulse" (see Fig. 5.6).

The RF energy is provided by an RF electromagnetic coil that transmits an oscillating RF wave at the Larmor frequency to cause nuclear excitation. After the RF pulse is turned off, the excited nuclei go through a relaxation phase. Under the nuclear relaxation phase, the net longitudinal magnetization vector returns to its original state in the thermal equilibrium and the net transverse magnetization vector disappears due to dephasing of the nuclei.

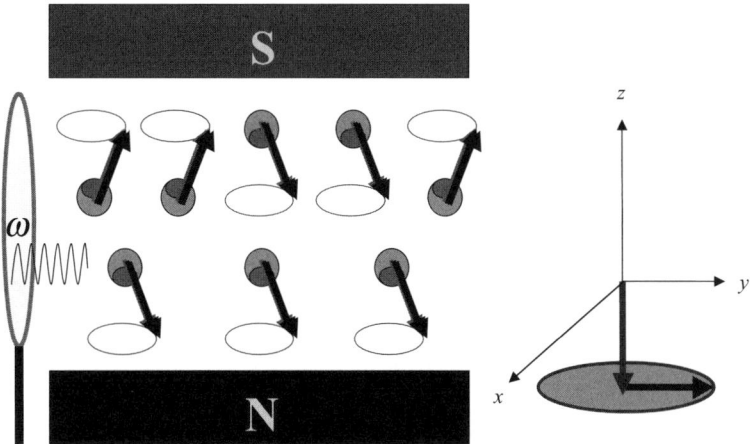

Figure 5.6 The 180-degree pulse causing nuclei to precess in phase with the longitudinal vector shifted clockwise by 180 degrees as a result of the absorption of RF energy at the Larmor frequency.

The energy emitted during the relaxation process induces an electrical signal in an RF coil tuned at the Larmor frequency. The free induction decay of the electromagnetic signal in the RF coil is the basic signal that is used to create MR images. Thus, under the NMR phenomenon, the RF energy received by the nuclei at the Larmor frequency causes characteristic excitation of nuclei. The nuclear excitation forces the net longitudinal and transverse magnetization vectors to move. The movement of longitudinal and transverse vectors can be explained through Bloch's equation as described below (Eq. 5.12) (1–5).

Assuming N to be the total number of spinning nuclei in the object being imaged, a stationary magnetization vector, $\vec{M}$, can be defined from the available magnetic moments as

$$\vec{M} = \sum_{n=1}^{N} \vec{\mu}_n. \tag{5.5}$$

Let us now define a rotating frame as a coordinate system with a transverse plane rotating at the angular frequency, ω. Let us define a stationary magnetization vector as $\vec{M}$ with its components in the unit direction vectors $\vec{i}$, $\vec{j}$, and $\vec{k}$ respectively, in the direction of the actual coordinate system, x, y, and z, that is also called the laboratory coordinate system. For a rotating frame, let us define the rotating magnetization vector $\vec{M}_r$ with the unit direction vectors $\vec{i}'$, $\vec{j}'$, and $\vec{k}'$, respectively, in the x, y, and z coordinate system as (3, 5, 6)

$$\vec{M} = M_x \vec{i} + M_y \vec{j} + M_z \vec{k}$$

and

$$\vec{M}_r = M_x \vec{i}' + M_y \vec{j}' + M_z \vec{k}'. \tag{5.6}$$

From the rotation transformation (given in Chapter 2), the stationary and clockwise rotating frames are related as

$$\vec{i'} = \cos(\omega t)\vec{i} - \sin(\omega t)\vec{j}$$
$$\vec{j'} = \sin(\omega t)\vec{i} + \cos(\omega t)\vec{j}$$
$$\vec{k'} = \vec{k}. \quad (5.7)$$

Thus, the magnetization vectors corresponding to the stationary (laboratory) and clockwise rotating frames can be written as

$$\begin{bmatrix} M_{x'} \\ M_{y'} \\ M_{z'} \end{bmatrix} = \begin{bmatrix} \cos\omega t & -\sin\omega t & 0 \\ \sin\omega t & \cos\omega t & 0 \\ 0 & 0 & 1 \end{bmatrix} \begin{bmatrix} M_x \\ M_y \\ M_z \end{bmatrix}. \quad (5.8)$$

The transverse magnetization vector in the rotating frame can be written as

$$M_{x',y'} = M_{x,y} e^{i\omega t}$$

where

$$M_{x,y} = M_x + iM_y \quad \text{and} \quad M_{x',y'} = M_{x'} + iM_{y'}. \quad (5.9)$$

Let us assume that H_{1r} and H_1 are, respectively, the RF field in the rotating frame and the stationary coordinate systems. Similar to Equation 5.7, an oscillating RF field causing nuclear excitation can be expressed as

$$H_{1r}(t) = H_1(t) e^{i\omega t}$$

with

$$H_1 = H_{1,x} + iH_{1,y} \quad \text{and} \quad H_{1r} = H_{1,x'} + iH_{1,y'}. \quad (5.10)$$

It is to be noted that H_1 is a short-term field produced by the oscillating RF pulse that is much weaker (of the order of a few tens of millitesla). It is turned on only for a few microseconds to milliseconds of nuclear excitation. The external magnetic field, H_0, is static in nature and much stronger (usually in the range of 0.5–1.5T).

The relationship between the rates of change of stationary magnetization vector $\vec{M}$ and rotating magnetization vector $\vec{M}_r$ can then be expressed as (5)

$$\frac{d\vec{M}}{dt} = \frac{\partial \vec{M}_r}{\partial t} + \omega \times \vec{M}_r. \quad (5.11)$$

From the above formulation, it can be shown that during the RF pulse (nuclear excitation phase), the rate of change in the net stationary magnetization vector can be expressed as (Bloch's equation):

$$\frac{d\vec{M}}{dt} = \gamma \vec{M} \times \vec{H} \quad (5.12)$$

where $\vec{H}$ is the net effective magnetic field.

Considering the total response of the spin system in the presence of an external magnetic field along with the RF pulse for nuclear excitation, followed by the nuclear relaxation phase, the change of the net magnetization vector can be expressed as (3)

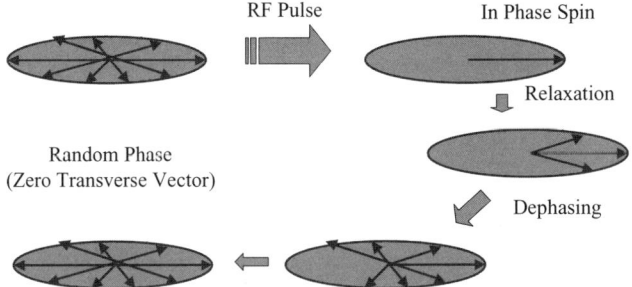

Figure 5.7 The transverse relaxation process of spinning nuclei.

$$\frac{d\vec{M}}{dt} = \gamma \vec{M} \times \vec{H} - \frac{M_x \vec{i} + M_y \vec{j}}{T_2} - \frac{(M_z - M_z^0)\vec{k}}{T_1} \quad (5.13)$$

where $\vec{M}_z^0$ is the net magnetization vector in thermal equilibrium in the presence of an external magnetic field H_0 only, and T_1 and T_2 are, respectively, the longitudinal (spin–lattice) and transverse (spin–spin) relaxation times in the nuclear relaxation phase when excited nuclei return to their thermal equilibrium state. In other words, the longitudinal relaxation time, T_1, represents the return of the net magnetization vector in z-direction to its thermal equilibrium state, while the transverse relaxation time, T_2, represents the loss of coherence or dephasing of spin leading to the net zero vector in the x-y plane. Figure 5.7 shows the transverse relaxation process through spin dephasing.

The solution to above Bloch equations for the transverse and longitudinal magnetization vectors can be obtained through relaxation processes while the system recovers to its thermal equilibrium state. The transverse magnetization equation solution is obtained through a clockwise precession-based spin–spin relaxation process with a decay rate of $1/T_2$ until $\vec{M}_{x,y}(t) \to 0$. The longitudinal magnetization vector $\vec{M}_z(t)$ decays with a rate of $1/T_1$ through the spin–lattice relation process until it returns to the net magnetization vector in thermal equilibrium, $\vec{M}_z^0$. The longitudinal and transverse magnetization vectors with respect to the relaxation times in the actual stationary coordinate system can be given by

$$\vec{M}_z(t) = \vec{M}_z^0(1 - e^{-t/T_1}) + \vec{M}_z(0)e^{-t/T_1}$$
$$\vec{M}_{x,y}(t) = \vec{M}_{x,y}(0)e^{-t/T_2}e^{-i\omega_0 t}$$
$$\text{with } \vec{M}_{x,y}(0) = \vec{M}_{x',y'}(0)e^{-i\omega_0 \tau_p} \quad (5.14)$$

where $\vec{M}_{x,y}(0)$ represents the initial transverse magnetization vector with the time set to zero at the end of the RF pulse of duration τ_p.

Equation 5.14 describes the nature of the change in the transverse and longitudinal magnetization vectors with respect to time after the RF pulse. The exponential decay of e^{-t/T_2} can be seen in the transverse magnetization relaxation shown in Figure 5.8a while the recovery of longitudinal magnetization vector after 90-degree and 180-degree pulses are shown, respectively, in Figure 5.8b,c.

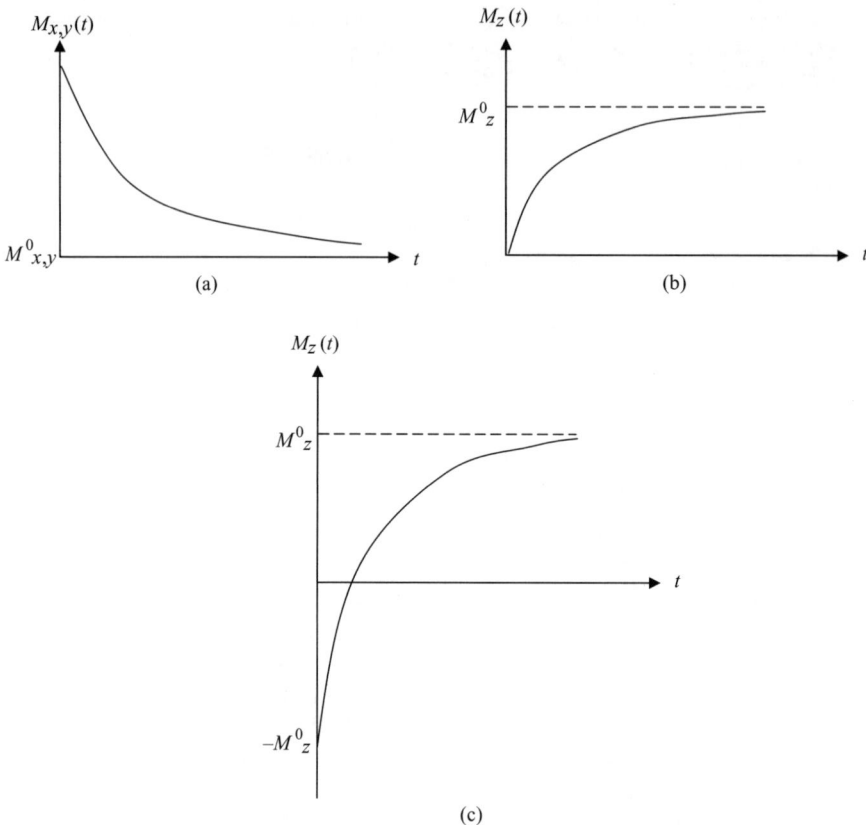

Figure 5.8 (a) Transverse relaxation and recovery to zero transverse magnetization vector after an RF pulse, (b) longitudinal magnetization relaxation and recovery to M_z^0 after the 90-degree RF pulse, and (c) longitudinal magnetization relaxation and recovery to M_z^0 after the 90-degree RF pulse.

As described above, the RF pulse, transmitted through an RF coil, causes nuclear excitation, changing the longitudinal and transverse magnetization vectors. After the RF pulse is turned off, the excited nuclei go through the relaxation phase, emitting the absorbed energy at the same Larmor frequency that can be detected as an electrical signal, called the free induction decay (FID). The FID is the raw NMR signal that can be acquired through the same RF coil tuned at the Larmor frequency.

Let us represent a spatial location vector $\mathbf{r}$ in the spinning nuclei system with a net magnetic field vector $\vec{H}_r(\mathbf{r})$ and the corresponding net magnetization vector $\vec{M}(\mathbf{r},t)$. The magnetic flux $\phi(t)$ through the RF coil can be given as (5)

$$\phi(t) = \int_{object} \vec{H}_r(\mathbf{r}) \cdot \vec{M}(\mathbf{r},t)\, d\mathbf{r} \qquad (5.15)$$

where $\mathbf{r} = x\vec{i} + y\vec{j} + z\vec{k}$.

5.1. MRI PRINCIPLES

The voltage induced in the RF coil, $V(t)$, is the raw NMR signal and can be expressed (using Faraday's law) as

$$V(t) = -\frac{\partial \phi(t)}{\partial t} = -\frac{\partial}{\partial t} \int_{object} \vec{H}_r(\mathbf{r}) \cdot \vec{M}(\mathbf{r},t) \, d\mathbf{r}. \tag{5.16}$$

The realization of a spatial location-dependent signal in Equation 5.16 is important to create an MR image that maps the MR response of the spinning nuclei available in that location. Since the Larmor or precession frequency is based on the net magnetic field, if an additional magnetic gradient field is superimposed on the static external magnetic field, the spatial locations within the object can be encoded with localized specific precession frequencies. Thus, spatial locations within the object that is placed inside a large magnet (producing the static external magnetic field) can be viewed as small volumes containing nuclei that can be excited using different RF frequencies. NMR signals generated by specific excited volumes within the object can thus be differentiated with respect to the individual RF frequencies. Access to the small volumes within the object to generate corresponding NMR signals is obtained through spatial encoding techniques. These techniques utilize different gradient methods for frequency- and phase-based spatial encoding. Once the spatial locations with an object being imaged are accessed, the corresponding NMR signals are acquired using specific RF pulse sequences for image reconstruction. NMR signals are mapped into the image of the object with the spatial relationship between the object and image spaces. An image reconstruction process assigns values to the image pixels (in case of two-dimensional [2-D] images) or voxels (in case of three-dimensional [3-D] images) displaying a particular feature associated with the NMR phenomenon of the nuclei present in the corresponding volume. The application of a specific pulse sequence determines the feature associated with the specific image pixels or voxels. The conventional MR images take advantage of three common parameters of nuclei: spin density (density of nuclei), longitudinal relaxation time T_1, and transverse relaxation time T_2. Several versions of the image with different weightings of the NMR parameters (spin density, T_1, and T_2) can be reconstructed using computer processing and reconstruction methods in association with selected pulse sequences.

Since the NMR signal is collected in the frequency domain, the spatial information of the image can be obtained by taking a Fourier transform with appropriate dimensions. More details on image reconstruction methods for MRI are described in Chapter 8. The basic form of MRI can be described using the 3-D Fourier transform-based reconstruction method. This method is also called the FID method in which the spin echoes are formed using RF pulse sequences for 3-D spatial location (volume) selection. Let us assume that three gradient fields, G_x, G_y, and G_z, are, respectively, applied in x-, y-, and z-directions for the selection and excitation of a spatial location (volume) with a spin nuclei density $\rho(x, y, z)$. The overall gradient $\mathbf{G}(t)$ for a spatial location, $\mathbf{r}$, is expressed as

$$\mathbf{G}(t) = G_x(t)\vec{i} + G_y(t)\vec{j} + G_z(t)\vec{k}. \tag{5.17}$$

From Equation 5.14, after some simplifications and assumptions such as field homogeneity and absence of chemical shifts, the NMR spin-echo signal, $S(t)$, from a specific location or volume of the object can be expressed as

TABLE 5.1 Typical T_1 and T_2 Relaxation Times and the Spin Density (SD) of Some of the Tissues and Fluids Present in the Human Body

Tissue	T_1 (ms)	T_2 (ms)	SD (%)
Fat	150	150	10.9
Liver	250	44	10.0
White matter	300	133	11.0
Gray matter	475	118	10.5
Blood	525	261	10.0
CSF	2000	250	10.8

$$S(t) = \int \vec{M}(\mathbf{r},t) \, d^3r \tag{5.18}$$

where $\vec{M}(\mathbf{r},t) = \vec{M}_0 \rho(\mathbf{r}) e^{-i\gamma \mathbf{r} \cdot \int_0^t G(t') dt'}$ and $\vec{M}_0$ is the magnetization vector in thermal equilibrium.

Let ω_x, ω_y, and ω_z be the angular frequencies corresponding to the gradient fields, G_x, G_y, and G_z, respectively, Equation 5.18 can be further simplified as (3):

$$S(\omega_x, \omega_y, \omega_z) = \vec{M}_0 \iiint \rho(x,y,z) e^{-i(\omega_x x + \omega_y y + \omega_z z)} dx\, dy\, dz. \tag{5.19}$$

The MR image of the spin density can then be reconstructed from the FID signal, $S(t)$, by taking a 3-D inverse Fourier transform (from frequency domain to the spatial domain) as (3)

$$\rho(x,y,z) = \vec{M}_0 \iiint S(\omega_x, \omega_y, \omega_z) e^{i(\omega_x x + \omega_y y + \omega_z z)} d\omega_x\, d\omega_y\, d\omega_z. \tag{5.20}$$

Table 5.1 shows typical T_1 and T_2 relaxation times and the spin density of some of the tissues and fluids present in the human body. It can be seen that there is considerable change in relaxation parameters of tissues and fluids of interest such as blood and cerebrospinal fluid (CSF). Once NMR raw signals are acquired and MR parameters are computed, the contrast in an image can be adjusted by changing the respective weights of the parameters. Normally the spin-density images are weighted by the T_1 parameter to improve contrast features of anatomical structures.

5.2. MR INSTRUMENTATION

The stationary external magnetic field for MRI of the human body is provided by a large superconducting magnet with a typical strength of 0.5 to 1.5 T. The magnet is required to have a 30–50 cm diameter spherical volume for the human body and housing of gradient coils as needed. A diagnostic-quality imaging system requires a magnet with good field homogeneity, typically on the order of 10–50 ppm. For high-quality spectroscopy and fMRI, a set of shim coils is used to provide an addi-

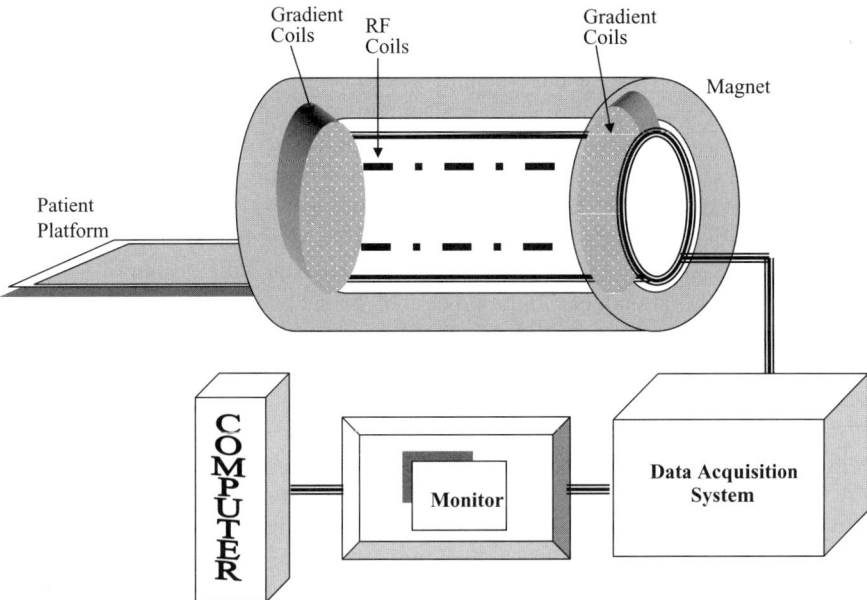

Figure 5.9 A general schematic diagram of an MRI system.

tional magnetic field to compensate for the field inhomogeneity of the main magnet. A general schematic of an MRI system is shown in Figure 5.9.

In typical MRI systems, three orthogonal gradient coils are used to provide gradient magnetic fields (1, 3). Although the gradient coils generate magnetic fields in the z-direction, they provide software-controlled displacements in the x-, y-, and z-directions. The simplest form of gradient coil generates a linear, spatially dependent magnetic field. Field strength, linearity, and switching time are three important considerations for the selection of gradient coils. The shape and placement of the coil are crucial for generating the field in the desired direction. The Golay-type coils are commonly used for x- and y-direction gradients, while a double loop-based Helmholtz coil is typically used for the z-direction gradient.

During the nuclear excitation phase, an RF coil with electronic circuitry is used to transmit time-varying RF pulses. The same RF coil with computerized programming and switching control is used to receive the RF emissions during the nuclear relaxation phase. The NMR signal, as described above, is recorded through FID in the RF coil at a selected RF. The computerized control of electronic circuitry allows the programming of the RF coil to transmit and receive specific RF pulses as required by the pulse sequences for image reconstruction. The RF transmitter section includes a wave synthesizer, RF modulator, RF amplifier, and a coupler that couples the RF signal to the RF coil. The RF receiver section uses the coupler to switch the signal from the RF coil to an assembly of pre-amplifiers and demodulators. The FID signal thus received is then sent to an analog-to-digital converter to record the data in digital format.

5.3. MRI PULSE SEQUENCES

To obtain MR images, a spatial encoding has to be established between the object and image coordinate systems. As described above, the spatially encoded locations or volumes are first excited though RF pulses and then accessed to acquire the FID signal during the relaxation phase for image reconstruction. Various sequences of RF pulses for spatial encoding and signal acquisition have been designed for MRI. These sequences are based on different methods that can be exploited to improve the SNR and scanning rate of a 3-D object. To understand the design of RF pulse sequences let us first understand the process of spatial encoding and the coordinate system. Figure 5.10a shows a 3-D object with an x-y-z object coordinate system that can be scanned to provide three different orientations of image views: axial, sagital, and coronal. Figure 5.10b shows axial, sagital, and coronal images of a human brain. Usually, a patient is oriented on the platform shown in Figure 5.9 for axial imaging with the spine aligned in the z-direction (1–5).

The encoding of the NMR signal has to be performed in all three dimensions to scan the object and reconstruct its 3-D images. This means that all three dimensions have to be encoded with spatially dependent coding of NMR signals. As with any other RF wave, the NMR signal has two basic features: the frequency and the phase. For this reason, there are two basic methods of spatial encoding in MRI: frequency encoding and phase encoding.

In frequency encoding, a linear gradient is applied throughout the imaging space along a selected direction (such as the z-direction). As described above, the precession or Larmor frequency is dependent on the net magnetic field at the location of the spinning nuclei. If a linear gradient is superimposed on the stationary magnetic field of the external magnet, the net magnetic field is spatially encoded along the direction of the gradient and consequently the effective Larmor frequency of spinning nuclei is also spatially encoded along the direction of the gradient as shown in Figure 5.11. Thus, a linear gradient can be used along the z-direction for slice selection for axial imaging.

After the slice selection through frequency encoding using a linear gradient along the z-direction, x- and y-directions need to be spatially encoded for 3-D imaging. This is accomplished by further encoding the phase of the spinning nuclei along the x-direction of the selected slice while the spatial encoding in the y-direction is provided by another linear frequency encoding gradient along the y-direction. In such a scanning method, a linear frequency encoding gradient along the y-direction is also used for reading out the NMR signal. This is further explained below for spin-echo pulse sequences.

The phase-encoding gradient is applied as a constant step gradient in the direction in which all of the spinning nuclei are spinning with the same Larmor frequency. A fixed magnitude of the gradient changes the phase of the spinning nuclei by a respective fixed amount. Since the spatial encoding in two directions is provided by linear frequency encoding gradients, a step function-based gradient field can be applied in the third direction for phase encoding to acquire NMR signals for 3-D scanning and imaging. Unlike frequency encoding, the phase-encoding gradient is applied in steps with repeated cycles. For example, if 256 steps are to be applied in

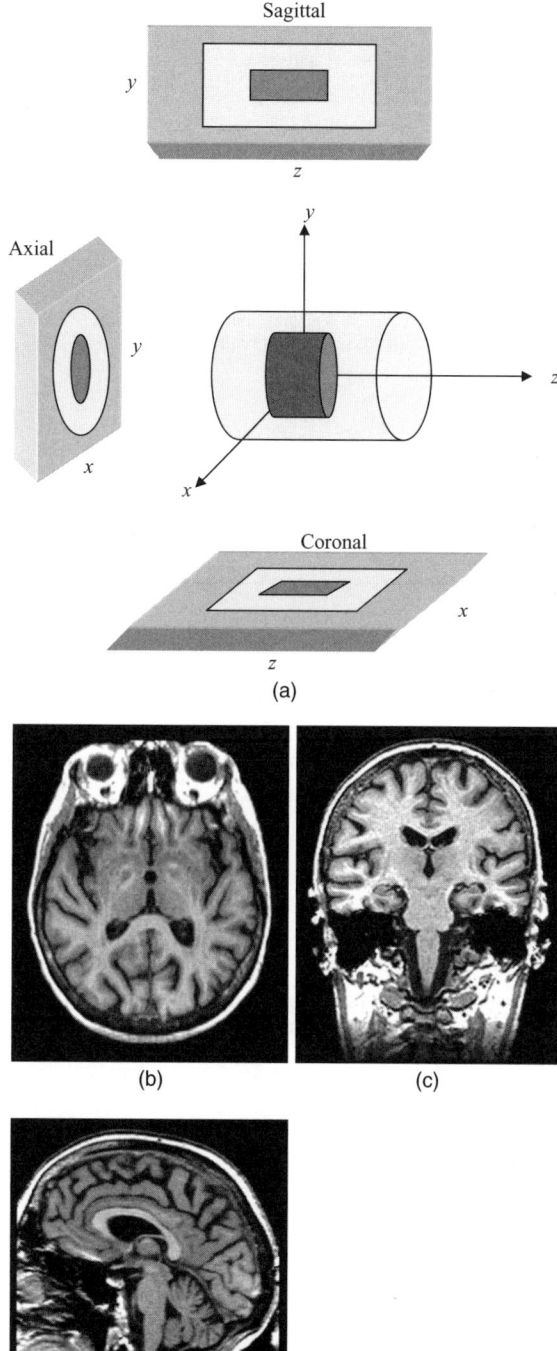

Figure 5.10 (a) Three-dimensional object coordinate system with axial, sagital, and coronal image views. (b) From top left to bottom right: Axial, coronal, and sagital MR images of a human brain.

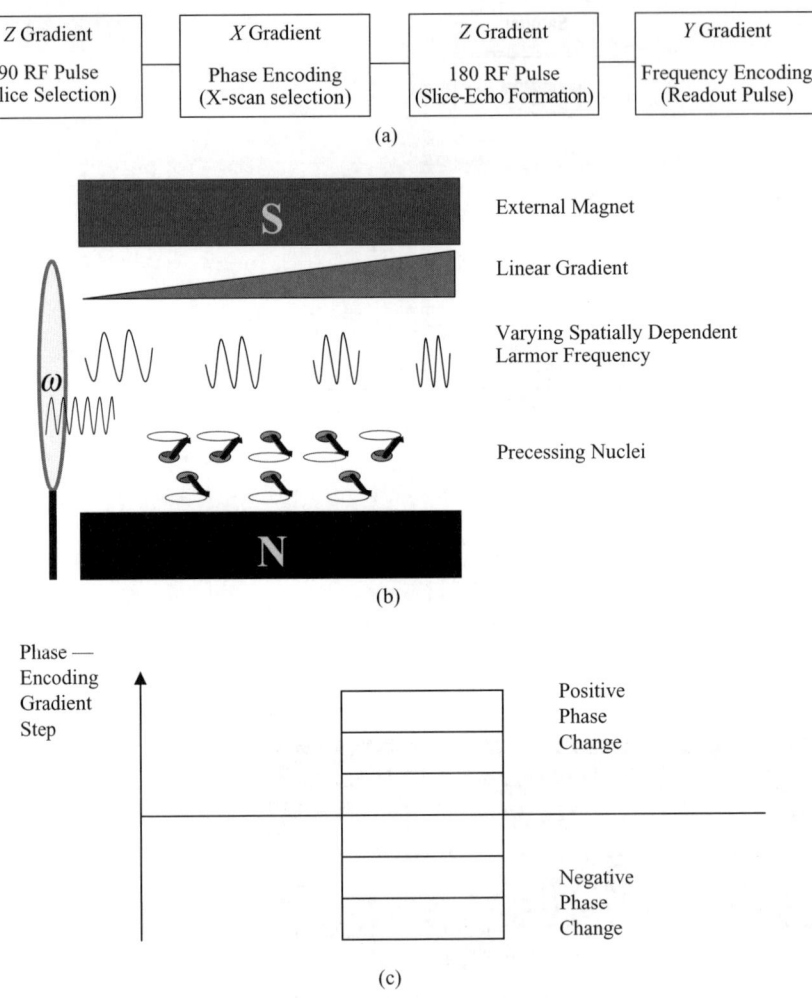

Figure 5.11 (a) Three-dimensional spatial encoding for spin-echo MR pulse sequence. (b) A linear gradient field for frequency encoding. (c) A step function-based gradient field for phase encoding.

the phase-encoding gradient, the readout cycle is repeated 256 times, each time with a specific amount of phase-encoding gradient.

5.3.1 Spin-Echo Imaging

Let us understand the formation of a spin echo, a commonly used method in NMR imaging. If an axial image of the human brain is to be reconstructed, an axial slice of the brain in the object coordinate system is selected by applying a linear frequency encoding gradient in the z-direction. Along with the gradient, a 90-degree pulse can be applied to cause nuclear excitation in the entire slice volume. During the time a

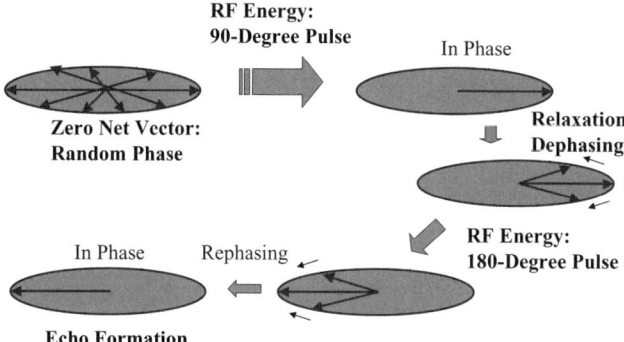

Figure 5.12 The transverse relaxation and echo formation of the spin-echo MR pulse sequence.

frequency encoding gradient is established and applied for slice selection along the z-direction, a phase shift is introduced in the selected volume. To avoid any loss of signal due to dephasing and phase shift, a rephasing gradient pulse is usually applied, as shown in Figure 5.12. To obtain a 2-D image of the selected slice, spatial encoding gradients are applied in the x- and y-directions. A phase-encoding gradient is applied in the x-direction after the 90-degree pulse has been applied for nuclear excitation in the slice volume. The 90-degree pulse causes the spinning nuclei to precess in phase. After the 90-degree pulse, the spinning nuclei start dephasing in the transverse direction while the net longitudinal magnetization vector starts returning to the state of thermal equilibrium. As shown in Figure 5.12, if a 180-degree pulse is applied along the z-direction before the spinning nuclei lose their coherence, the transverse magnetization vector is flipped in the reverse direction and the spinning nuclei start rephasing themselves to produce an echo exactly after the time lag between the 90-degree and 180-degree pulses. Thus, the time for echo formation, T_E, is defined between the application of the 90-degree pulse and the formation of echo (rephasing of nuclei). The time between the 90-degree pulse and 180-degree pulse is $T_E/2$, which is the same as the time between the 180-degree pulse and the formation of echo. At the formation of spin echo, the NMR signal is read through the readout frequency encoding gradient (along the y-direction). It should be noted that to implement a phase-encoding gradient with N steps, the readout cycle is repeated N times to collect phase-encoded echoes from different locations along the x-direction.

The frequency-encoded spin echoes can be mapped into a raw data space, called a "k-space." The k-space represents the placement of raw frequency data collected through the pulse sequences in a multidimensional space in which an image is to be reconstructed. The transformation from the frequency signal-based k-space to the image space is one of the most commonly used methods for MR image reconstruction. Thus, by taking the inverse Fourier transform of the k-space data, an image of the object can be reconstructed in the spatial domain. For example, a 2-D k-space can be used to map the raw spin-echo data for a selected slice along the z-direction. This k-space then represents the echo signals that are encoded with frequency and phase along the respective x–y directions. The NMR signals collected as frequency-encoded echoes can be placed as horizontal lines in the corresponding 2-D k-space. As multiple frequency encoded echoes are collected with different phase-encoding gradients, they are placed as horizontal lines in the corresponding k-space with the vertical direction representing the phase-encoding gradient values. After all spin echoes are collected, the k-space is complete with the raw frequency data. A 2-D inverse Fourier transform of the k-space data can provide a 2-D MR image of the selected slice.

It is clear from the above discussion that spin-echo pulse sequences are repeatedly applied to scan the entire object or, in other words, to complete the k-space frequency information. Before the next pulse sequence for echo formation and signal readout is started, the spinning nuclei are provided some time for longitudinal and transverse relaxations, bringing them close to the thermal equilibrium. The time period between the applications of two consecutive spin-echo pulse sequences is called the cycle repetition time, T_R. The manipulation of T_E and T_R times provides different weighting of T_1 and T_2 relaxation times as the longitudinal and transverse relaxation processes are directly affected by the selection of echo formation and cycle repetition times. It can be seen from Figures 5.12 and 5.13, if the time between the 90-degree pulse and 180-degree pulse is long, the spinning nuclei would almost lose their coherence depending on the T_2 relaxation time. Thus, the NMR signal at

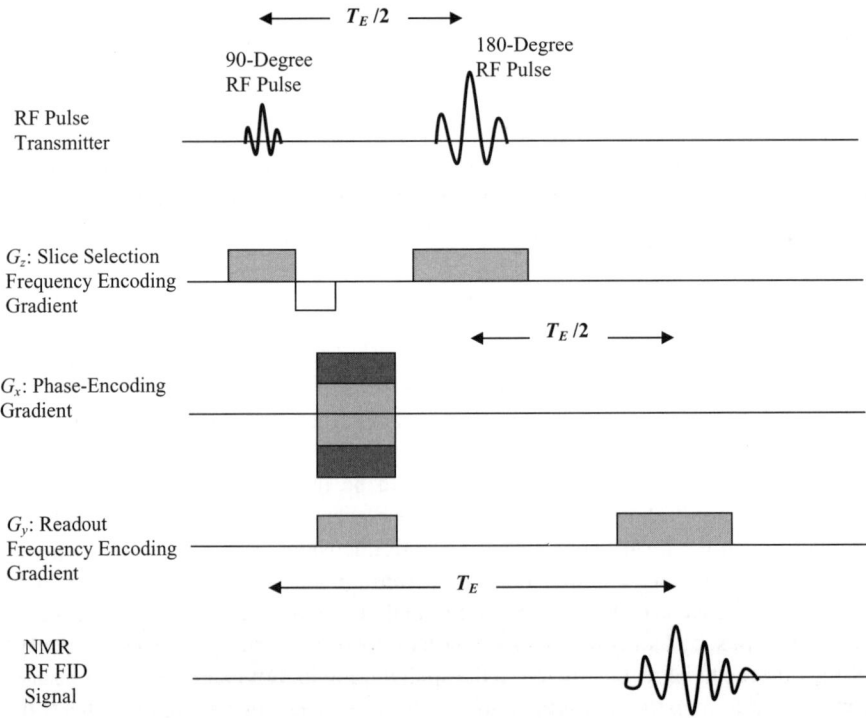

Figure 5.13 A spin-echo pulse sequence for MRI.

the formation of the echo would be largely influenced by the T_2 relaxation time if the 90-degree pulse was applied when the spinning nuclei were in (or were close to) thermal equilibrium. This means that T_2-weighted MRI requires a long T_R and a long T_E-based spin-echo pulse sequence. On the other hand, a short T_R and a short T_E-based spin-echo pulse sequence would provide T_1-weighted MRI. In this case, a short T_R would not allow the spinning nuclei to complete longitudinal relaxation, leaving the NMR signal at the short-time-based echo formation with T_1 influence. From these concepts, it can be easily understood that a long T_R- and a short T_E-based spin-echo pulse sequence would provide neither T_1- nor T_2- weighted MRI. As a matter of fact, in the absence of T_1 and T_2 influences, the long T_R and short T_E-based spin-echo pulse sequences provide spin-density (also called proton density) MR images. A short T_R- and a long T_E-based spin-echo pulse sequence are not used for MRI for obvious reasons. Equations 5.13 and 5.14, as described earlier in this section, present the mathematical representation of the dependency of longitudinal and transverse magnetization vectors on T_1 and T_2 relaxation times. Following Equations 5.13–5.19, the relationship of echo signal intensity and T_1 and T_2 relaxation times can be expressed as

$$\rho(x, y, z) = \rho_0(x, y, z) \left\{ e^{-\frac{T_E}{T_2}} \right\} \left\{ 1 - e^{-\frac{T_R}{T_1}} \right\} \tag{5.21}$$

where $\rho_0(x, y, z)$ is the initial spin density function.

The exponential decay terms of T_E/T_2 and T_R/T_1 in Equation 5.21 confirms that a short T_R and short T_E would lead to T_1-weighted imaging, while long T_R and long T_E would provide T_2-weighted imaging. As can be seen in Figure 5.1, T_1-weighted, T_2-weighted, and spin-density MR images of the same slice provide different tissue contrast in the respective images. This is a very useful feature in diagnostic radiology for lesion detection and characterization.

There are several factors that affect the MR signal acquisition, causing artifacts or degradation in the reconstructed image. These factors include field inhomogeneities, flow of nuclei, and change in resonance parameters due to chemical shifts within the object. Magnetic field inhomogeneities and gradient fields cause a direct dephasing effect to the transverse relaxation process. The effective transverse relaxation time, T_2^* from the field inhomogeneities can be expressed as

$$\frac{1}{T_2^*} = \frac{1}{T_2} + \frac{\gamma \, \Delta H}{2} \tag{5.22}$$

where ΔH is the field inhomogeneities representing the maximum deviation of the field strength over the imaging volume. When a spatial encoding gradient is applied along any direction to localize the distribution of nuclei, the transverse relaxation time is further reduced to T_2^{**} and can be expressed as

$$\frac{1}{T_2^{**}} = \frac{1}{T_2^*} + \frac{\gamma \, Gd}{2} \tag{5.23}$$

where G is the strength of the gradient field applied over the region of diameter d.

Magnetic susceptibility caused by the presence of other substances in the imaging medium is another important factor influencing relaxation times. For example, blood products such as deoxyhemoglobin, intracellular methemoglobin, ferritin, and other substances such as calcium present in the human body can cause inhomogeneities in the local magnetic field. Also as a result of the diffusion of protons within the tissue, the local magnetic fields are altered within the imaging volume. The loss in signal due to magnetic susceptibility can cause artifacts in the T_2-weighted and spin-density images. These effects could be significant in blood flow imaging.

The complex effects caused by the flow of protons and other substances in and out of the imaging volumes due to diffusion, perfusion, and blood flow could be turned around to allow visualization of moving protons leading to useful imaging methods such as MR perfusion imaging and MR angiography (3–5). A random diffusion of protons causes a loss of signal due to phase cancellation in the dephasing mechanism. Thus, useful information about water proton diffusion and its direction can be observed through appropriate MR pulse sequences. In MRI, the diffusion is defined as a random motion of water protons with a slower motion on the order of a few microns per millisecond. Perfusion is described by one of three mechanisms. A perfusion can involve the transition of a nondiffusible contrast agent through the microvasculature, or it can be described as the fast flow of water protons into a selected imaging volume. These perfusion processes can define the physiological behavior of a tissue or lesion and can be detected through the relaxation time parameters. However, perfusion can be forced into a tissue through a diffusible tracer in the extravascular space. The performance of perfusion imaging depends on the contrast agent (such as fluorine) and usually provides a low SNR. Volume averaging becomes necessary to improve the SNR for better image quality that limits the image resolution. However, the use of a perfusion contrast agent can provide important information about changes in the tissue behavior in the early stages of many critical brain diseases.

Another important factor that causes alterations in relaxation times is the presence of a molecular or chemical environment that can change the characteristic magnetic influence on the protons. This effect, called chemical shift, can cause minor deviations in the Larmor frequency of spinning protons depending on their molecular environment. For example, water protons present in fat will precess at a slightly different frequency than the protons in water. To minimize artifacts caused by the chemical shift phenomenon, larger bandwidth frequency encoding is done in MR pulse sequences with short echo times.

5.3.2 Inversion Recovery Imaging

As described above, MR FID signal can be generated in the relaxation (also called inversion recovery [IR]) process after applying the 180-degree pulse. Spin-echo imaging sequence as described in Figure 5.13 can also be applied in the inversion recovery process. In spin-echo imaging sequence, a slice is selected through frequency encoding gradient with a 90-degree pulse that creates a spin–lattice magnetization with all protons in the selected slice. IR imaging pulse sequence allows relaxation of some or all of T_1 before spins are rephased through 90-degree pulse and therefore emphasizes the effect of longitudinal magnetization. In IR imaging pulse sequence, 180-degree pulse is first applied along with the slice selection

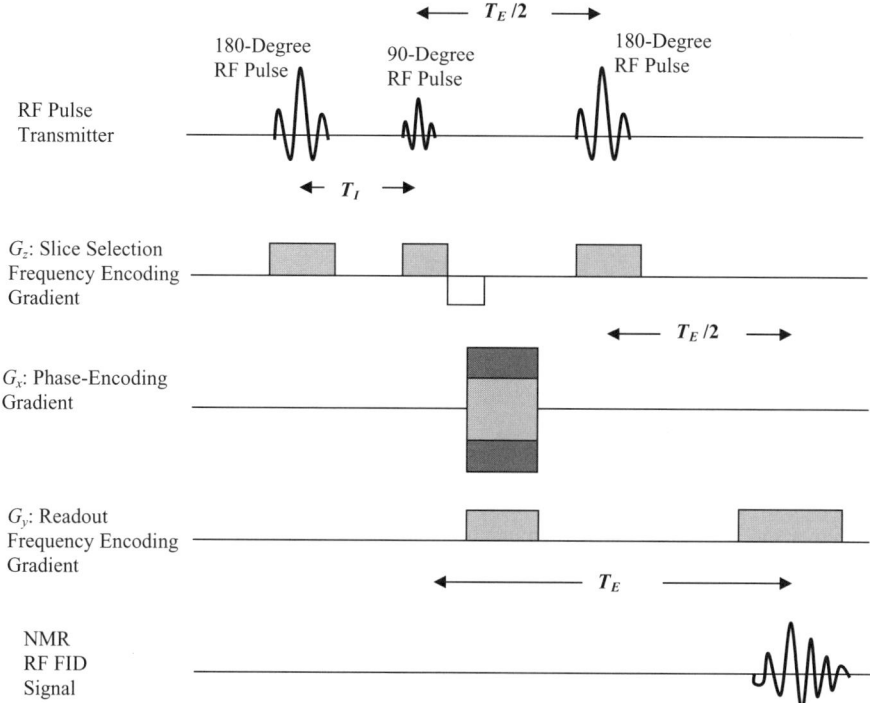

Figure 5.14 Inversion recovery (IR) pulse sequence for MR imaging.

frequency encoding gradient as shown in Figure 5.14. After the time T_I equivalent to the recovery of T_1 time ($T_I = T_1 \ln 2$), a 90-degree pulse is applied to start the spin-echo imaging pulse sequence. The rest of the imaging sequence is the same as described above in spin-echo imaging as 180-degree pulse is applied after $T_E/2$ time to create an echo. In the mean time, phase-encoding gradient is applied along the x-direction. The readout frequency encoding gradient is applied along the x-direction to record the echo FID (Fig. 5.14). Figure 5.15 shows a coronal image of the brain with IR imaging pulse sequence. The emphasized effect of longitudinal magnetization can be seen in the IR image.

5.3.3 Echo Planar Imaging

Echo planar imaging (EPI) is a fast scanning method for 2-D and 3-D MRI. Multiple echo-based measurements are obtained within one T_R cycle time. Multiple echoes are obtained with a single 90-degree RF selective pulse through an oscillating gradient rather than through application of a 180-degree phase reversal pulse as done in the spin-echo pulse sequences. Figure 5.16 shows the EPI pulse sequence for 2-D MRI. The slice selection is obtained through the frequency encoding gradient along the z-direction along with the 90-degree RF selective pulse. An oscillating gradient along the x-direction causes the phase reversal of the spinning nuclei to create periodic echoes. A small readout gradient is applied along the y-direction. This

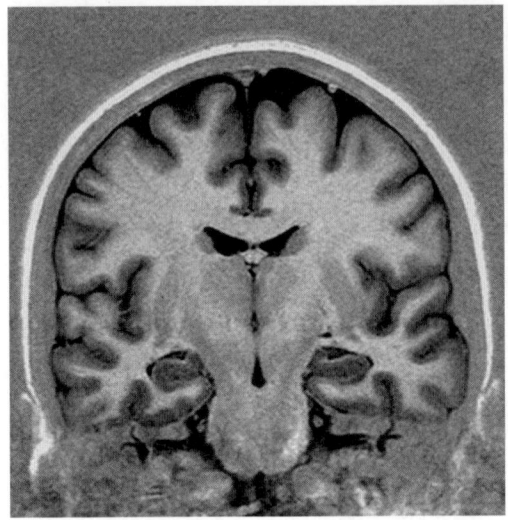

Figure 5.15 A coronal image of human brain obtained through MR inversion recovery imaging pulse sequence.

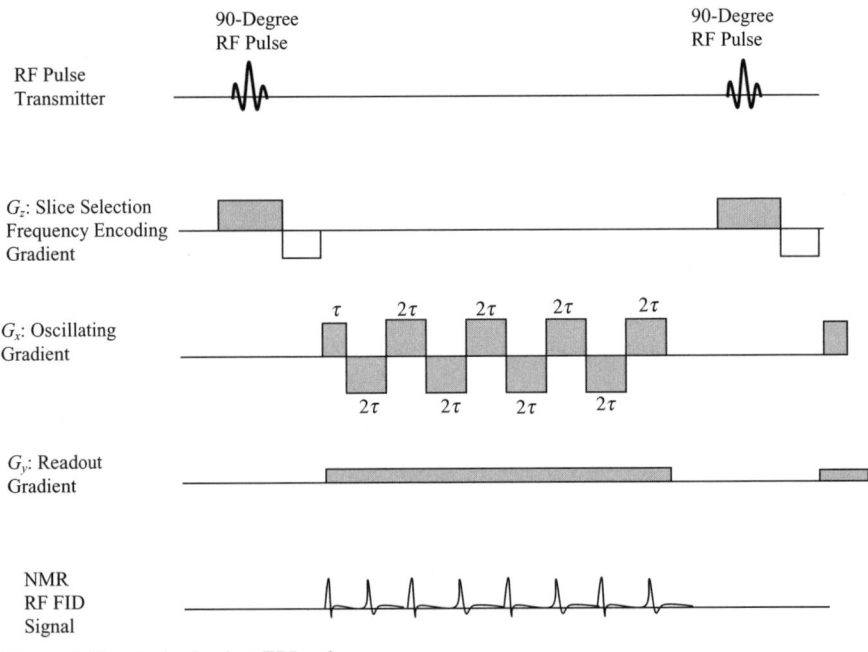

Figure 5.16 A single-shot EPI pulse sequence.

method creates a trajectory in the k-space to provide raw data points. The k-space trajectory of the EPI method as shown in Figure 5.17 creates subsampling of the frequency space. However, the entire image can be obtained in a single shot. Due to the signal decay by the T_2 relaxation time, the number of sampling points in the

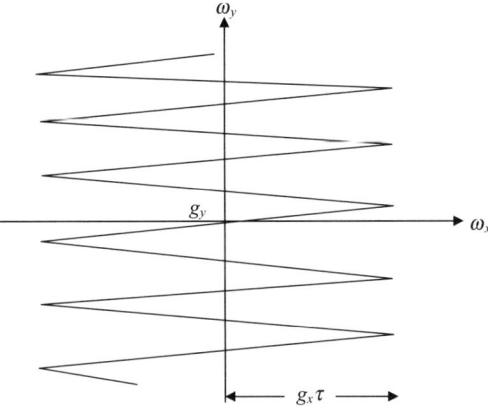

Figure 5.17 The k-space representation of the EPI scan trajectory.

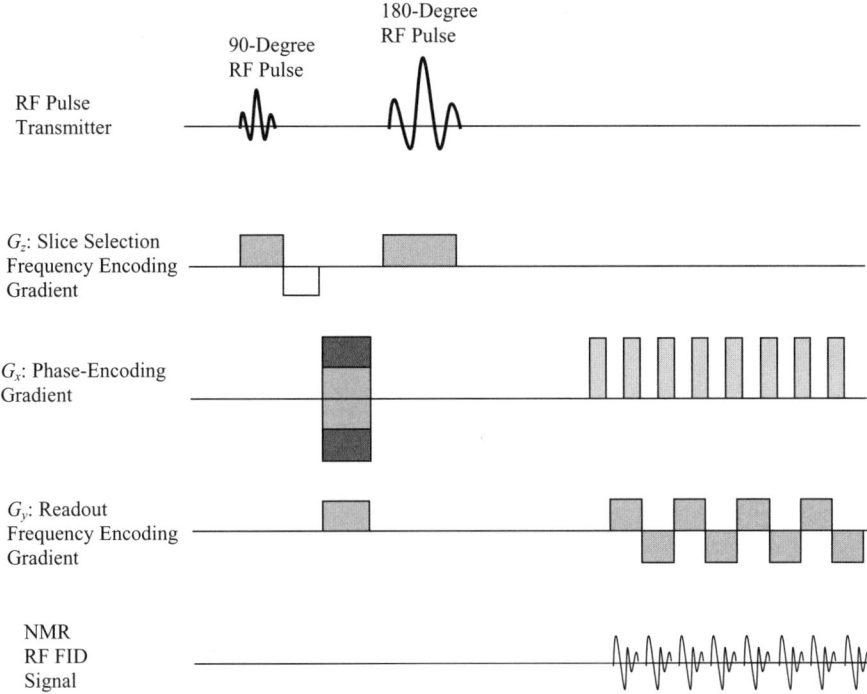

Figure 5.18 An echo planar imaging (EPI) sequence for MR imaging.

k-space is limited. This limitation causes low-resolution images with some degradation. As can be interpreted from k-space representation, the single-shot EPI sequence requires a rapidly oscillating gradient with a large magnitude, which is often difficult to achieve in practice (3, 5).

A variant to single shot EPI pulse sequence shown in Figure 5.18 utilizes the 90- to 180-degree pulse sequence commonly used in spin-echo imaging. After spin

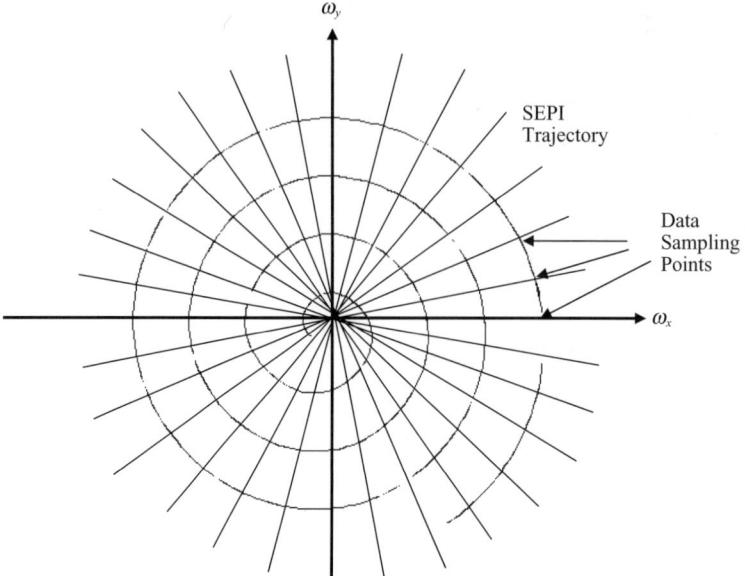

Figure 5.19 The spiral scan trajectory of SEPI pulse sequence in the k-space.

rephasing by 180-degree pulse, this EPI pulse sequence uses periodic phase gradient impulses synchronized with readout frequency encoding gradient impulses to record multiple echoes. A phase-encoding gradient can be placed between 90- and 180-degree pulses to adjust echo time T_E or even can be placed after the 180-degree pulse to minimize T_E.

An alternate approach for fast MRI without the need of a large oscillating gradient is called spiral echo planar imaging (SEPI). In this method, the entire k-space is covered with a spiral scan yielding a circularly symmetric response function that reduces the artifacts in the image. The more uniform distribution of frequency sampling in the k-space can be obtained by the spiral scan as shown in Figure 5.19. It can be shown that for such a spiral scan trajectory in the k-space, the required gradient in the x- and y-directions can be expressed as

$$G_x(t) = \frac{1}{\gamma} \frac{d}{dt} \omega_x(t)$$
$$G_y(t) = \frac{1}{\gamma} \frac{d}{dt} \omega_y(t)$$

where

$$\omega_x(t) = \gamma \lambda t \cos \xi t$$
$$\omega_y(t) = \gamma \lambda t \sin \xi t \tag{5.24}$$

where the spiral scan is obtained through two sin and cosine waves with an angular frequency ξ and amplitude λ.

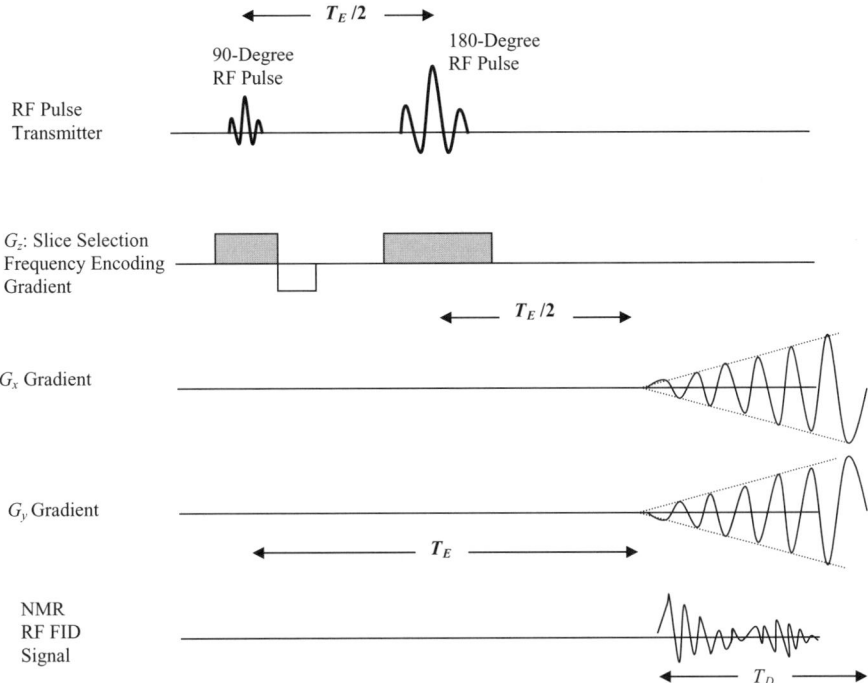

Figure 5.20 A spiral EPI pulse sequence.

In the SEPI pulse sequence (Fig. 5.20), a 90-degree selective RF pulse is applied with the frequency encoding slice selection gradient along the z-direction. This is followed by the 180-degree pulse to prepare the system for the generation of echoes. After the T_E time, that is twice the time duration between the 90-degree and 180-degree RF pulses, a sinusoidal gradient is applied in the x-direction. At the same time, a phase-shifted version or a cosine gradient is applied in the y-direction. The wave gradients in the x- and y-directions cause the required phase reversal for generating the raw data in the k-space with a spiral sampling scan (3, 6). The data are collected through the data collection time, T_D, as shown in Figure 5.20.

Figure 5.21 shows a sequence of 16 brain images obtained through a single-shot SEPI sequence. These slices were obtained in 1.5 s with a resolution of 105 × 100 pixel and slice thickness of 6 mm. The lower resolution and artifacts can be noticed in these images.

5.3.4 Gradient Echo Imaging

The EPI pulse sequences provide multiple echoes for obtaining NMR signals for image reconstruction through a single shot, that is, a single RF excitation pulse. The collection of data for an entire image through a single excitation pulse has a major disadvantage of yielding low-resolution images because of the T_2 relaxation time decay. Gradient echo imaging methods as applied to a fast low angle shot

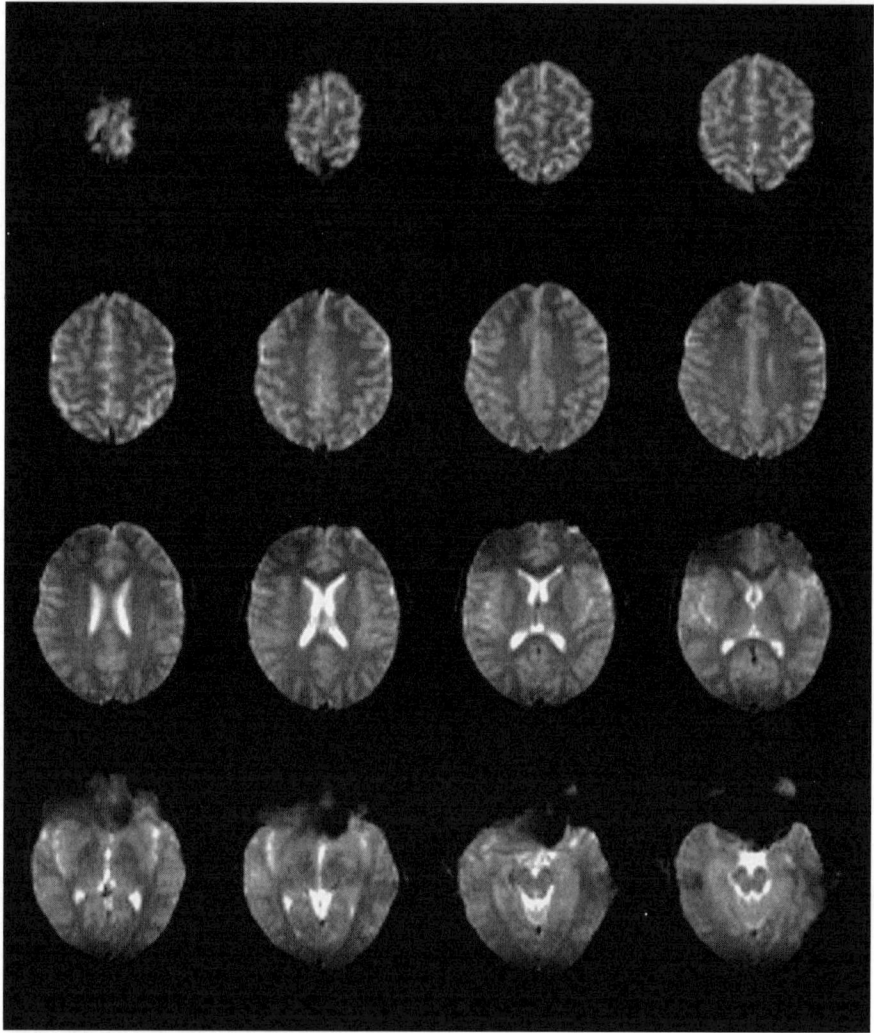

Figure 5.21 MR images of a human brain acquired through SEPI pulse sequence.

(FLASH) imaging sequences utilize low-flip angle RF pulses to create multiple echoes in repeated cycles to collect the data required for image reconstruction (3, 5). Thus, there are more sampling points in the k-space available to reconstruct images at higher resolution. The FLASH pulse sequence, as shown in Figure 5.22, uses a low-flip angle (as low as 20 degrees) RF selective pulse for nuclear excitation. The frequency encoding gradient is applied along the z-direction for slice selection. The slice selection gradient G_z is inverted after the RF pulse to help rephase the spinning nuclei. Since a phase-encoding gradient is applied in the x-direction, the pulse sequence has to be repeated for the number of steps used in phase-encoding. The readout gradient, similar to spin-echo sequence, is applied

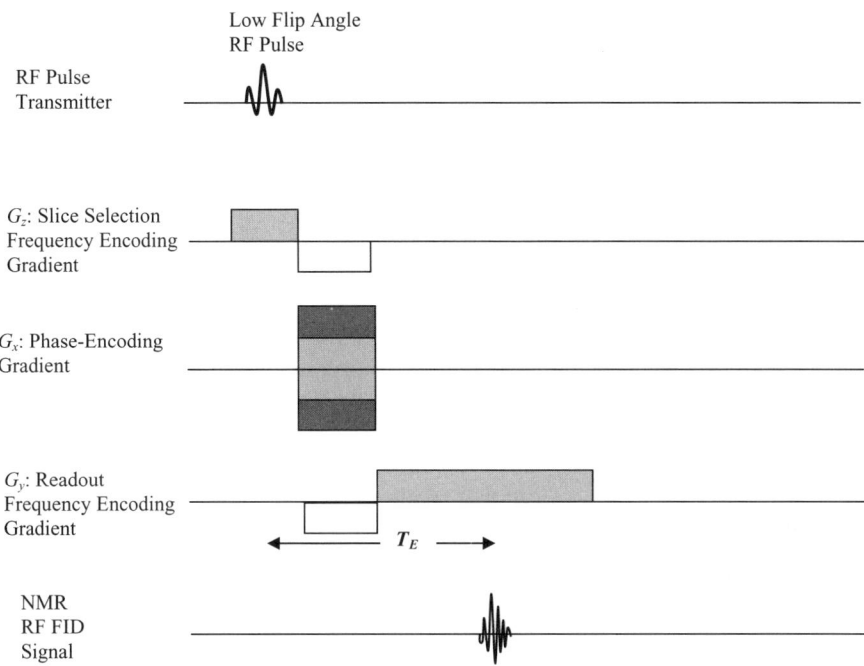

Figure 5.22 The FLASH pulse sequence for fast MR imaging.

along the y-direction. The major difference between spin-echo and gradient echo pulse sequences is that the longitudinal magnetization is not flipped by 90 degrees for nuclear excitation. Instead, a low-flip angle is used to affect the longitudinal magnetization by a small fraction. In addition, there is no 180-degree pulse in the gradient echo cycle, forcing a complete reversal of the spinning nuclei to create an echo. In a FLASH pulse sequence, the readout gradient is inverted to rephase nuclei leading to the gradient echo during the data acquisition period. Since a small flip in the longitudinal magnetization vector is used, the entire pulse sequence time is much shorter than the spin-echo pulse sequence, typically in the range of 10–20 ms.

5.4. FLOW IMAGING

One of the major advantages of MRI is the ability to track flow during image acquisition leading to diffusion (incoherent flow) and perfusion (partially coherent flow) imaging. Equation 5.17 defines the net time-varying gradient at a location vector **r** as a vector sum of 3-D gradients (3, 5). There are additional time varying magnetization effects and fields generated by time-varying RF fields, the flow of nuclei being imaged, and other paramagnetic substances. The effect of a bipolar gradient pulse after the 90-degree RF nuclear excitation pulse in generating an FID signal can be split into two parts. The first part is the FID signal generated in the RF receiver coil by the fixed nuclei and position-independent factors. Such a signal provides a net zero value when it is integrated over a symmetric bipolar gradient pulse without any consideration of relaxation processes. The second part is the FID signal generated in the RF receiver coil by the moving nuclei and velocity-dependent factors. It can be shown that a similar effect is obtained when a unipolar gradient pulse is applied during the 180-degree pulse in the spin-echo sequence. Such a flux, $\phi_v(t)$, can be expressed as (1, 3)

$$\phi_v(t) = \gamma \, \vartheta \int_0^\tau G_z(t) t \, dt \qquad (5.25)$$

where τ is the duration of the unipolar gradient pulse and ϑ is the flow velocity.

Figure 5.23 shows a spin-echo sequence for flow imaging. The slice selection gradient, G_z, is applied along the z-direction during the 180-degree phase to provide the flow velocity component in the FID signal. The phase-encoding gradient G_x and readout frequency encoding gradient G_y are similar to the conventional spin-echo pulse sequence. It should be noted that additional gradient pulses need to be incorporated along the x- and y-directions if the flow velocity components in these directions are to be compensated in imaging.

As shown above, the velocity component of spinning nuclei along the direction of the magnetic field gradient induces a proportional phase shift in the transverse

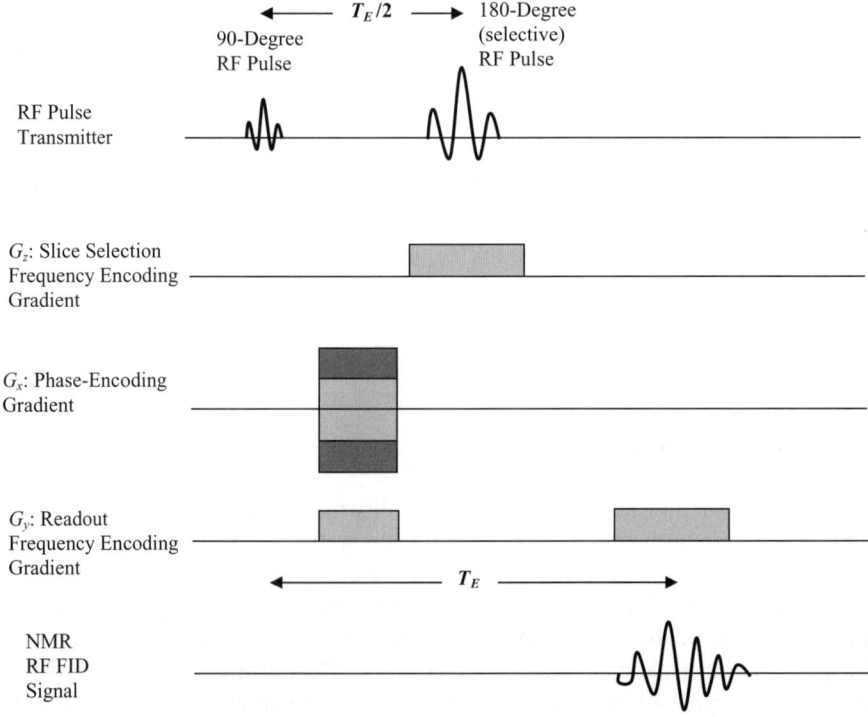

Figure 5.23 A flow imaging pulse sequence with spin echo.

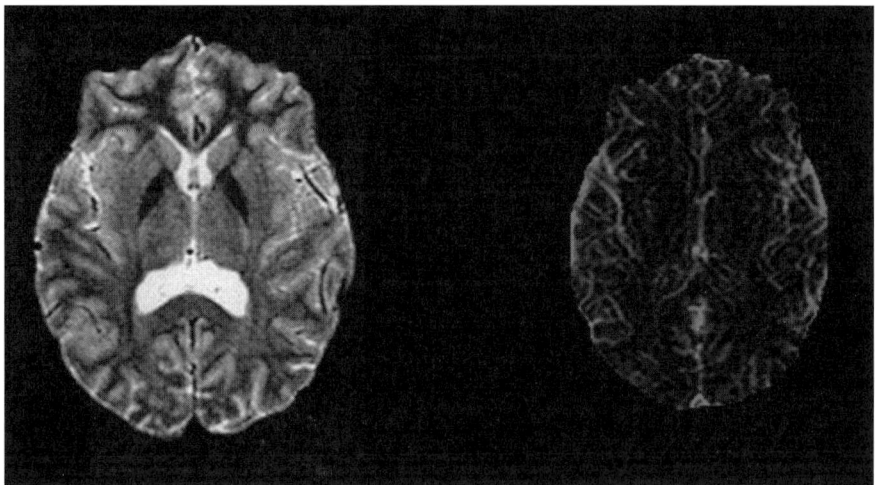

Figure 5.24 Left: A proton density image of a human brain. Right: The corresponding perfusion image.

magnetization. Any change in the velocity component causes dispersion in the phase that leads to unequal signal losses. Thus, phase sensitivity due to the flow is inherent in MR signal generation and is exploited in MRI for conventional flow measurements. Figure 5.24 shows an axial proton density image of a human brain with the corresponding perfusion image showing the vascular structure and flow.

The phase-sensitive methods for conventional flow measurement as described above do not provide accurate imaging and assessment of in-flow. When a specific slice or volume under flow is imaged through repeated pulse sequences, the phase sensitivity causes a loss in the signal but the in-flow of fresh nuclei leads to an increase in the signal intensity at the same time. In in-flow-sensitive or time-of-flight methods, longitudinal magnetization is exploited, making the signal insensitive to flow-induced phase shifts transverse magnetization. The ability to measure specific in-flow in predetermined directions leads to MR angiography. For example, time-of-flight angiography can be performed using a spin-echo imaging sequence where the slice selective 90- and 180-degree pulses have different frequencies. The 90-degree pulse excites protons in one plane while the 180-degree pulse excites protons in another plane. With blood flow, the protons move from a 90-degree plane to a 180-degree plane because of flow, they are rephased and an echo is formed. If there is no blood flow, the protons in the 180-degree plane will not go through echo formation. Contrast-enhanced angiography is performed using a paramagnetic contrast agent that is injected in the blood. The contrast agent reduces spin–lattice relation time T_1 in blood vessels. MR contrast-enhanced angiography uses fast volume imaging pulse sequences with a short TR. There have been a number of recent developments in 3-D MR volume angiography utilizing fast gradient echo and static signal suppression techniques. A pulse sequence for 3-D volume MR angiography is shown in Figure 5.25. The sequence is based on the 2-D planar

128 CHAPTER 5 MRI

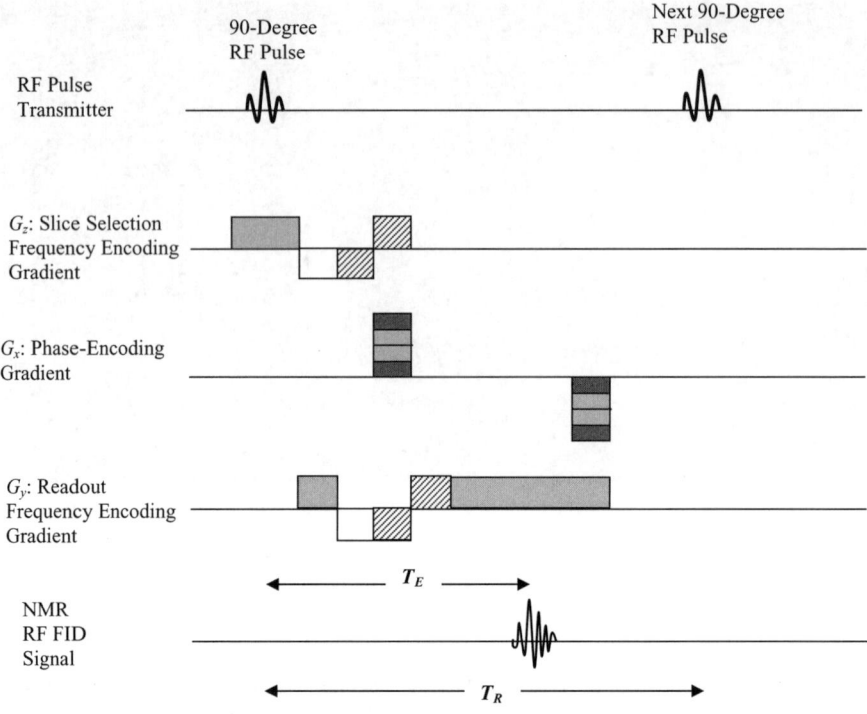

Figure 5.25 Gradient echo-based MR pulse sequence for 3-D MR volume angiography.

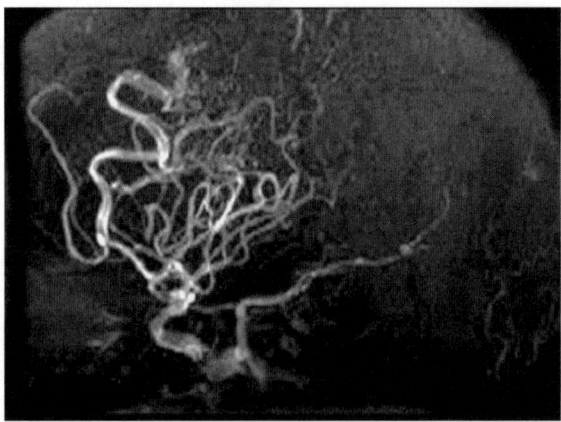

Figure 5.26 An MR angiography image.

imaging method and is repeated for the number of slices and the number of steps used in the phase encoding (3–7). The hatched regions in the gradient pulses provide necessary fields to compensate for phase sensitivity of the flow. An MR angiogram image is shown in Figure 5.26.

5.5. FMRI

Neural activity-based functions are critical for the survival of human beings as well as animals. For example, central and peripheral nervous systems of the human body contains hundreds of billions of neuronal cells that form different neural tissues in the brain and other parts of the body. Electrical signals or impulses such as action potentials are generated by neuronal cells in neural tissue for the proper physiological functioning of the body. The central nervous system involving the brain and spinal cord performs complex functions based on integration, generation, and transmission of electrical impulses. Neuronal cells generate electrical impulses in response to synaptic integration or sensory stimulations and consume oxygen in this process. Oxygenated hemoglobin molecules provide oxygen to enable cellular functions. As a neural tissue is stimulated for neural activity (firing of action potentials), oxygen is rapidly consumed by the cells, resulting in a decrease in the oxygen level in the blood. As the cells continue to demand oxygen for their functions, more oxygenated hemoglobin cells are rapidly needed, causing an increase in local blood flow. This phenomenon of increased blood flow and volume for high neural activity is known as hemodynamic response because of which the oxygenation level in the local region is increased as the blood flow is increased. Thus, the physiological functions of neural tissue such as that of the brain can be examined through its hemodynamic response, as neural activity can be representatively translated into increase of local blood flow and volume, which in turn shows an increase in oxygenation level. fMRI imaging methods measure blood oxygen level during sensory stimulation or any task that causes a specific neural activity. For example, visual or auditory stimulation, finger movement, or a cognitive task can cause neural activities in specific parts of cortical structures in the brain, causing increased cerebral blood flow. The blood oxygen level, or, simply put, blood flow, during neural stimulation is considered strongly correlated with glucose metabolism of the tissue. The neural activities or functions can be examined through blood oxygen level measurement by fMRI using blood oxygenated level dependent (BOLD) contrast (8, 9).

It is well known that oxygenated hemoglobin (HbO_2) is diamagnetic while deoxygenated hemoglobin (Hb) is paramagnetic. Thus, magnetic susceptibility is increased with the increase in oxygenated hemoglobin. This leads to an increase in MR signal with the increase in oxygen level in the blood or blood flow. This is effectively measured by BOLD imaging sequence. A reduction of the relative de-oxy-hemoglobin concentration due to an increase of blood flow and hence increased supply of fresh oxy-hemoglobin during neural activity is measured as an increase in T_2 or T_2 weighted MR signals. The difference in MR signals through BOLD in stimulated condition than the normal (or baseline) situation is usually very small. Therefore, the stimulation (or task) has to be repeated several times and MR signal measurements are taken through the repetition of BOLD sequence. The brain is scanned at a lower resolution with a fast pulse sequence such as gradient echo. Statistical correlation methods are applied to determine the specific area of the brain that reliably shows the significant difference in oxygen levels and is therefore considered to be involved in the respective neural activity. Figure 5.27

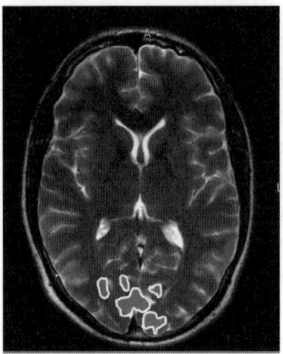

Figure 5.27 Functional magnetic resonance (fMR) image of a human brain acquired through BOLD contrast sequence with visual stimulation. The activated areas in the visual cortex are outlined.

shows an MR image of a human brain with BOLD contrast activation areas in the visual cortex region that resulted from the visual stimulation task during imaging.

5.6. DIFFUSION IMAGING

As MRI uses hydrogen protons for creating FID signal to reconstruct images of proton density as well as spin–lattice and spin–spin relaxation parameters, specialized imaging pulse sequences can be designed to follow water molecules involved in diffusion around a cell. It is interesting to note that a neuronal cell in the neural tissue has a cell body known as soma with a dendrite tree carrying synaptic junctions for integration of electrical signals from other neurons, and a long axon that delivers the electrical signal to other neuronal synapses once the output action potential or impulse is generated by the cell. The cell uses a permeable membrane for ionic transport to modify its electrical potential to generate, receive, and transmit electrical signal. The biochemical functions of the membrane of the cell body and axon involves water diffusion (10–13). The water molecules can be tracked by diffusion-weighted MRI pulse sequences to characterize neural tissue. Neural tissue (such as brain tissue) in living beings is categorized largely into two categories: (1) gray matter containing cell bodies, and (2) white matter containing nerve fibers (axons with the protective myelin sheath that speeds up electrical transmission through the axon). It is clear that different regions of neural tissue (such as brain cortex) are interconnected through axonal pathways involving a huge number of synaptic junctions. A human body is believed to have as many as 300 billion neurons with several hundreds of trillions of synaptic junctions. It is important to image neural tissue characterizing gray and white matters for physiological functions such as water diffusion in the diagnosis, treatment, and rehabilitation of neurological disorders such as Parkinson's, Alzheimer's, and diseases involving loss of neural functions. DWI and DTI allow in vivo measurement of diffusivity of water molecules in the neural tissue.

5.6. DIFFUSION IMAGING

In the diffusion process, water molecules spread out over time that is represented by Brownian motion. The displacement of diffused molecules can be modeled as an anisotropic Gaussian distribution along a given spatial axis such that the spread of the position of molecules after a time T along a spatial axis x can be represented with a variance of

$$\sigma_x^2 = 2DT \qquad (5.26)$$

where D is diffusion coefficient in the tissue.

The directional displacement of diffused molecules is parameterized by the diffusion tensor. The diffusion tensor allows computation of diffusion anisotropy (directional activity) through the analysis of underlying eigenvalues of each voxel tensor field. The diffusion model assumes homogeneity and linearity of the diffusion within each image voxel. Axonal structure covered with myelin sheath, as shown in Figure 5.28, facilitates the diffusion of the water molecules preferentially along the direction of axons, providing anisotropic diffusion in the white matter. However, the gray matter lacks a specific orientation and therefore accounts for relatively isotropic diffusion.

The DTI through a specialized MRI pulse sequence provides information about the cellular organization in the tissue factor based on the state of the membrane permeability, myelination, compactness and axonal packing structure. DTI pulse sequence utilizes motion probing gradients (MPG) to examine the motion of water molecules in the diffusion process in a specific direction. As the data are collected while applying MPG in different directions, a diffusion tensor matrix is obtained and eigenvalues are computed to determine an anisotropy factor known as fractional anisotropy (FA), along with the diffusion magnitude and direction. DTI is performed with the application of MPGs in multiple gradient directions (e.g., 6 or more) to compute the diffusion tensor. In diffusion weighted imaging (DWI), three gradient directions are used to estimate the trace of the diffusion tensor or average diffusivity within each voxel.

Figure 5.29 shows a DWI/DTI pulse sequence for MRI. The pulse sequence is similar to spin-echo pulse sequence except that it uses two additional gradient pulses before and after 180-degree RF pulse to detect the motion of diffused molecules. For a faster scan, EPI pulse sequence can be used with two gradient pulses in a similar way. These two gradients are called motion probe gradients MPGs.

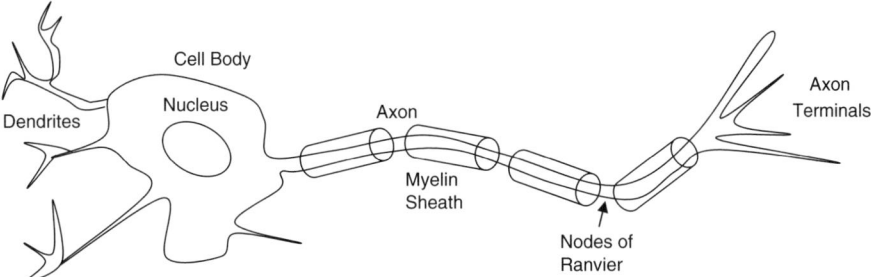

Figure 5.28 A schematic diagram of a neuron cell structure.

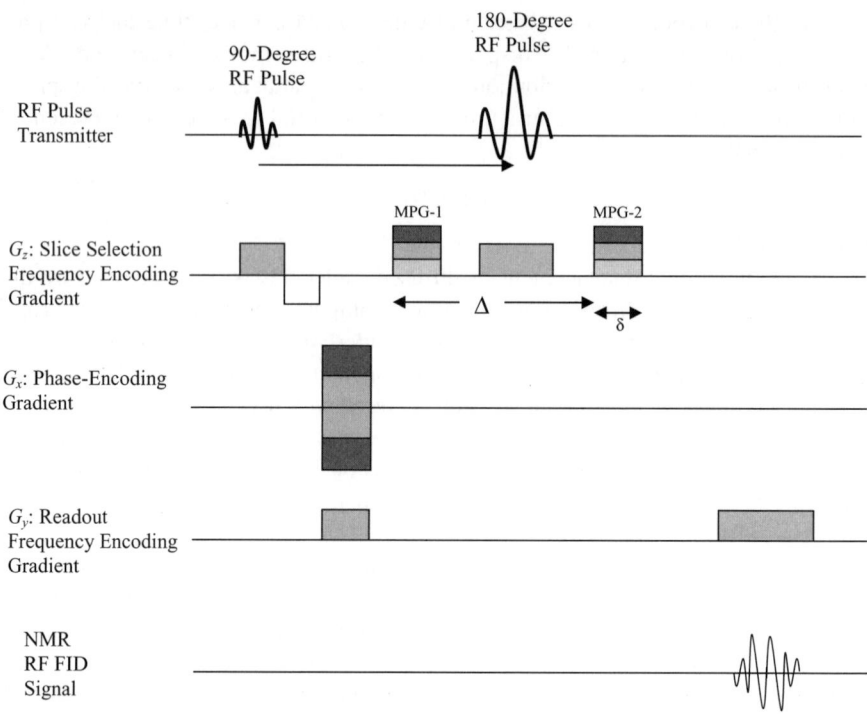

Figure 5.29   A DWI/DTI pulse sequence for MR diffusion imaging.

MPGs can be applied in any combination of predetermined directions to detect molecules diffusing in different directions. The first gradient pulse of MPG that is applied before the 180-degree RF pulse dephases the protons of water molecules, while the second gradient pulse in the same direction but with opposite polarity rephases their spins with respect to their displacement. In Figure 5.29, two gradient pulses of MPG each of δ duration are applied with Δ time difference. If the protons have moved between the times of application of these two gradient pulses, the rephasing does not take place completely resulting in the loss of signal. If the protons are stationary and do not move between the two gradient pulses, they are rephased with the spin-echo cycle and therefore yield a higher intensity signal. Thus, for healthy tissue with water diffusion, the MR FID signal is decreased while the tissue with trapped-in water molecules (as in the case of swelling of damaged tissue), the MR FID signal is increased. Let us assume that S and S_0, respectively, represent MR FID signal intensities with and without diffusion weighting, then for a pulse sequence shown Figure 5.29, it can be shown as (14):

$$S = S_0 e^{-\gamma^2 G^2 \delta^2 (\Delta - \delta/N) D} \qquad (5.27)$$

where γ is the gyromagnetic ratio, D is diffusion coefficient, and G is the strength of two MPG gradients each with δ duration separated by Δ applied in N spatial directions (e.g., for DWI imaging three spatial directions, x, y, and z, are used).

Equation 5.27 can be simply written as:

$$S = S_0 e^{-bD}$$

with $b = \gamma^2 G^2 \delta^2 (\Delta - \delta/N) D$ providing $D = \dfrac{1}{b} \ln \dfrac{S}{S_0}.$ (5.28)

It should be noted that D is a scalar quantity (average diffusivity) in case of DWI but is a tensor in case of DTI data. For example, if MPGs are applied with $u_x = (1, 0, 0)$; $u_y = (0, 1, 0)$; $u_z = (0, 0, 1)$ directions, a 3×3 tensor can be represented as

$$D = (u_x, u_y, u_z) \begin{bmatrix} D_{xx} & D_{xy} & D_{xz} \\ D_{yx} & D_{yy} & D_{yz} \\ D_{zx} & D_{zy} & D_{zz} \end{bmatrix} \begin{pmatrix} u_x \\ u_y \\ u_z \end{pmatrix}. \quad (5.29)$$

While the vector $\bar{U}$ can be extended with a higher number of directions in which motion probe gradients are applied to collect the data, the tensor matrix is symmetric along the diagonal for which eigenvalues $\lambda_1, \lambda_2, \lambda_3$ and trace of $[D]$ can be computed as

$$\bar{\Lambda} = \begin{bmatrix} \lambda_1 & & \\ & \lambda_2 & \\ & & \lambda_3 \end{bmatrix} \quad (5.30)$$

$$\begin{aligned} \text{trace}[D] &= D_{xx} + D_{yy} + D_{zz} \\ &= \lambda_1 + \lambda_2 + \lambda_3. \end{aligned} \quad (5.31)$$

It should be noted that trace of $[D]$ is a scalar quantity providing diffusion weighted (DWI) images. Figure 5.30 shows an axial slice of DWI MR image of the brain with acute stroke. The medial cerebral artery (MCA) watershed infarction can be seen in the image.

In case of DTI data analysis, each eigenvalue is compared. If they are similar to each other for a given voxel, the voxel is considered belonging to the gray

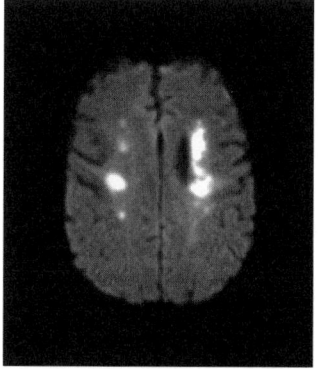

Figure 5.30 A diffusion weighted image (DWI) MR image of the brain with middle cerebral artery (MCA) watershed infarction.

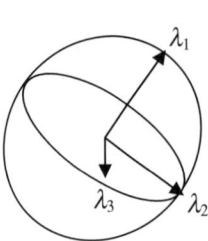 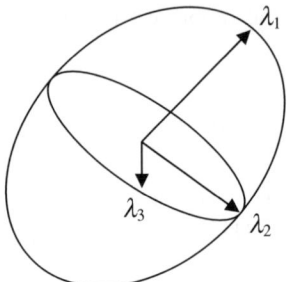

Figure 5.31 A schematic diagram of eigenvalue analysis for isotropic diffusion ($\lambda_1 \approx \lambda_2 \approx \lambda_3$) representing a gray matter voxel at the left, and anisotropic diffusion in the direction of λ_1 while $\lambda_1 > \lambda_2 > \lambda_3$ representing a white matter voxel at the right.

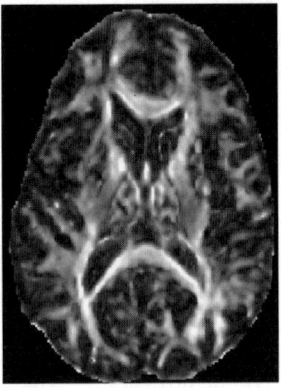

Figure 5.32 A color axial fiber orientation map of a diffusion tensor image (DTI) of a human brain in three eigenvector directions, x, y, and z, coded, respectively, in red, green, and blue colors.

matter (as there is no specific directional sensitivity in the data), but if they are different and can be arranged in a descending order, the diffusion directional sensitivity is determined in the direction of largest value of eigenvalue λ_1 as shown in Figure 5.31.

In case of anisotropic diffusion related to white matter of the neural tissue, FA is computed as

$$\text{FA} = \frac{1}{\sqrt{2}} \sqrt{\frac{(\lambda_1 - \lambda_2)^2 + (\lambda_2 - \lambda_3)^2 + (\lambda_3 - \lambda_1)^2}{\lambda_1^2 + \lambda_2^2 + \lambda_3^2}}. \quad (5.32)$$

The FA values as assigned to each voxel can be used to code connectivity among the voxels. Also, the FA values can be used in estimation of white matter tract orientations to show connectivity in white matter tractography (13, 14). A color-coded FA map of an axial brain image in three eigenvector directions, x, y, and z, coded, respectively, in red, green, and blue colors, is shown in Figure 5.32.

DWI/DTI show a great potential in diagnosis and treatment evaluation of diseases that disrupt normal organization and integrity of cerebral tissue such as multiple sclerosis, strokes, tumors, Parkinson's and Alzheimer's disease. DTI is useful to study diseases of the white matter and connectivity of brain pathways. Patients with attention deficit hyperactivity disorder (ADHD) have been observed with abnormal fiber pathways in frontal cortex, basal ganglia, and cerebellum through DTI.

5.7. CONTRAST, SPATIAL RESOLUTION, AND SNR

The contrast in MR images comes from the differentiation of MR signal with respect to spin (proton) density, and T_1 and T_2 relaxation times. One of the major advantages of MRI is its sensitivity to soft tissue contrast. The actual contrast-to-noise ratio depends on the data collection method (pulse sequence or spatial sampling and signal averaging), imaging parameters (strength of magnetic field, spin density, T_1 and T_2 relaxation times, coil sensitivity) and any flow as applicable. Table 5.1 shows spin-density and relaxation time parameters for specific issues. The faster scans such as single-shot EPI may not provide good contrast in the image as the data collection process compromises signal intensity with spatial sampling in a single cycle. In general, the contrast between two specific tissues can be estimated by the difference of respective signal intensities that are determined through the applied imaging pulse sequence as

$$S = k\rho \left(1 - e^{-\frac{T_R}{T_1}}\right)\left(e^{-\frac{T_E}{T_2}}\right) \quad \text{for spin-echo imaging pulse sequence.} \quad (5.33)$$

$$S = k\rho \left(\left(1 - 2e^{-\frac{T_I}{T_1}}\right) + e^{-\frac{T_R}{T_1}}\right)\left(e^{-\frac{T_E}{T_2}}\right)$$

for inversion recovery (180-90-180) imaging pulse sequence. (5.34)

$$S = k\rho \frac{\left(1 - e^{-\frac{T_R}{T_1}}\right)\sin\theta \left(e^{-\frac{T_E}{T_2^*}}\right)}{\left(1 - \cos\theta \, e^{-\frac{T_R}{T_1}}\right)} \quad \text{for gradient echo imaging pulse sequence.} \quad (5.35)$$

where S is the signal intensity of FID in frequency domain, ρ is spin density, and k is a proportionality constant.

Spectral response of various tissues provides more dispersion at higher field strengths. It means that spectral peaks are better separated at higher field strengths and therefore certain lesions such as gray matter lesions in brain images can be better seen. It should also be noted that the SNR is significantly improved with higher field strength. However, higher field strength also increases T_1 relaxation time, which decreases overall contrast sensitivity because of the saturation effect in spin–lattice magnetization.

To improve the contrast of vascular structures, a paramagnetic contrast agent such as gadolinium (Gd) can be used to change the susceptibility of the net magnetization vector. Such a paramagnetic contrast agent reduces T_1 relaxation time and therefore increases the signal intensity of T_1-weighted images. As the contrast agent is injected in the vascular system, MRI is performed with the appropriate pulse sequence. MR angiography is a good example of MR contrast imaging. Gd-enhanced T_1-weighted MR brain imaging is often used in diagnostic radiology.

There are several sources of noise and field inhomogeneities that cause artifacts and affect tissue contrast in MR images. Among them, the most prominent are RF noise, field inhomogeneities, motion, and chemical shift. RF shields are used to prevent external signals into RF coil. However, any failure in RF shield may cause bright artifacts such as spots or lines in the image due to RF noise. Nonuniformity of the external magnetic field and gradient coils can cause artifacts in the reconstructed image as the spatial frequency and phase encodings are adversely affected. Motion artifacts such as blurring and the appearances of ghost edges are caused by the motion of the tissue due to patient's movements or breathing during imaging.

Under an external magnetic field, each atom in the molecular structure of the tissue experiences its own small magnetic field (due to the circulation of electrons) in the direction opposite to the external magnetic field. Thus, the effective field strength at each nucleus varies depending on the molecular bonding and structure in the surrounding tissue. The chemical shift of a nucleus is determined as the deviation of its effective resonance frequency in the presence of other nuclei from a standard reference without any other nuclei with their local magnetic fields present. The chemical shift δ is expressed in ppm and computed as

$$\delta = \frac{(\omega - \omega_{ref}) \times 10^6}{\omega_{ref}}. \tag{5.36}$$

It can be seen from Equation 5.35 that chemical shift is proportionally impacted by the strength of external magnetic field that determines the Larmor frequency. It is also inversely proportional to the sampling rate in the direction of frequency encoding. Thus, chemical shifts affecting the Larmor frequency distribution, and therefore signal localization, cause artifacts in the presence of other nuclei in the tissue such as fat and water.

The SNR of a tissue in an image is the ratio of the average signal for the tissue to the standard deviation of the noise in the background of the image. In addition to the parameters above, SNR depends on signal acquisition methods and can be improved by signal averaging. With the assumption of a random noise in signal acquisition, the increase in SNR is proportional to the square root of number of images averaged. However, such image averaging to improve SNR is done at the expense of imaging time, which is often not a practical solution.

In conclusion, MRI is a relatively a noninvasive imaging method and uses no external radiation. It provides high-resolution multicontrast images due to its inherent capability of multiparameter signal acquisition methods that can be adopted and tuned to the imaging requirements with respect to pathology. Recent advances in functional and diffusion imaging have opened new doors to complex potential applications in neuroimaging.

5.8. EXERCISES

5.1. What is the principle of magnetic resonance imaging (MRI)? Which imaging modality would you choose to obtain images with better soft-tissue contrast? Explain your answer.

5.2. Under the external magnetic field strength of 1.5 T, what is the Larmor frequency for the nuclei: (i) ^{1}H, (ii) ^{23}Na, and (iii) ^{31}P?

5.3. What are the major advantages of MRI?

5.4. Explain Bloch's equation with respect to a rotating magnetization frame for longitudinal and transverse magnetization vectors.

5.5. Describe the longitudinal and transverse magnetization decays. How are these decays used in MRI?

5.6. What are the characteristic features of RF coils used in MRI?

5.7. Explain the various factors influencing the MR signal intensity and its shape.

5.8. How are the longitudinal and transverse relaxation times computed?

5.9. Let us assume that a tissue has a spin–lattice relaxation time of 100 ms. How long will it take for the longitudinal relaxation time to recover by 90%? (Consider the initial net magnetization vector to be zero.)

5.10. Let us assume that a tissue has a spin–spin relaxation time of 100 ms. Find the time of transverse magnetization vector to decay to 30% of its initial value.

5.11. Describe a general spin-echo imaging pulse sequence. What are the major issues in implementing it for 3-D imaging?

5.12. Describe fast EPI imaging sequence for 3-D imaging. What are its advantages and disadvantages over spin-echo pulse sequence?

5.13. Describe a gradient echo imaging pulse sequence with the explanation of sampling in the *k*-space. What are its advantages and disadvantages over EPI pulse sequence?

5.14. Draw a timing diagram for an inversion recovery imaging sequence that uses a 90-FID sequence to detect the signal present T_1 after the inversion (180-degree) pulse.

5.15. How are the activation areas determined in fMRI?

5.16. What T_E should be used to maximize contrast between two tissues with spin–spin relaxation times of 30 and 40 ms in spin-echo pulse sequence?

5.17. What is diffusion imaging? Describe an imaging pulse sequence and discuss its differences from flow imaging.

5.18. What is the difference between DWI and DTI?

5.19. What is fractional anisotropy and how is it computed?

5.20. Display in MATLAB the axial MR brain images with a stroke. Display proton density, T_1-weighted, T_2-weighted, and DWI images in separate windows. Compare and contrast the spatial resolution of each image with respect to lesions, white matter, gray matter, and CSF space.

5.9. REFERENCES

1. J.T. Bushberg, J.A. Seibert, E.M. Leidholdt, and J.M. Boone, *The Essentials of Medical Imaging*, Williams & Wilkins, Philadelphia, 1994.
2. Z.H. Cho, J.P. Jones, and M. Singh, *Fundamentals of Medical Imaging*, John Wiley & Sons, New York, 1993.
3. Z. Liang and P.C. Lauterbur, *Principles of Magnetic Resonance Imaging*, IEEE Press, Piscataway, NJ, 2000.
4. M.H. Lev and F. Hochberg, "Perfusion magnetic resonance imaging to assess brain tumor responses to new therapies," *J. Moffit Cancer Cent.*, Vol. 5, pp. 446–450, 1998.
5. D.D. Stark and W.G. Bradley, *Magnetic Resonance Imaging*, 3rd Edition, Mosby, New York, 1999.
6. F. Schmitt, M.K. Stehling, and R. Turner (Eds), *Echo Planar Imaging Theory, Techniques and Applications*, Springer-Verlag, Berlin, 1998.
7. K.K. Shung, M.B. Smith, and B. Tsui, *Principles of Medical Imaging*, Academic Press, San Diego, CA, 1992.
8. C.T.W. Moonen and P.A. Bandettini, *Functional MRI*, Springer-Verlag, Berlin, 2000.
9. P. Jezzard, P.M. Mathews, and S.M. Smith (Eds), *Functional Magnetic Resonance Imaging: An Introduction to Methods*, Oxford University Press, Oxford, 2001.
10. M.E. Moseley, J. Kucharczyk, J. Mintorovitch, Y. Cohen, J. Kurhanewicz, N. Derugin, H. Asgari, and D. Norman, "Diffusion-weighted MR imaging of acute stroke: Correlation with T_2-weighted and magnetic susceptibility-enhanced MR imaging in cats," *AJNR Am. J. Neuroradiol.*, Vol. 11, No. 3, pp. 423–429, 1990.
11. P.J. Basser, J. Mattiello, et al., "Estimation of the effective self-diffusion tensor from the NMR spin echo," *J. Magn. Reson. B*, Vol. 103, No. 3, pp. 247–254, 1994.
12. C.H. Sotak, "The role of diffusion tensor imaging in the evaluation of ischemic brain injury—a review," *NMR Biomed.*, Vol. 15, No. 7–8, pp. 561–569, 2002.
13. M.E. Moseley, J. Kucharczyk, J. Mintorovitch, Y. Cohen, J. Kurhanewicz, N. Derugin, H. Asgari, and D. Norman. Diffusion-weighted MR imaging of acute stroke: correlation with T_2-weighted and magnetic susceptibility-enhanced MR imaging in cats. *AJNR Am J Neuroradiol*, Vol. 11, pp. 423–429, 1990.
14. D.S. Kim and I. Ronen, "Recent advances in diffusion magnetic resonance imaging," in A.P. Dhawan, H.K. Hunag, and D.S. Kim (Eds), *Principal and Advanced Methods in Medical Imaging and Image Analysis*, World Scientific Press, Singapore, pp. 289–309, 2008.

CHAPTER 6

NUCLEAR MEDICINE IMAGING MODALITIES

Radiological imaging modalities such as X-ray radiographic imaging, mammography, and computed tomography (CT) are based on the transmission of X-ray radiation through the body and therefore provide anatomical information about the body. As briefly described in Chapter 1, the anatomical imaging modalities are limited to structural information and do not provide any functional or metabolic information about an organ or a tissue in the body. Since physiological processes are dependent on the metabolic and functional behavior of the tissue, it is important to involve tissue itself in the imaging process. Magnetic resonance imaging (MRI) methods do involve tissue through its chemical composition and therefore are capable of providing some functional and/or metabolic information in addition to anatomical information. However, radionuclide imaging methods directly involve an organ and associated tissue in the body in such a way that the tissue itself becomes a source of radiation that is used in the imaging process. Such methods are also called emission imaging methods and primarily utilize radioactive decay. In the process of radioactive decay, an unstable nucleus disintegrates into a stable nucleus by releasing nuclear energy and emitting photons such as gamma photons and/or specific particles such as positrons and alpha particles (1–5).

6.1. RADIOACTIVITY

A nucleus in an atom contains neutrons and protons. Since protons are positively charged, there is a repulsive force within the nucleus that is also packed with neutrons in a small space. In addition, there are attractive forces between neutrons and protons. The stability of a nucleus depends on the balance of all repulsive and attractive forces within the nucleus. For atomic mass less than 50, nuclei with an equal number of neutrons and protons are usually stable. For atomic mass greater than 50, a higher number of neutrons than protons is required to have a stable nucleus. An unstable nucleus disintegrates through radioactivity in its quest to achieve a stable configuration. The radioactivity is defined as the number of nuclear disintegrations per unit time. The radioactive decay may occur in many ways. However, the decays of significant interest are described below.

Medical Image Analysis, Second Edition, by Atam P. Dhawan
Copyright © 2011 by the Institute of Electrical and Electronics Engineers, Inc.

(1) **Alpha Decay:** Decay occurs through emission of alpha (α) particles. An alpha particle, with a typical energy of 4–8 MeV, consists of a helium nucleus with two protons and two neutrons. The penetration of an alpha particle in human tissue is very small, within a few millimeters.

(2) **Beta Decay:** Beta (β) decay occurs in one of the two ways, either through emission of electrons or through emission of positrons (a positron is a positively charged antiparticle of the electron). Electron emission increases the atomic number by 1 while positron emission decreases the atomic number by 1. The emission of beta particles also ranges a few MeV. Depending on the energy of the beta particle, its penetration in human tissue is also restricted to a few millimeters at the most. Positron emission is particularly interesting and used in the nuclear medical imaging modality called positron emission tomography (PET).

(3) **Gamma Decay:** Radioactive decay is through the emission of gamma (γ) rays. This type of decay may involve an electron capture process in which an electron from the K- or L-shell is captured by the nucleus, creating a gap in the respective orbit. Electrons from outer shells fill the gap, resulting in emission of characteristic X rays along with γ-rays. Decays by emission of γ-rays with an energy range of 100–200 keV (although higher energy γ-ray photons have also been investigated) are very useful and commonly used for nuclear medical imaging modality in γ-ray imaging or single photon emission computed tomography (SPECT).

Radioactive decay can be described by an exponential decay process with respect to time as

$$N(t) = N(0)e^{-\eta t} \qquad (6.1)$$

where $N(0)$ is the number of initial radionuclides, $N(t)$ is the number of radionuclides at time t and η is the radioactive decay constant.

The half-life of a radionuclide decay T_{half} is defined by the time required for half of the radionuclides to transform into stable nuclei, and can be expressed as

$$T_{half} = \frac{0.693}{\eta}. \qquad (6.2)$$

As mentioned above, the radioactivity of a radionuclide is defined as the average decay rate that can be computed from the derivative of $N(t)$ with respect to time t and thus is equal to the decay constant times number of $N(t)$. The radioactivity can be measured by one of the two commonly used units: curie or becquerel. A curie (CI) is equal to the 3.7×10^{10} disintegrations or decays per second (dps). A becquerel (Bq) is equal to one decay per second.

6.2. SPECT

In 1934, Jean Frederic Curie and Irene Curie discovered radiophosphorous ^{32}P, a radioisotope that demonstrated radioactive decay. In 1951, radionuclide imaging of

TABLE 6.1 Gamma Photon Emitter Radionuclides with Their Half-Life Duration and Clinical Applications

Radionuclide	Photon energy (keV)	Half-life (h)	Clinical applications
Technetium ^{99m}Tc	140	6	General and tumor
Thallium ^{201}Tl	135	73	Cardiovascular
Iodine ^{123}I	159	13	Thyroid, tumor
Gallium ^{67}Ga	93, 185, 300, 304	78	Infections
Indium ^{111}In	171, 245	68	Infection, tumor

the thyroid was demonstrated by Cassen through administration of iodine radioisotope ^{131}I (1). Hal Anger in 1952 developed a scintillation camera, later known as the Anger camera, with sodium iodide crystals coupled with photomultiplier tubes (PMTs) (2). Kuhl and Edwards developed a transverse section tomography gamma-ray scanner for radionuclide imaging in the early 1960s (3). Their imaging system included an array of multiple collimated detectors surrounding a patient with rotate–translation motion to acquire projection for emission tomography. With the advances in computer reconstruction algorithms and detector instrumentation, gamma-ray imaging now known as SPECT is used for 3-D imaging of human organs, extended even to full body imaging. Radioisotopes are injected into the body through administration of radiopharmaceutical drugs, which metabolize with the tissue, making the tissue a source of gamma-ray emissions. The gamma rays from the tissue pass through the body and are captured by the detectors surrounding the body to acquire raw data for defining projections. The projection data is then used in reconstruction algorithms to display images with the help of a computer and high-resolution displays. In SPECT imaging, the commonly used radionuclides are thallium (^{201}Tl), technetium (^{99m}Tc), iodine (^{123}I), and gallium (^{68}Ga). These radionuclides decay by emitting gamma rays for imaging with photon energies up to a few hundreds of keV (4–11). Table 6.1 shows the photon energy and half-life of the radioactivity decay for radionuclides used in SPECT imaging.

The attenuation of gamma rays is similar to that of X rays and can be expressed as:

$$I_d = I_0 e^{-\xi x} \qquad (6.3)$$

where I_0 is the intensity of gamma rays at the source, I_d is the intensity at the detector after the gamma rays have passed the distance x in the body and a linear attenuation coefficient that depends on the density of the medium, and ξ is the energy of gamma-ray photons.

The radionuclides required for SPECT such as technetium are artificially generated with appropriate radiopharmaceuticals suitable for administration in the body. After the tissue or organ to be imaged becomes radioactive, the patient is positioned in a scanner with detectors placed surrounding the patient. In modern scanners, the detectors are placed in a ring surrounding the patient covering a full 360-degree range. However, scanners involving a finite array of detectors with

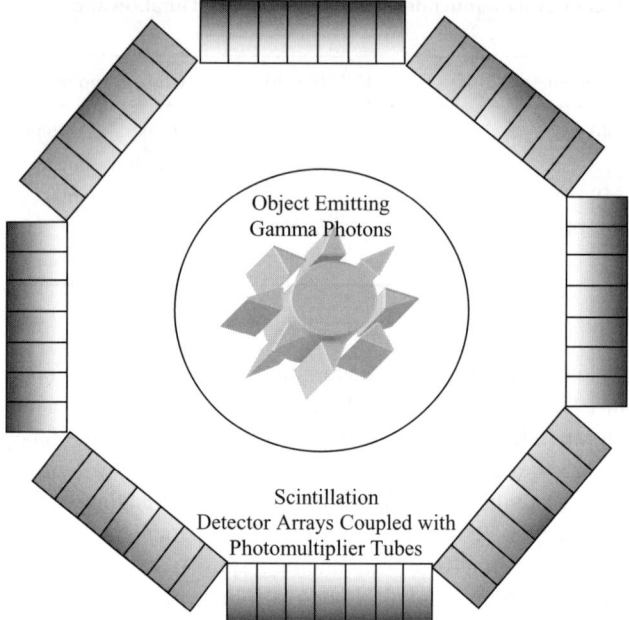

Figure 6.1 A schematic diagram of detector arrays of SPECT scanner surrounding the patient area.

rotational motion are also used. Figure 6.1 shows a schematic representation of a SPECT scanner.

6.2.1 Detectors and Data Acquisition System

The SPECT imaging systems used today are based on the Anger scintillation camera (8), which uses a collimator to reject scatter events and maps scintillation events on the attached scintillation crystal. The scintillation material converts γ-ray photon energy into light photons that are received by a photocathode of a position-sensitive PMT, which converts light photons into electrons that are amplified through a series of dynodes (as described in Chapter 4).

Finally, an amplified electrical voltage signal is digitized using an analog-to-digital convertor and stored in a computer memory with the information about the energy magnitude and position of the detected γ-ray photon. This basic principle is illustrated with details in Figure 6.2.

As illustrated in Figure 6.2, γ-ray photons are emitted from the tissue with the uptake of a radioactive pharmaceutical such as ^{99m}Tc. The emission distribution is isotropic in 3-D space around the patient body. The direct straight-line path between the emission source and detector is important to determine the point of emission for image reconstruction. Not all photons that reach the detector come directly from the emission source of tissue. As shown in Figure 6.2, photon 1 is not detected by the camera as it is not in the direction of the detector. Photon 2 is absorbed within

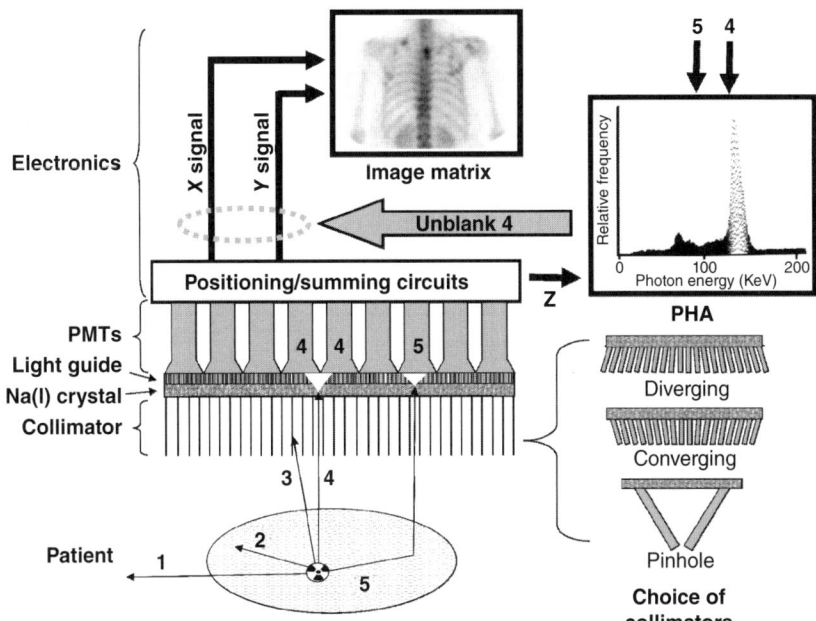

Figure 6.2 A detailed schematic diagram of SPECT imaging system (used with permission from L.S. Zuckier (11); Dr. Lionel Zuckier is gratefully acknowledged).

the body. Photon 3 intersects the detector at an angle other than parallel to the collimator and therefore gets absorbed by the lead septa (walls) of the parallel-hole collimator. Photon 4 travels in a direction such that it is able to pass through a collimator aperture and is detected by the Na(I) scintillation crystal. The energy of the photon is transformed to visible light photons that are received by PMTs, which produce an electronic pulse that is amplified and then analyzed by the positioning and summing circuits to determine the apparent position of scintillation. Figure 6.3 shows a matrix of 8×8 PMTs that are connected with horizontal and vertical summing networks X^+, X^-, Y^+, and Y, as originally designed by Hal Anger (8). The position of the scintillation event can be detected by analyzing the location of the pulse height in each of the summing network outputs. For example, as shown in Figure 6.3, the scintillation event in box (3,2) will provide higher output current in Y^+ and X^- than in X^+ and Y^- at respective locations since the scintillation event is closer to top (Y^+) and left (X^-) summing networks. The four composite outputs of the summing networks are appropriately amplified and then summed together to provide the total electric current that is converted into respective voltage signal Z. The amplitude of the voltage signal Z is proportional to the energy of the scintillated photon. A pulse-height analyzer (PHA) circuit then examines the amplitude of the voltage signal Z to determine whether to accept and store it in the data matrix or reject it. If the total energy as represented by the amplitude of voltage Z signal (as shown in Fig. 6.2 for photon 4) falls within the full width at half maximum (FWHM) of the energy spectrum of the γ-ray emission of the radioisotope (such as ^{99m}Tc), the scintillation event is accepted and data are stored with its energy level and X-Y

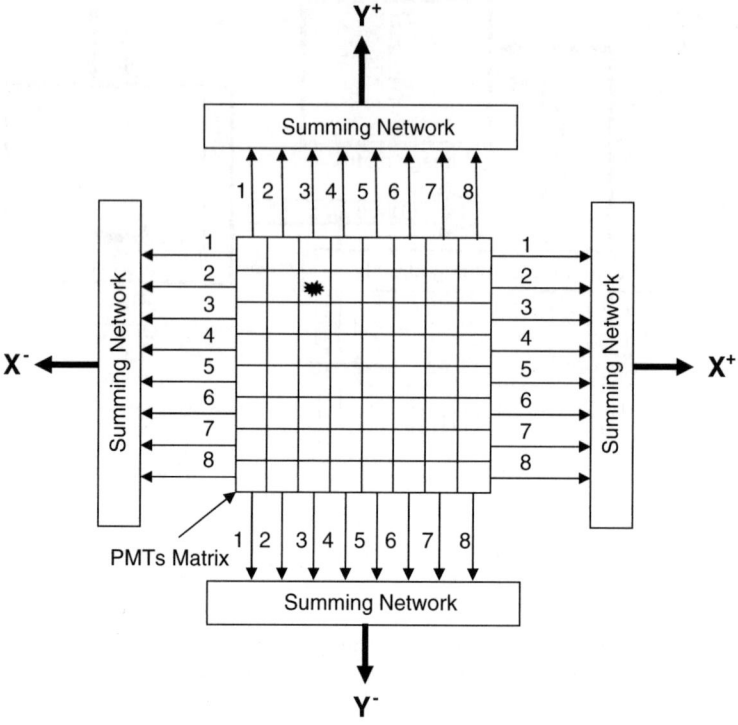

Figure 6.3 A schematic diagram of PMT matrix and summing networks for localization of scintillation events in SPECT imaging systems.

position coordinate information. For ^{99m}Tc radioisotope-based imaging, usually a window of 20% centered on the 140 keV energy peak is used to accept a scintillation event. If a γ-ray photon is scattered within the patient as shown by photon 5 in Figure 6.2, the lower energy of its pulse will cause its rejection by PHA, and the photon will not be included in the data matrix. Parallel-hole collimators are most common in nuclear medicine imaging systems. However, diverging, converging, or pin-hole collimators may be used in place of the parallel-hole collimator as shown in Figure 6.2 to focus on imaging various types and shapes of tissue and organs. The length of the septa of collimator L and the distance d between the septa, and distance Z between the source and the front of the collimator determine the spatial resolution R in the acquired image as

$$R = \frac{d(L+Z)}{L}. \tag{6.4}$$

As can be seen from the above equation, the spatial resolution is improved if the length of the collimator is increased and the detectors are brought closer to the emission source, in other words, closer to the body.

Sodium iodide NaI(Tl) crystal-based scintillation detectors coupled with PMTs are most commonly used for detection of gamma rays to acquire raw data.

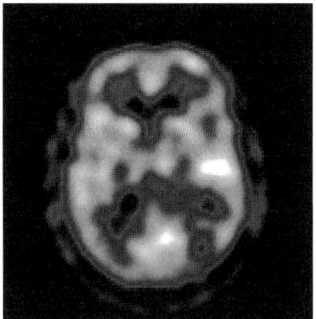

Figure 6.4 A ^{99}Tc SPECT image of a human brain.

Other detector material such as barium fluoride (BaF$_2$), cesium iodide (CsI(Tl)), and bismuth germinate (BGO) have also been used for scintillation. After the detection of gamma photons, the projection data is assembled from the raw data and fed into the computerized 3-D reconstruction algorithms. The reconstructed images are displayed on display terminals. Figure 6.4 shows an axial ^{99m}Tc SPECT image of a human brain. Note that SPECT images are poor in resolution and anatomical structure as compared with CT or MR images. The SPECT images show metabolism information related to a radioactive tracer with specific photon energy. Recently, multiple photon energy imaging has been found very useful in clinical diagnostic radiology by using a single radioisotope that can emit multiple γ-ray energy photons or more than one radioisotope with different γ-ray photon energy emissions. For example, gallium (^{67}Ga) can provide γ-ray photons at 93, 185, 300, and 394 keV (Table 6.1). This becomes possible because of the wide spectral response of scintillation detectors and appropriate PHA. Dual radioisotopes can be used in the body if there is a significant difference in the way they metabolize with the tissue and provide different γ-ray photon energies (11, 12). For example, one can be targeted at metastases while the other could provide information about specific infections in the body. Figure 6.5 shows a dual energy full body scan of the same patient using ^{99m}Tc and ^{111}In radioisotopes. Two scans specifically provide different information about the marrow and infection in the body.

6.2.2 Contrast, Spatial Resolution, and Signal-to-Noise Ratio in SPECT Imaging

The contrast of SPECT images depends on the signal intensity, which depends on the emission activity of the source. The source intensity is based on the dose, metabolism, and absorption in the body, and the half-life of the radionuclide used for imaging. Low photon statistics and scattering are major problems associated with SPECT imaging. Scattering events cause loss of source information as it is difficult to identify the path of travel for the photon originating from the source. Lead-based collimators are used to reduce detection of scattered events to improve the signal-to-noise ratio (SNR) and detection of actual radiation from the localized source. As described above, the spatial resolution is determined by the design of the

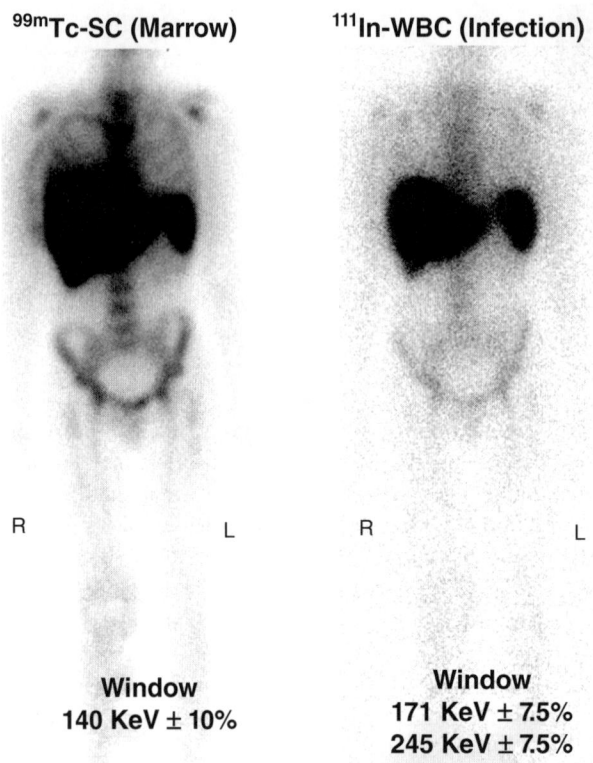

Figure 6.5 Dual-isotope acquisition: 24 h prior to imaging, 0.5 mCi of ^{111}In-labeled autologous white blood cells (^{111}In-WBCs) were injected intravenously into the patient to localize sites of infection. Thirty minutes prior to imaging, 10 mCi of ^{99m}Tc-sulfur colloid were injected intravenously to localize marrow. Co-imaging of the ^{99m}Tc window (140 ± 20% keV) and dual ^{111}In windows (171 ± 15% keV and 245 ± 15% keV) was performed, thereby producing simultaneous images of the marrow (left panel) and WBC distribution (right panel). Marrow, liver, and spleen are visible on both marrow and WBC studies. The ^{99m}Tc study is used to estimate WBC activity that is due to normal marrow distribution and of no pathologic consequence. To signify infection, ^{111}In-WBC activity must be greater than the visualized marrow distribution. (Dr. Lionel Zuckier, Director of Nuclear Medicine, University of Medicine and Dentistry of New Jersey, Newark, is gratefully acknowledged for providing the above images (11)).

collimator (septa length and diameter for circular parallel channels) and the distance between the source and collimator. This is the reason that images taken from one direction may not have the same image quality and resolution as an image taken from the opposite side when the source object is not in the middle. The images taken from the direction providing closer distance between the source object and collimator will provide better resolution and image quality.

The SNR depends on signal intensity (source activity as reflected by the dose), tissue metabolism or uptake, total time over which the data are acquired, attenuation within the body, scatter rejection, and detector sensitivity and efficiency.

The nonlinearities caused by the detectors and PMTs make the SPECT imaging process spatially variant. Thus, images would show degradations and geometric artifacts such as cushion and barrel artifacts because the registered detector count fluctuates from the actual count depending on the detector location. Usually, intensity nonuniformaties are corrected by using phantom data of uniform emission activity in the region of imaging. The geometric artifacts are difficult to correct, as these corrections require statistical preprocessing methods such as maximum likelihood estimation. Assessment of point spread and line spread functions help in developing preprocessing methods to compensate for detector nonlinearities and sensitivity variations due to geometrical configuration.

Since the source of radiation is inside the body, the gamma photons interact with the matter inside the body for attenuation and scattering processing, including photoelectric absorption and Compton scattering. Such interactions lead to the loss of a photon or significant changes in its direction, in case of Compton scattering events. The distribution of the data (gamma photons) collected by the array of detectors from spatial locations within an object may be different from the actual distribution of emission source activity within the object. The attenuation correction methods incorporate weighting factors that are based on the average regional or pixel-level activity. The scatter correction methods are based on estimation techniques using photon statistics derived from distribution models or experimental measurements. The distribution model-based estimation methods involve Monte Carlo simulations and are computationally expensive. Experimental measurement methods involving comparison of photon counts collected by detectors at different times with different activity levels are commonly used. Figure 6.6 shows the reconstructed SPECT ^{99m}Tc axial images without attenuation correction (left) and with attenuation correction (right) of a brain. The improved structure visibility is evident in the image with attenuation correction while the image without attenuation correction has significant

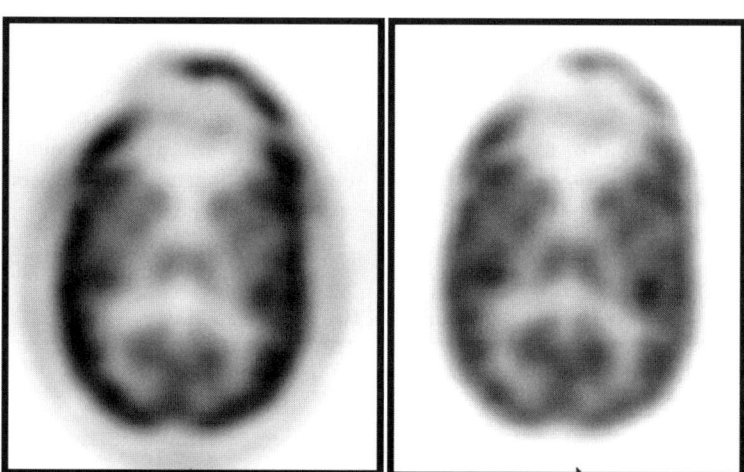

Figure 6.6 SPECT images of a brain reconstructed without attenuation correction (left) and with attenuation correction (right).

blurring of edges. Image reconstruction and estimation algorithms are described in Chapter 8.

Even though SPECT images are poor in structural information because of attenuation and scattering problems, they show important biochemical information tagged with specific physiology. SPECT imaging is a proven tool in the assessment of metastases or characterization of a tumor. Also, SPECT imaging is a low-cost imaging modality compared with PET because of the lower preparation cost of the radioisotopes used in SPECT imaging.

6.3. PET

Positron emission tomography imaging methods were developed in 1970s by a number of researchers including Phelps, Robertson, Ter-Pogossian, and Brownell (9–13). The concept of PET imaging is based on the simultaneous detection of two 511 keV energy photons traveling in the opposite direction. The distinctive feature of PET imaging is its ability to trace radioactive material metabolized in the tissue to provide specific information about its biochemical and physiological behavior.

Some radioisotopes decay by emitting positively charged particles called positrons. Table 6.2 shows some commonly used positron-emitting radionuclides and their half-life duration. The emission of a positron is accompanied by a significant amount of kinetic energy. After emission, a positron travels typically for 1–3 mm, losing some of its kinetic energy. The loss of energy makes the positron suitable for interaction with a loosely bound electron within a material for annihilation. The annihilation of the positron with the electron causes the formation of two gamma photons with 511 keV traveling in opposite directions (close to 180 degrees apart). The two photons can be detected by two surrounding scintillation detectors simultaneously within a small time window. This simultaneous detection within a small time window (typically on the order of nanoseconds) is called a coincidence detection, indicating the origin of annihilation along the line joining the two detectors involved in coincidence detection. Thus, by detecting a large number of coincidences, the source location and distribution can be reconstructed through image reconstruction algorithms. It should be noted that the point of emission of a positron is different from the point of annihilation with an electron. Although the imaging process is aimed at the reconstruction of source representing locations of emission of positrons, it is the locations of annihilation events that are reconstructed as an

TABLE 6.2 Positron Emitter Radionuclides and Their Half-Life Duration

Positron emitting radionuclides	Two-photon energy (keV)	Half-life time (min)
Fluorine ^{18}F	511	109
Oxygen ^{15}O	511	2
Nitrogen ^{13}N	511	10
Carbon ^{11}C	511	20

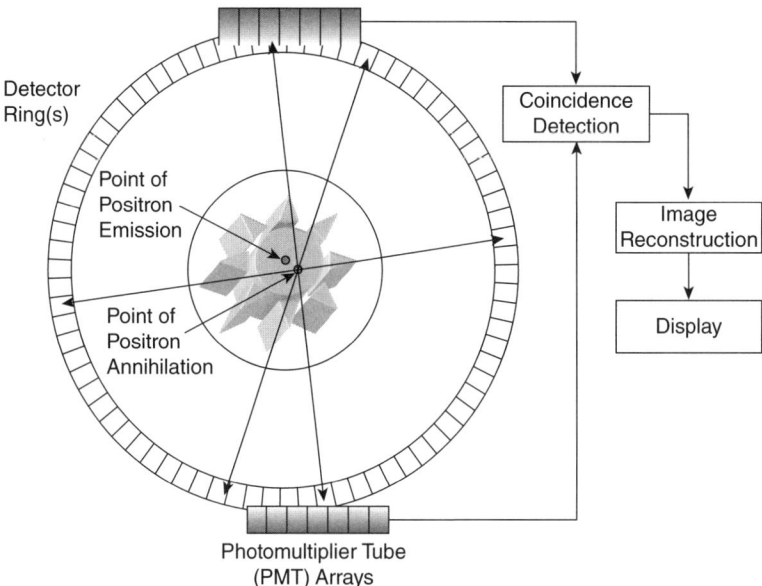

Figure 6.7 A schematic diagram of a PET imaging system.

image in the PET. However, the distribution of emission events of positrons is considered close enough to the distribution of annihilation events within a resolution limit.

As shown in Figure 6.7, coincidence detection forms the basic raw data in PET imaging. The finite time window used in coincidence detection involving two surrounding detectors placed opposite to each other provides an efficient mechanism of electronic collimation. Since the scattered photons have to travel a longer path, they may not reach the detector within a specified time window. Thus, the scattered radiation is likely to be rejected if the coincidence detection time window is appropriately set. Nevertheless, lead-based collimators are also used to reject scattered photons with an angular trajectory. Scintillation detectors coupled with PMTs are used in a single or multiple circular rings surrounding the patient for data acquisition. Commonly used scintillation detectors include sodium iodide (NaI(Tl)), barium fluoride (BaF_2), cesium iodide (CsI(Tl)), and bismuth germinate (BGO) crystals, but recently semiconductor detectors have also been used in PET imaging scanners.

The main advantage of PET imaging is its ability to extract metabolic and functional information of the tissue because of the unique interaction of the positron with the matter of the tissue. The most common positron emitter radionuclide used in PET imaging is fluorine (^{18}F), which is administered as fluorine-labeled radiopharmaceutical called fluorodeoxyglucose (FDG). The FDG images obtained through PET imaging show very significant information about the glucose metabolism and blood flow of the tissue. Such metabolism information has been proven to be critical in determining the heterogeneity and invasiveness of tumors. Figure 6.8 shows a set of axial cross-sections of brain PET images showing glucose

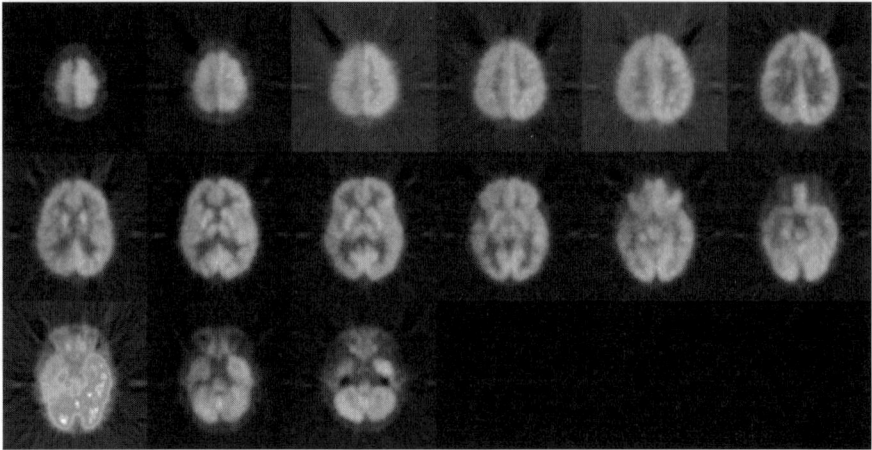

Figure 6.8 Serial axial images of a human brain with FDG-PET imaging.

metabolism. The streaking artifacts and low-resolution details can be noticed in these images. The artifacts seen in PET images are primarily because of the low volume of data caused by the nature of radionuclide–tissue interaction and electronic collimation necessary to reject the scattered events.

6.3.1 Detectors and Data Acquisition Systems

Since the coincidence detection method provides an excellent method of electronic collimation, the degradation effects of scattering are reduced in the data collection process. However, random coincidence and scatter coincidences can still degrade the data, causing poor quality images. The time window for the coincidence detection can be tightened to reduce random coincidences. Another method to reject scattered photons in the coincidence detection is the use of minimum energy level criteria. The scattered photons are of lower energy levels. By applying a threshold to the photon's energy level, photons with lower energy are considered to be coming from scattering interactions and are therefore not included in the coincidence detection. Since the photon's energy level is higher in PET imaging than in SPECT imaging, the attenuation problems in PET imaging are less severe. Several geometrical configuration-based ad hoc correction methods are used in PET imaging. A transmission scan can also be used for a more accurate attenuation correction. The transmission scan can be obtained by using an external positron source for imaging. However, such methods are often sensitive to statistical noise.

6.3.2 Contrast, Spatial Resolution, and SNR in PET Imaging

Contrast, spatial resolution, and sensitivity of PET imaging are significantly better than SPECT imaging mainly because of electronic collimation provided by the coincidence detection method. The coincidence detection method provides a more sensitive and accurate count of the photon-emission events. In addition, resolution of PET images does not depend on the distance between the emission source and detector. The time window (usually 6–12 ns) can be adjusted to sensitize to the coincidence detection response. A larger time window will allow greater data statistics but at the expense of higher random coincidences. A narrow energy range in the PHA will decrease the scattered photons to be detected in coincidences and provide higher sensitivity to detection of true emission events. However, it will also reduce the number of coincidence events detected by the system, causing a lower amount of data. The pair of 511 keV photons interacts with the body matter in a different way from lower energy photons in SPECT, providing less attenuation. But the spatial resolution is inherently limited by the distance between the emission of positron and its annihilation that emits two 511 keV photons. The SNR is superior in PET images to SPECT but is still affected by the detector efficiency, intensity distribution of source emission, and dose of the positron emitter nuclide. In addition, the SNR is further improved by using retractable septa of the external collimator in multislice imaging when multiple rings of detectors are used. Each detector ring with extended septa receives data directly only from respective parallel planes of slices. This mode rejects any cross-plane event detection, reducing the data to only true coincidence events within the selected plane without any scattering. When the septa are retracted to a specific position, cross-plane events can be allowed. In a full 3-D multi slice imaging mode, the septa may be completely removed to allow cross-planar data acquisition. It should be noted that the removal of septa would provide high sensitivity but with the acceptance of more scattered events, which would impact the spatial resolution.

The most significant advantage of PET imaging is the ability to tag a very specific biochemical activity and trace it with respect to time. PET imaging is an effective radiological imaging tool in metabolic, blood-flow, functional, and neuroreceptor imaging. However, the preparation of radiopharmaceuticals used in PET imaging is much more expensive than those used in SPECT imaging. Also, due to the limitations on detector size and sensitivity, and low emission statistics, the reconstructed images are relatively noisy and poor in resolution compared with MR and CT imaging modalities.

6.4. DUAL-MODALITY SPECT–CT AND PET–CT SCANNERS

X-ray CT and nuclear medicine imaging modalities (SPECT and PET) provide complimentary anatomical and metabolic information about the tissues and organs in the body. For several years patients have been scanned individually in both scanners at different times. Anatomical images from X-ray CT and metabolic images from SPECT or PET have been fused through postprocessing image registration methods using fiducial or internal landmarks. Multimodality image fusion has allowed examination of the metabolism and blood perfusion within an anatomically labeled tissue volume. This is an extremely important issue in diagnostic, treatment, and therapeutic evaluations. However, postprocessing image registration and fusion methods (described in Chapter 12) are not guaranteed to be completely accurate with

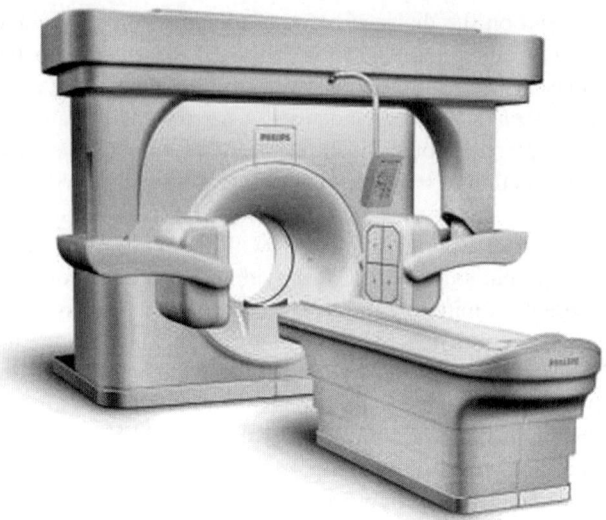

Figure 6.9 A picture of Philips Precedence SPECT–Xray CT scanner.

limitations on spatial and contrast resolutions. Recent advances in detector instrumentation, fast data acquisition, and high-capacity storage capabilities have led to hybrid or dual-modality imaging scanners combining SPECT or PET with X-ray CT systems. In these hybrid systems, the γ-ray camera and CT scanner share the same gantry to allow scanning of the patient efficiently by both modalities providing registered sets of X-ray and nuclear medicine images. The registered images can be displayed for any cross-sectional view and through a fused color display, providing visualization of both anatomical and metabolic information. For example, intensity of the gray scales in the fused image can be provided from X-ray anatomical images, but the color shades can be coded with metabolic information. In addition to the availability of accurately registered image sets, the dual-modality imaging system also provides accurate data for attenuation correction from the CT scan to be used in the reconstruction of SPECT or PET images improving their contrast resolution and sensitivity. Furthermore, a dual-modality scanner saves time and health care costs as the patient does not have to be moved or rescheduled for another scan.

Figure 6.9 shows a picture of the Philips Precedence SPECT–X-ray CT imaging system with a flexible γ-ray camera and 16-slice X-ray CT scanner. The Precedence imaging system with 16-slice high-resolution CT and complementary SPECT capabilities provides combined coronary computed tomography angiography (CTA), coronary calcium scoring, and attenuation-corrected SPECT myocardial perfusion imaging in a single imaging session. The accuracy of radionuclide therapy planning using the dual-modality scanners has been widely investigated and claimed to be improved by using the CT attenuation-corrected SPECT data. A wide spectrum of clinical applications includes combined coronary CT angiography and myocardial perfusion imaging.

Figure 6.10 shows a SPECT image (on the left), a CT image (in the middle), and a fused SPECT–CT image of a human brain. It is evident that the metabolic

6.4. DUAL-MODALITY SPECT–CT AND PET–CT SCANNERS

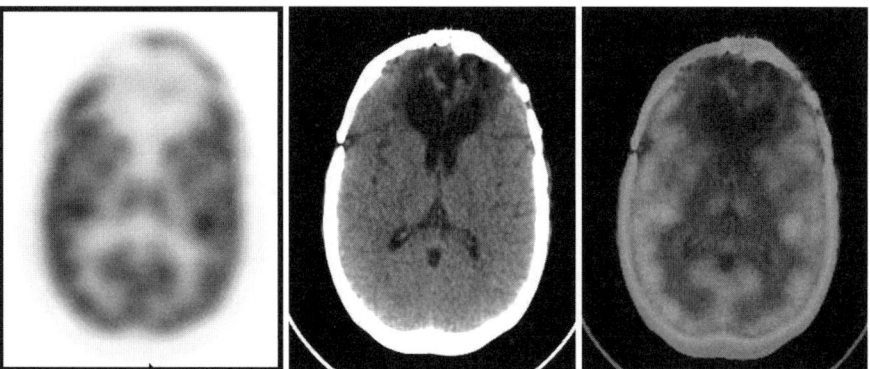

Figure 6.10 A ^{99m}Tc SPECT image (left), X-ray CT image (middle), and the fused SPECT–CT image (right) of the same axial section of a brain.

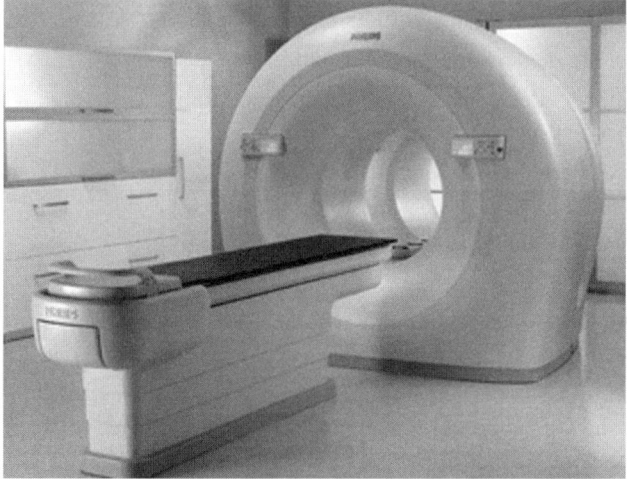

Figure 6.11 A picture of Philips GEMINI TF Big Bore PET–CT imaging system.

information in anatomical cortical structures can be better examined and evaluated from the fused image.

Philips dual-modality PET–CT GEMINI imaging system (shown in Fig. 6.11) provides a combined multislice advanced PET imaging with high-resolution X-ray CT using the same large gantry with 85 cm bore diameter. The dual-modality imaging technology allows consolidation of radiation oncology procedures with better accuracy and scheduling. The PET imaging scanner in the GEMINI system also uses time-of-flight (TOF) information in iterative reconstruction methods for better quality reconstructed images. During the coincidence detection when two photons are detected in two detectors across the line of coincidence, the time interval between the detections with their respective order of detection is called TOF information. If an annihilative event is closer to one detector than the other along the line of coincidence, the photon detection in the nearest detector is followed by the second detection event in the farthest detector with a longer delay. If the annihilation is in the middle of line of coincidence, both photons will reach their respective detectors at almost the same time, giving a very short time interval between two detection events. Thus TOF information can be used in estimating the point of photon emission (annihilation event) along the line of coincidence to improve the sensitivity, spatial resolution, and quality of reconstructed images. Advantages of dual-modality Philips PET-CT imaging system include automatic registration, image fusion, and tracking of anatomically labeled segmented regions of specific metabolism. It also provides a seamless data transfer capability to radiation treatment and planning systems. The dual-imaging capability improves patient scheduling and lowers health care costs.

6.5. EXERCISES

6.1. What are the principles of SPECT and PET imaging modalities?

6.2. How γ-ray photons are generated by a radioisotope?

6.3. Why do some radionuclides such as ^{67}Ga produce multiple energy γ-rays? Describe the emission spectra of ^{67}Ga.

6.4. Assume that a radioisotope reduces its radioactivity by 1/3 every hour. What is the decay constant?

6.5. What is the advantage of dual-energy photon SPECT imaging?

6.6. What scintillation detectors are used in SPECT imaging?

6.7. Describe the function of Anger's summing networks for position and pulse-height analysis.

6.8. A parallel-hole collimator is designed to have 4 mm diameter holes with the 8 mm long septa. Find the maximum spatial resolution if the distance between the body of the patient and front of the collimator is 10 cm.

6.9. Find and compare the spatial resolution, if the distance between the body of the patient and front of the collimator is (a) reduced to 4 cm, and (b) increased to 13 cm.

6.10. Find the spatial resolution of a pin-hole collimator with a front hole of 4 mm diameter, 8 mm long septa, and 10 cm distance between the patient body and the pinhole.

6.11. Find the impact on the spatial resolution if there is a 1.5 mm gap between the back of the septa and front of the scintillation crystal.

6.12. What are the advantages of PET over MRI and fMRI modalities?

6.13. Describe the advantages and disadvantages of PET over SPECT.

6.14. Describe the relationship among the detector size, signal-to-noise ratio, and image resolution for SPECT and PET imaging modalities.

6.15. What should be the preferred characteristics of a detection system in PET imaging modality?

6.16. What is time-of-flight information in PET imaging and how can it help in improving image quality?

6.17. Display ^{99m}Tc-SPECT and MR brain images for the same axial slice in MATLAB. Apply edge enhancement methods to both images and compare the definitions of the cortical structure in SPECT and MR images.

6.18. Display FDG-PET and MR brain images for the same axial slice in MATLAB. Apply edge enhancement methods on both images and compare the definitions of the anatomical structure in PET and MR images.

6.19. Compare the resolution, structure details, and image quality of ^{99m}Tc-SPECT and FDG-PET images displayed in Exercises 6.17 and 6.18.

6.6. REFERENCES

1. B. Cassen, L. Curtis, C. Reed, and R. Libby, "Instrumentation for ^{131}I used in medical studies," *Nucleonics*, Vol. 9, pp. 46–48, 1951.
2. H. Anger, "Use of gamma-ray pinhole camera for in-vivo studies," *Nature*, Vol. 170, pp. 200–204, 1952.
3. E. Kuhl and R.Q. Edwards, "Reorganizing data from transverse sections scans using digital processing," *Radiology*, Vol. 91, pp. 975–983, 1968.
4. H. Barrett and W. Swindell, *Radiological Imaging: The Theory of Image Formation, Detection and Processing*, Volumes 1–2, Academic Press, New York, 1981.
5. J.T. Bushberg, J.A. Seibert, E.M. Leidholdt, and J.M. Boone, *The Essentials of Medical Imaging*, Williams & Wilkins, Philadelphia, 1994.
6. Z.H. Cho, J.P. Jones, and M. Singh, *Fundamentals of Medical Imaging*, John Wiley & Sons, New York, 1993.
7. K.K. Shung, M.B. Smith, and B. Tsui, *Principles of Medical Imaging*, Academic Press, San Diego, CA, 1992.
8. G.N. Hounsfield, "A method and apparatus for examination of a body by radiation such as X or gamma radiation," Patent 1283915, The Patent Office, London, 1972.
9. G. Brownell and H.W. Sweet, "Localization of brain tumors," *Nucleonics*, Vol. 11, pp. 40–45, 1953.
10. A. Webb, *Introduction to Biomedical Imaging*, Wiley Interscience-IEEE Press, Hoboken, NJ, 2003.
11. L.S. Zuckier, "Principles of nuclear medicine imaging modalities," in A.P. Dhawan, H.K. Hunag, and D.S. Kim (Eds), *Principal and Advanced Methods in Medical Imaging and Image Analysis*, World Scientific Press, Singapore, pp. 63–98, 2008.
12. M.E. Casey, L. Eriksson, M. Schmand, M. Andreaco, M. Paulus, M. Dahlborn, and R. Nutt, "Investigation of LSO crystals for high spatial resolution positron emission tomography," *IEEE Trans. Nucl. Sci.*, Vol. 44, pp. 1109–1113, 1997.
13. A.P. Dhawan, "A review on biomedical image processing and future trends," *Comput. Methods Programs Biomed.*, Vol. 31, Nos. 3–4, pp. 141–183, 1990.

CHAPTER 7

MEDICAL IMAGING MODALITIES: ULTRASOUND IMAGING

Sound or acoustic waves were successfully used in sonar technology in military applications in World War II. The potential of ultrasound waves in medical imaging was explored and demonstrated by several researchers in the 1970s and 1980s, including Wild, Reid, Frey, Greenleaf, and Goldberg (1–7). Today ultrasound imaging is successfully used in diagnostic imaging of anatomical structures, blood flow measurements, and tissue characterization. Safety, portability, and low-cost aspects of ultrasound imaging have made it a successful diagnostic imaging modality (5–9).

7.1. PROPAGATION OF SOUND IN A MEDIUM

Sound waves propagate mechanical energy, causing periodic vibration of particles in a continuous elastic medium. Sound waves cannot propagate in a vacuum since there are no particles of matter in the vacuum. The initial energy creates the mechanical movement of a particle through compression and rarefaction that is propagated through the neighbor particles depending on the density and elasticity of the material in the medium.

Sound waves are characterized by wavelength and frequency. Sound waves audible to the human ear are comprised of frequencies ranging from 15 to 20 kHz. Sound waves with frequencies above 20 kHz are called ultrasound waves. The velocity of a sound wave c in a medium is related to its wavelength λ and frequency v by

$$c = \lambda v. \tag{7.1}$$

Since the frequency remains constant in the medium even when there is a change in the medium such as from soft tissue to fat, the propagation speed or velocity of the sound determines the wavelength. For example, the velocity of a sound in air, water, soft tissue, and fat are, respectively, 331, 1430, 1540, and 1450 m/s. Thus, a 5 MHz ultrasound beam has a wavelength of 0.308 mm in soft tissue with a velocity

---

Medical Image Analysis, Second Edition, by Atam P. Dhawan
Copyright © 2011 by the Institute of Electrical and Electronics Engineers, Inc.

of 1540 m/s. Because the frequency remains unchanged when a sound wave enters from one medium to another, the resultant change is experienced in the wavelength and the direction of the propagation determined by the principle of refraction. Like light waves, sound waves follow the principles of reflection, refraction, and superposition. The amplitude of a sound wave is the maximum particle displacement in the medium determined by the pressure applied by the sound energy. The intensity, I, is proportional to the pressure and is measured by power per unit area. For example, the intensity of sound waves can be expressed in milliwatts/per square centimeter (mW/cm^2). Another term, decibel (dB), is often used in expressing the relative intensity levels and is given by

$$\text{Relative Intensity in dB} = 10 \log_{10} \frac{I_1}{I_2} \tag{7.2}$$

where I_1 and I_2 are intensity values of sound energy that are being compared.

For example, an incident ultrasound pulse of intensity I_1 loses its intensity when it travels through soft tissue. If its intensity in the soft tissue is I_2, the loss can be computed from Equation 7.2 and is expressed in decibels. Thus, a $100 \, mW/cm^2$ acoustic pulse would be at $0.1 \, mW/cm^2$ after a 30 dB loss.

As mentioned above, sound waves propagate through displacement of particles in a medium. Let us assume that the medium is linear and lossless to the propagation of a sound wave that applies a mechanical force ∂F to cause a particle displacement ∂u (in the range of a few nanometers) in the direction z (depth in the tissue while the x–y coordinates represent the two-dimensional [2-D] plane of the surface of the tissue). The particle displacement in the direction z can then be represented by a second-order differential equation as (1–5, 8)

$$\frac{\partial^2 u}{\partial z^2} = \frac{1}{c^2} \left(\frac{\partial^2 u}{\partial t^2} \right) \tag{7.3}$$

where c is the velocity of sound propagation in the medium that is assumed to be linear and lossless.

Equation 7.3 is known as the wave equation where the velocity of sound wave is given by

$$c = \sqrt{\frac{1}{k\rho}} \tag{7.4}$$

where k and ρ are, respectively, the compressibility (inverse of the bulk modulus) and density of the medium.

The solution to the second-order differential wave equation (Eqn 7.3) can be given by an appropriate selection of the function $u(t, z)$ as a function of time t and space z as

$$u(t,z) = u_0 e^{j\omega(ct-z)} \text{ with } \omega = \frac{2\pi}{\lambda} \tag{7.5}$$

where ω and λ represent, respectively, wave number and wavelength.

The particle displacement causes a pressure wave $p(t, z)$ in the medium that can be represented by

$$p(t,z) = p_0 e^{j\omega(ct-z)}. \quad (7.6)$$

It can be realized that

$$u = \frac{p}{Z} \quad (7.7)$$

where Z represents the acoustic impedance of the medium at the point of propagation.

The pressure at a particular point is related to the displacement and density of the medium by

$$p = \rho c u. \quad (7.8)$$

From Equations 7.7 and 7.8, it follows that

$$Z = \rho c. \quad (7.9)$$

Thus, the acoustic impedance of a medium is defined as the product of the density and sound propagation velocity in the medium. Since the intensity is also defined by the average flow of energy per unit area in the medium perpendicular to the direction of propagation, the intensity of the propagating wave is given as

$$I = \frac{p_0^2}{2Z}. \quad (7.10)$$

The density and elastic properties of the medium play a significant role in the propagation of sound. Stress–strain relationships of the medium are used to define elasticity and compressibility and can be described in a mathematical form to show the precise dependency of the propagation of sound waves in an inhomogeneous medium. However, the common properties of the propagation of sound waves in terms of reflection, refraction, scattering, and attenuation are similar to those experienced with light waves. Ultrasound waves can be reflected, refracted, and attenuated depending on the changes in the acoustic impedance in the medium.

In medical imaging applications, shorter wavelengths provide deeper penetration and better spatial resolution. Since the velocity of sound in a specific medium is fixed, the wavelength is inversely proportional to the frequency. In medical ultrasound imaging, sound waves of 2–10 MHz can be used, but 3–5 MHz frequencies are the most common. Higher frequencies are used for low-depth high-resolution imaging.

7.2. REFLECTION AND REFRACTION

As the incident sound waves reach a boundary surface that defines a change of the medium with an angle not perpendicular to the surface, a part of the acoustic energy is reflected and the remaining is transmitted into the second medium. With the change in medium, the transmitted wave changes its direction. Like the refraction

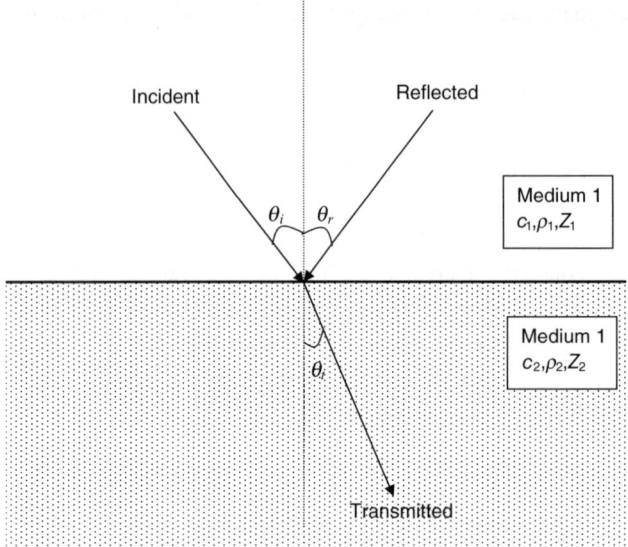

Figure 7.1 Reflection and refraction of ultrasound waves as incident from medium 1 to medium 2.

phenomenon of light waves, the angle of incidence is equal to the angle of reflection (Fig. 7.1). The angle of a transmitted wave is given by Snell's law and is dependent on the propagation speeds of the two mediums. Let us assume that c_1 and c_2 are, respectively, the propagation speeds of the incident sound wave in the two mediums across the incident boundary. According to Snell's law,

$$\theta_i = \theta_r$$
$$\frac{c_1}{c_2} = \frac{\sin \theta_i}{\sin \theta_t} \qquad (7.11)$$

where θ_i and θ_t are the incident and transmitted waves, respectively, in medium 1 and medium 2 (Fig. 7.1).

It should be noted that a critical incident angle θ_{ci} exists for which the incident wave is completely reflected without any transmission as

$$\theta_{ci} = \sin^{-1}\left(\frac{c_1}{c_2}\right) \text{ with } c_2 > c_1. \qquad (7.12)$$

7.3. TRANSMISSION OF ULTRASOUND WAVES IN A MULTILAYERED MEDIUM

When a sound wave enters from one medium to another such as in the case of a boundary of a tissue, the acoustic impedance changes and therefore the direction of the wave is altered. The difference in the acoustic impedance of the two media causes

7.3. TRANSMISSION OF ULTRASOUND WAVES IN A MULTILAYERED MEDIUM

reflection of a fraction of the incident sound energy. If a sound wave in incident with an angle θ_i at the interface of two mediums with acoustic impedance, Z_1 and Z_2, the pressure reflection coefficient or simply called reflection coefficient R is given by (1–3, 8)

$$R = \frac{p_r}{p_i} = \frac{Z_2 \cos\theta_i - Z_1 \cos\theta_t}{Z_2 \cos\theta_i + Z_1 \cos\theta_t}. \tag{7.13}$$

As the pressure waves generated by reflection and transmission are in opposite direction, it can be realized that

$$p_t = p_i + p_r. \tag{7.14}$$

Thus, the transmitted pressure coefficient T is given by

$$T = \frac{p_t}{p_i} = \frac{p_i + p_r}{p_i} = 1 + \frac{p_r}{p_i} = 1 + R$$

which gives

$$T = \frac{2Z_2 \cos\theta_i}{Z_2 \cos\theta_i + Z_1 \cos\theta_t}. \tag{7.15}$$

Using the above formulations, intensity reflection coefficients R_I and intensity transmission coefficients T_I can be expressed as

$$R_I = \frac{I_r}{I_i} = R_p^2 = \frac{(Z_2 \cos\theta_i - Z_1 \cos\theta_t)^2}{(Z_2 \cos\theta_i + Z_1 \cos\theta_t)^2}$$

$$T_I = 1 - R_I = \frac{4Z_2 Z_1 \cos^2\theta_i}{Z_2 \cos\theta_i + Z_1 \cos\theta_t}. \tag{7.16}$$

If the incident ultrasound wave is focused at the interface of medium 1 and medium 2 in the direction perpendicular to the boundary, the above expressions for reflection and transmission coefficients can be simplified as

$$R_{1,2} = \frac{Z_2 - Z_1}{Z_1 + Z_2}$$

and

$$T_{1,2} = \frac{2Z_2}{Z_1 + Z_2} \tag{7.17}$$

where $R_{1,2}$ is the reflection from the second medium to the first medium and $T_{1,2}$ is the transmission from the first medium to the second medium.

In medical ultrasound imaging, the sound waves propagate through multilayered structures. A simplified multilayered structure with acoustic impedance Z_i; $i = 1, 5$ is shown in Figure 7.2. Generalizing the above equations for normal incidence cases, the transmission and reflection coefficients can be expressed as

$$R_{ij} = \frac{Z_j - Z_i}{Z_i + Z_j}$$

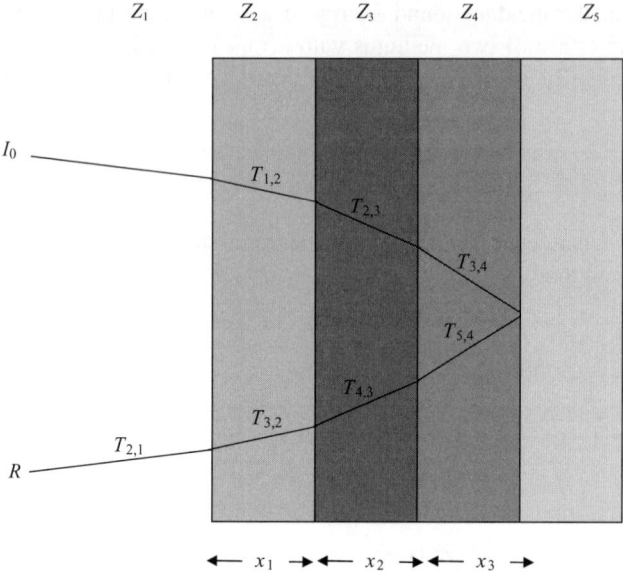

Figure 7.2 A path of a reflected sound wave in a multilayered structure.

and

$$T_{ij} = \frac{2Z_j}{Z_i + Z_j}. \quad (7.18)$$

Applying Equation 7.18 to the multilayer structure shown in Figure 7.2, the final reflected wave can be expressed as

$$R_0 = I_0 T_{12} T_{23} T_{34} T_{54} T_{43} T_{32} T_{21}. \quad (7.19)$$

Since $1 + R_{ij} = T_{ij}$, the above can be simplied as

$$R_0 = I_0 (1 - R_{12}^2)(1 - R_{23}^2)(1 - R_{34}^2) R_{45}. \quad (7.20)$$

7.4. ATTENUATION

Various mechanical properties such as density, elasticity, viscosity, and scattering properties cause attenuation of the sound waves in a medium. As with electromagnetic radiation, the loss of energy of sound waves occurs as the waves propagate in a medium. Extending Equation 7.5 to include viscosity and compressibility of the medium, the displacement can be related to the attenuation coefficient α of the ultrasound wave as (1, 8, 9)

$$u(t, z) = u_0 e^{-\alpha z} e^{j\omega(ct-z)}$$

$$\text{with } \alpha = \frac{\left(\frac{4\gamma}{3} + \xi\right)\omega^2}{2\rho c} \quad (7.21)$$

TABLE 7.1 Attenuation Coefficients and Propagation Speeds of Sound Waves

Tissue	Average attenuation coefficient in dB/cm at 1 MHz	Propagation velocity of sound in m/s	Average acoustic impedance in $\times 10^5$ $(g/cm^2/s)$
Fat	0.6	1450	1.38
Soft tissue	0.7–1.7	1540	1.7
Liver	0.8	1549	1.65
Kidney	0.95	1561	1.62
Brain	0.85	1541	1.58
Blood	0.18	1570	1.61
Skull and bone	3–10 and higher	3500–4080	7.8
Air	10	331	0.0004

where γ and ξ, respectively, are shear viscosity and compressional viscosity coefficients.

As defined in Equation 7.10, the intensity of the propagating wave can now be expressed in terms of attenuation coefficient α as

$$I(t,z) = \frac{p_0^2}{Z} e^{-2\alpha z} e^{2j\omega(ct-z)}. \quad (7.22)$$

The attenuation coefficient is characterized in units of decibels per centimeter and is dependent on the frequency of the sound waves. As frequency increases, the attenuation coefficient also increases. Table 7.1 shows attenuation coefficients of some biological tissues.

7.5. ULTRASOUND REFLECTION IMAGING

Let us assume that a transducer provides an accoustic signal of $s(x, y)$ intensity with a pulse $\phi(t)$ that is transmitted in a medium with an attenuation coefficient, μ, and reflected by a biological tissue of reflectvity $R(x, y, z)$ with a distance z from the transducer. The recorded reflected intensity of a time varying accoustic signal, $J_r(t)$ over the region $\Re$ can then be expressed as

$$J_r(t) = K \left| \iiint_\Re \left(\frac{e^{-2\mu z}}{z} \right) R(x,y,z) s(x,y) \phi\left(t - \frac{2z}{c}\right) dx\,dy\,dz \right| \quad (7.23)$$

where K, $\phi(t)$, and c, respectively, represent a normalizing constant, received pulse, and the velocity of the acoustic signal in the medium.

Using an adaptive time-varying gain to compensate for the attenuation of the signal, Equation 7.23 for the compensated recorded reflected signal from the tissue, $J_{cr}(t)$, can be simplified to

$$J_{cr}(t) = K \left| \iiint_\Re R(x,y,z) s(x,y) \phi\left(t - \frac{2z}{c}\right) dx\,dy\,dz \right|$$

or, in terms of a convolution, as

$$J_{cr}(t) = K \left| R\left(x, y, \frac{ct}{2}\right) \otimes s(-x, -y)\phi(t) \right| \tag{7.24}$$

where $\otimes$ represents a three-dimensional (3-D) convolution. This is a convolution of a reflectivity term characterizing the tissue and an impulse response characterizing the source parameters.

7.6. ULTRASOUND IMAGING INSTRUMENTATION

A piezoelectric crystal-based transducer can be used as a source to form an ultrasound beam as well as a detector to receive the returned signal from the tissue. A schematic diagram of a typical single crystal-based ultrasound transducer is shown in Figure 7.3. In a plastic casing, a piezoelectric crystal is used along with a damping material layer and acoustic insulation layer inside the plastic casing. An electromagnetic tuning coil is used to apply a controlled voltage pulse to produce ultrasound waves. In the receiver mode, the pressure wave of the returning ultrasound signal is used to create an electric signal through the tuned electromagnetic coil. The piezoelectric crystal has a natural resonant frequency f_0 that can be expressed as

$$f_0 = \frac{c_1}{2d} \tag{7.25}$$

where c_1 is the velocity of sound in the crystal material and d is the thickness of the crystal.

While higher harmonics of the natural resonant frequency of the piezoelectric crystal can be created, multiple crystals can be grouped together to form a specific

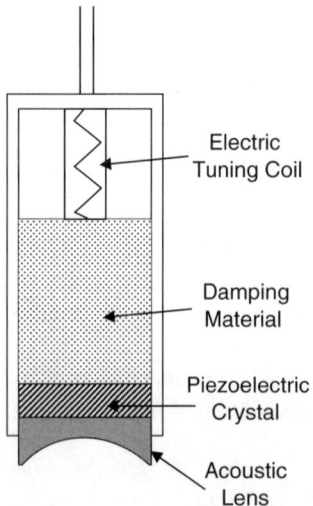

Figure 7.3 A schematic diagram of an ultrasound single-crystal transducer.

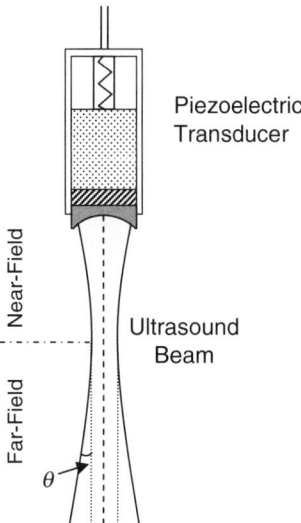

Figure 7.4 Ultrasound beam from a piezoelectric transducer.

ultrasound beam of desired shape and focus. The ultrasound beam (as shown in Fig. 7.4) transmits energy into three zones: (1) a near-field transmission (also called Fresnel region) of the energy of the ultrasound pulse; (2) a far-field transmission (also called Fraunhofer region); and (3) an unwanted side-lobe resulting from the radial expansion of the piezoelectric crystal appearing on the sides of the main direction of the beam. The length of the near-field region L_{nf} is determined by the radius of the crystal r and the wavelength λ of ultrasound beam as

$$L_{nf} = \frac{r^2}{\lambda}. \tag{7.26}$$

The far-field effect of the ultrasound beam is diverging as shown in Figure 7.4 with an angle that is given by

$$\theta = \arcsin\left(\frac{0.61\lambda}{r}\right). \tag{7.27}$$

A conventional ultrasound imaging system is comprised of a piezoelectric crystal-based transducer that works as a transmitter as well as receiver based on an electronic transmitter/receiver switching circuit, a control panel with pulse generation and control, and a computer processing and display system. Figure 7.5 shows a schematic diagram of a conventional ultrasound imaging system.

In the transmitter mode, a piezoelectric crystal converts an electrical signal to sound energy. The same crystal can convert sound waves into an electrical signal in the receiver mode. The transducers for medical imaging are tuned for the specific frequency range (2–10 MHz). A backing block absorbs the backward-directed vibrations and sound energy to eliminate undesired echoes from the housing enclosure of the piezoelectric crystal. Additional acoustic absorbers are used to improve the performance of ultrasound pulses with the desired mode and timings.

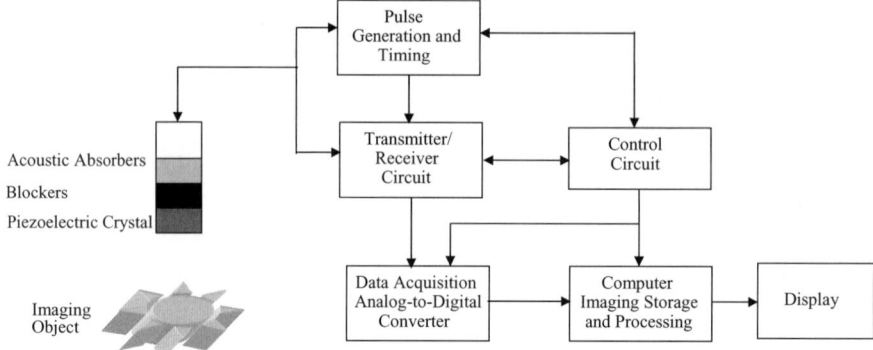

Figure 7.5 A schematic diagram of a conventional ultrasound imaging system.

Usually, an ultrasound transducer provides brief pulses of ultrasound when stimulated by a train of voltage spikes of 1–2 μs duration applied to the electrodes of the crystal element. An ultrasound pulse can be a few cycles long, typically on the order of two to three cycles. As the same crystal element is used as the receiver, the time between two pulses is used for detecting the reflected signal or echo from the tissue. The PRF is thus dependent on the time to be devoted to listening for the echo from the tissue. In a typical mode of operation, the transducer is positioned at the surface of the body or an object. The total travel distance traveled by the ultrasound pulse at the time of return to the transducer is twice the depth of the tissue boundary from the transducer. Thus, the maximum range of the echo formation can be determined by the speed of sound in the tissue multiplied by half of the pulse-repetition period. When the echoes are received by the transducer crystal, their intensity is converted into a voltage signal that generates the raw data for imaging. The voltage signal then can be digitized and processed according to the need to display on a computer monitor as an image.

Since the acoustic echoes are position-dependent, the spatial resolution and quality of ultrasound images are somewhat different from the conventional radiographic images. Typically, ultrasound images appear noisy with speckles, lacking a continuous boundary definition of the object structure. The interpretation and quantification of the object structure in ultrasound images is more challenging than in X-ray computed tomography (X-ray CT) or magnetic resonance (MR) images.

7.7. IMAGING WITH ULTRASOUND: A-MODE

The "A-mode" of ultrasound imaging records the amplitude of returning echoes from the tissue boundaries with respect to time. In this mode of imaging, the ultrasound pulses are sent in the imaging medium with a perpendicular incident angle. Unlike X-ray CT and MR imaging (MRI), the operator in ultrasound imaging has a great ability to control the imaging parameters in real time. These parameters include positioning, preamplification, time gain compensation and rejection of noisy echoes to improve the signal-to-noise ratio (SNR), leading to an improvement in image quality.

A-mode-based data acquisition is the basic method in all modes of diagnostic ultrasound imaging. Depending on the objectives of imaging and tissue characterization and the nature of the imaging medium, only relevant information from the A-mode-based signal acquisition is retained for further processing and display.

Since the echo time represents the acoustic impedance of the medium and depth of the reflecting boundary of the tissue, distance measurements for the tissue structure and interfaces along the ultrasound beam can be computed. This is a great advantage in ultrasound imaging. The intensity and time measurements of echoes can provide useful 3-D tissue characterization. Thus, shape and position measurements can be obtained from ultrasound images.

7.8. IMAGING WITH ULTRASOUND: M-MODE

The "M-mode" of ultrasound imaging provides information about the variations in signal amplitude due to object motion. A fixed position of the transducer, in a sweep cycle, provides a line of data that is acquired through A-mode. The data is displayed as a series of dots or pixels with brightness level representing the intensity of the echoes. In a series of sweep cycles, each sequential A-line data is positioned horizontally. As the object moves, the changes in the brightness levels representing the deflection of corresponding pixels in the subsequent sequential lines indicate the movement of the tissue boundaries. Thus, the x-axis represents the time, while the y-axis indicates the distance of the echo from the transducer.

M-mode is a very effective method in tracking the object motion such as the movement of a valve in a beating heart. Figure 7.6 shows the M-mode display of an ultrasound cardiac signal showing mitral stenosis with anterior motion of the posterior mitral leaflet.

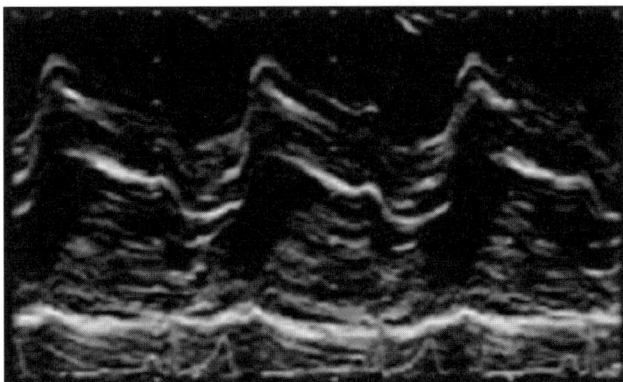

Figure 7.6 M-Mode display of mitral valve leaflet of a beating heart.

7.9. IMAGING WITH ULTRASOUND: B-MODE

The "B-Mode" of ultrasound imaging provides 2-D images representing the changes in acoustic impedance of the tissue. The brightness of the B-Mode image shows the strength of the echo from the tissue structure. To obtain a 2-D image of the tissue structure, the transducer is pivoted at a point about an axis and is used to obtain a V-shaped imaging region. Alternately, the transducer can be moved to scan the imaging region. Using position encoders and computer processing, several versions of the acquired data can be displayed to show the acoustic characteristics of the tissue structure and its medium.

As with the A-mode method, the returned echoes are processed with proper preamplification and adaptive gain amplifiers for acquiring the raw data that are converted into a 2-D image for display. Dynamic B-mode scanners provide real-time ultrasound images using multiple transducer arrays and computer control-based data acquisition and display systems. Several types of transducer arrays such as linear, annular, and linear phased arrays can be used in dynamic real-time ultrasound scanners. In such array-based scanners, the ultrasound beam is electronically steered with pulse generators that are synchronized with the clock for automatic data acquisition. The operator-based dependency is thus minimized in such ultrasound imaging systems. Figure 7.7 shows a B-scan of the mitral valve area of a beating heart.

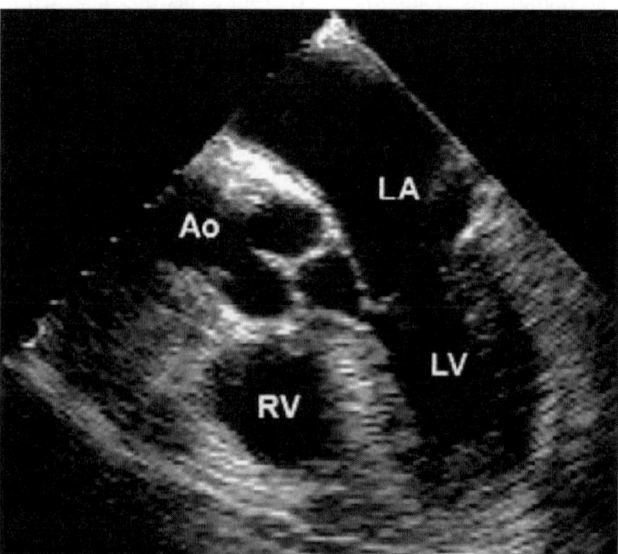

Figure 7.7 The B-Mode image of a beating heart for investigation of mitral stenosis. Left atrium (LA), left ventricle (LV), right ventricle (RV), and aorta (Ao) are labeled in the image.

7.10. DOPPLER ULTRASOUND IMAGING

Blood flow can be effectively imaged with ultrasound imaging using the Doppler method. According to the Doppler effect, a change in the frequency from a moving source is observed by a stationary observer. The change in the perceived or observed frequency is called the Doppler frequency, $f_{doppler}$, and is given by

$$f_{doppler} = \pm \frac{2v \cos \theta \ f}{c+v} \qquad (7.28)$$

where v is the velocity of the moving source or object, f is the original frequency, c is the velocity of the sound in the medium, and θ is the incident angle of the moving object with respect to the propagation of the sound.

Since the velocity of the moving object is much less than the velocity of the sound, the above equation is simplified in medical imaging as

$$f_{doppler} = \pm \frac{2v \cos \theta \ f}{c}. \qquad (7.29)$$

Since the above term of Doppler shift includes a cosine of the angle of incidence wave, it should be noted that there will be no shift in Doppler frequency if the angle of incidence is 90 degrees. The Doppler shift is a very popular method of measuring blood flow with ultrasound pulses typically at 5 MHz. It is not possible to align the ultrasound transducer parallel to the flow at 90-degree incidence angle. The preferred angles are between 30 and 60 degrees to obtain a good discriminatory signal for Doppler shift.

In Doppler scanners, the received signal is amplified and mixed with the reference frequency (transmitter signal). The demodulated signal is then passed through a series of filters zero-crossing detectors to estimate the deviation from the reference signal. Thus, the Doppler shift representing the flow is measured and displayed against the time. With a single transducer, a pulse-echo format is used for Doppler ultrasound imaging. A spatial pulse width of usually 5–25 cycles is used to achieve a narrow-band frequency response. Depth selection is achieved through electronic gating of the echo time. For a given depth, the round-trip echo time is determined and used to select the correct echo from the selected depth, as all other echoes are rejected in the gating process. The sampling of the echo signal with the selection of a specific depth is accomplished by the operator who manipulates the pulse-repetition frequency (PRF) to be greater than the twice the maximum Doppler frequency shift (following the Nyquist criterion) for accurate measurements. Alternately, two transducers can be used in a continuous mode where one transducer transmits the incident ultrasound waves and the second continuously receives the echoes. Using the demodulator and spectrum analyzer, all similar frequencies from stationary objects are filtered out to extract the Doppler shift information from the returned echoes.

Modern imaging systems convert the Doppler shift into a 2-D image through spatial scanning and mapping of the Doppler frequency shift into color or brightness levels. Figure 7.8 shows a diastolic color Doppler flow convergence in the apical four-chamber view of mitral stenosis.

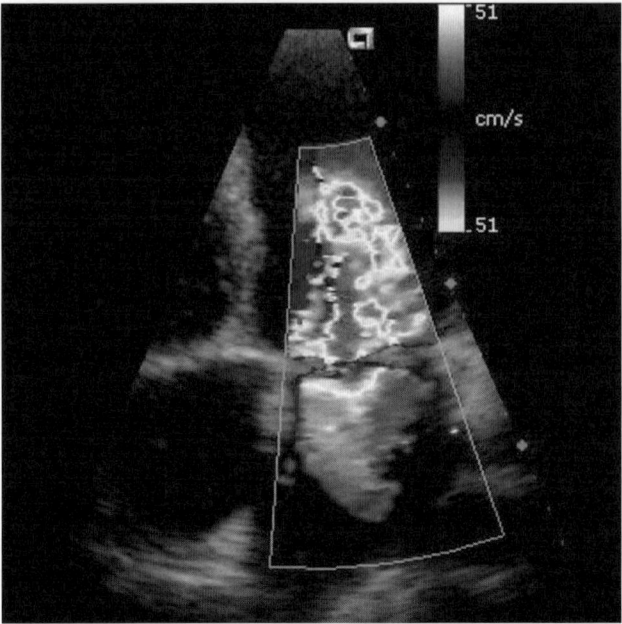

Figure 7.8 A Doppler image of the mitral valve area of a beating heart.

7.11. CONTRAST, SPATIAL RESOLUTION, AND SNR

Contrast in ultrasound images depends on the ability of detection of small differences in acoustic signals for discrimination between the tissue types. Since ultrasound imaging is based on the returned echoes, the contrast is determined by the SNR in detection of weak echoes. Contrast can be improved by increasing the intensity or power of the ultrasound source and also by increasing the PRF, as it allows better lateral resolution and signal averaging. However, any ultrasound imaging system may have limitations on increasing the power level as well as the PRF depending on the piezoelectric crystal, amplifier and mixer/demodulator subsystems, and depth of scanning. Moreover, interferences of multiple echoes from other objects in the turbid biological medium cause considerable noise and artifacts in the received signal (returned echoes).

The spatial resolution in ultrasound images is analyzed in axial and lateral directions. The axial resolution (also called range, longitudinal, or depth resolution) is determined by the spatial discrimination of two separate objects in the direction parallel to the incident ultrasound beam. The depth positions of reflecting surfaces or objects have to be resolved through returned echoes. The minimum separation distance between reflecting surfaces is determined by the half of the spatial pulse width, which is represented by the Q factor. Thus, a narrower pulse width should be used to improve axial resolution. For example, an ultrasound beam at 5 MHz may provide an axial resolution up to 0.3 mm with appropriate electronic subsystems.

A lateral resolution (also called azimuthal resolution) is determined by the ability to discriminate two spatial objects perpendicular to the direction of the incident ultrasound beam. Lateral resolution depends on the diameter of the ultrasound beam. As shown in Figure 7.4, the diameter of an ultrasound beam varies with the distance between the transducer and object. In the near-field (Fresnel region), the best lateral resolution can be considered equal to the radius of the transducer. As the beam enters into the far-field or Fraunhofer region, the lateral resolution worsens with the diverging diameter of the beam. To improve lateral resolution, acoustic lenses can be used to focus the beam and reduce its diameter. It can be noted that in order to reduce the diameter of the beam, the range or focus of the beam has to be sacrificed for a smaller depth. Phased array transducers can be used to achieve variable depths of focus in the lateral direction (5, 7).

In dynamic imaging mode, the PRF is determined by the product of frame rate and number of scan lines per image. Increasing the PRF provides an increased number of scan lines per image for better lateral resolution. However, as mentioned above, the increase in PRF is limited because of the depth of scanning and the frequency response of the associated hardware subsystems.

The SNR of an ultrasound imaging system depends on the differentiation of the meaningful echoes from the noise that may be created by the interferences of multiple echoes from the surrounding objects and also by the system components. The first type of noise, because of interferences of coherent waves in the medium, appears as speckles in the image. The electronics associated with the detection system adds noise to ultrasound images, causing appearances of noisy speckles with granular structures. In addition, the spectral response of the ultrasound transducer and the side lobes also contribute to the noise and clutter in the signal. Increasing the frequency of the ultrasound source increases the attenuation coefficients and lowers the SNR for higher depths of penetration. An acoustic focusing lens improves the SNR within the near-field region, as discussed above, but lowers the SNR outside the focus regions because of sharp divergence in the far-field (Franhaufer region). As discussed above, to improve the SNR of an ultrasound imaging system, the intensity and PRF should be increased. However, an increase in power and PRF may be limited due to the depth of scanning and limitations on the associated hardware.

7.12. EXERCISES

7.1. Describe the fundamental principles of ultrasound imaging that make it capable of tissue characterization.

7.2. For ultrasound imaging at 3 MHz, what will be the wavelength in a soft tissue? Assume that the speed of ultrasound in soft tissue is 1540 m/s.

7.3. Describe what changes will be experienced when an ultrasound wave of 5 MHz will travel through fat and then enter into kidney. Assume the speed of ultrasound in fat and kidney, respectively, is 1450 m/s and 1561 m/s.

7.4. Describe the desired characteristics of an ultrasound transducer.

7.5. If an ultrasound crystal is 1.8 mm thick, considering that the speed of sound in the crystal is 4000 m/s, what is the natural frequency generated by the ultrasound transducer?

7.6. What are the significant factors in determining the contrast of ultrasound images?

7.7. What factors can improve signal-to-noise ratio (SNR) in ultrasound B-mode imaging?

7.8. Describe the M-mode operation for ultrasound imaging.

7.9. What is the Doppler effect and how is it used in ultrasound imaging?

7.10. Consider an ultrasound imaging system at 5 MHz that is used in imaging a blood flow with a velocity of 30 cm/s. If the ultrasound transducer is targeted at blood vessels at 45 degrees, calculate the Doppler shift.

7.11. Can an acoustic lens provide a higher SNR in ultrasound imaging for near-field and far-field regions? Explain your answer.

7.12. What is the limit of axial resolution in the near-field region for a 4 MHz ultrasound beam?

7.13. Display an ultrasound image of a cardiac cavity in MATLAB. Also display an X-ray CT image of the cardiac region. Apply an edge enhancement operation on both images. Can you define structural boundaries in ultrasound image? Explain your answer.

7.14. Display an ultrasound image of a cardiac cavity in MATLAB. Threshold the image using various gray levels of 50, 75, 100, 150, 200, and 225. Do you see any meaning meaningful region from thresholded images? Explain your answer.

7.13. REFERENCES

1. J.T. Bushberg, J.A. Seibert, E.M. Leidholdt, and J.M. Boone, *The Essentials of Medical Imaging*, Williams & Wilkins, Philadelphia, 1994.
2. Z.H. Cho, J.P. Jones, and M. Singh, *Fundamentals of Medical Imaging*, John Wiley & Sons, New York, 1993.
3. P. Fish, *Physics and Instrumentation of Diagnostic Medical Ultrasound*, John Wiley & Sons, Chichester, 1990.
4. P.N.T. Wells, *Biomedical Ultrasonics*, Medical Physics Series, Academic Press, London, 1977.
5. F.W. Kremkau, *Diagnostic Ultrasound Principles and Instrumentation*, Saunders, Philadelphia, 1995.
6. F.W. Kremkau, *Doppler Ultrasound: Principles and Instruments*, Saunders, Philadelphia, 1991.
7. D. Hykes, *Ultrasound Physics and Instrumentation*, Mosby, New York, 1994.
8. E. Konofagou, "Principles of ultrasound imaging," in A.P. Dhawan, H.K. Hunag, and D.S. Kim (Eds), *Principal and Advanced Methods in Medical Imaging and Image Analysis*, World Scientific Press, Singapore, pp. 129–149, 2008.
9. A. Webb, *Introduction to Biomedical Imaging*, IEEE-Wiley Interscience, Hoboken, 2003.

CHAPTER 8

IMAGE RECONSTRUCTION

Medical imaging modalities with instrumentation have been described in Chapters 4–7. As imaging instrumentation and computing capabilities evolved for data acquisition in two and three dimensions, computerized algorithms for multidimensional image reconstruction were developed. The historical perspective of image reconstruction algorithms started with J. Radon (1), who laid the mathematical foundation of image reconstruction from projections in his classic paper that was published in 1917. But the implementation of the Radon transform for reconstructing medical images was only realized in the 1960s. In 1972, G.N. Hounsfield developed the first commercial X-ray computed tomography (X-ray CT) scanner that used a computerized image reconstruction algorithm based on the Radon transform. G.N. Hounsfield and A.M. Cormack jointly received the 1979 Nobel prize for their contributions to the development of CT for radiological applications (2–4).

The classic image reconstruction from projection method based on the Radon transform is popularly known as the backprojection method. The backprojection method has been modified by a number of investigators to incorporate specific data collection schemes and to improve the quality of reconstructed images. Fourier transform and iterative series expansion-based methods have been developed for reconstructing images from projections. With the fast-growing developments in computer technology, advanced image reconstruction algorithms using statistical and estimation methods were developed and implemented for several medical imaging modalities. Recently, wavelet transform and other multiresolution signal processing methods have been applied in multidimensional image reconstruction.

Image reconstruction algorithms use the raw data collected from the imaging scanner to produce images that can provide information about internal physiological structures and associated properties. Reconstructing images from raw data is similar to solving a large number of simultaneous equations with unknown variables as it is mathematically proven that the number of simultaneous equations (analogous to measurements) should be at least equal to the number of unknown variables for determining a unique solution. In medical imaging, images are required to be reconstructed with high spatial resolution from the limited raw data. The number of measurements in the data collected during the scanning of a patient is much smaller than the number of unknown variables (pixels in two-dimensional [2-D] space; voxels in three-dimensional [3-D] space) to be solved for image reconstruction. As is evident from the imaging instrumentation discussed in Chapters 4–7, the measurements in

---

Medical Image Analysis, Second Edition, by Atam P. Dhawan
Copyright © 2011 by the Institute of Electrical and Electronics Engineers, Inc.

the data acquisition process are limited because of the limitations of detector subsystems, imaging geometry, physics of imaging, and patient scanning time. Furthermore, the measurements are degraded due to noise, scattering, geometrical occlusions, and errors in the data acquisition process. Thus, image reconstruction is an ill-posed problem as it is not possible to determine a unique solution from such an underdetermined system. However, advanced mathematical methods and algorithms have been successfully developed to reconstruct reasonably good images that have been proven to be of great value in diagnostic radiology.

8.1. RADON TRANSFORM AND IMAGE RECONSTRUCTION

As described in Chapter 2, the Radon transform defines a projection of an object as a collection of ray integrals. Figure 2.15 shows a line integral that is computed along the parallel arrow lines that are sampled along the p axis and are defined by the angle θ. A set of line integrals or projections can be obtained for different θ angles. A projection, $J_\theta(p)$, is periodic in θ with a period of 2π and is also symmetric.

The Radon transform of an object $f(x, y)$ is expressed as the projection $J_\theta(p)$ and is defined as

$$R\{f(x, y)\} = J_\theta(p) = \int_{-\infty}^{\infty} f(p\cos\theta - q\sin\theta, p\sin\theta + q\cos\theta)\, dq \quad (8.1)$$

where p and q form a rotated coordinate system with an angle θ with respect to the x-y coordinate system such that

$$p = x\cos\theta + y\sin\theta$$
$$q = -x\sin\theta + y\cos\theta$$

and

$$x = p\cos\theta - q\sin\theta$$
$$y = p\sin\theta + q\cos\theta. \quad (8.2)$$

8.1.1 The Central Slice Theorem

The central slice theorem, also called the projection theorem, provides a relationship between the Fourier transform of the object function and the Fourier transform of its Radon transform or projection. Let us continue to assume the object function $f(x, y)$ in two dimensions with one-dimensional (1-D) projections $J_\theta(p)$ defined as the Radon transform of the object function shown in Equation 8.1.

The Fourier transform of the Radon transform of the object function $f(x, y)$ can be written as (5–7)

$$F\{R\{f(x, y)\}\} = F\{J_\theta(p)\} = \int_{-\infty}^{\infty}\int_{-\infty}^{\infty} f(p\cos\theta - q\sin\theta, p\sin\theta + q\cos\theta)e^{-j2\pi\omega p}\, dq\, dp \quad (8.3)$$

where ω represents the frequency component in the Fourier domain.

8.1. RADON TRANSFORM AND IMAGE RECONSTRUCTION

The Fourier transform, $S_\theta(\omega)$ of the projection $J_\theta(p)$ can also be expressed as

$$S_\theta(\omega) = \int_{-\infty}^{\infty} J_\theta(p) e^{-j2\pi\omega p} dp. \tag{8.4}$$

Substituting Equations 8.2 and 8.3 in Equation 8.4, the Fourier transform of the Radon transform of the object function can be written as

$$S_\theta(\omega) = \int_{-\infty}^{\infty}\int_{-\infty}^{\infty} f(x,y) e^{-j2\pi\omega(x\cos\theta + y\sin\theta)} dx\, dy = F(\omega, \theta). \tag{8.5}$$

Equation 8.5 can be considered as the 2-D Fourier transform of the object function $f(x, y)$ and can be represented as $F(u, v)$ with

$$u = \omega\cos\theta$$
$$v = \omega\sin\theta \tag{8.6}$$

where u and v represent frequency components along the x- and y-directions in a rectangular coordinate system.

It should be noted that $S_\theta(\omega)$ represents the Fourier transform of the projection $J_\theta(p)$ that is taken at an angle θ in the space domain with a rotated coordinate system (p, q). The frequency spectrum $S_\theta(\omega)$ is placed along a line or slice at an angle θ in the frequency domain of $F(u, v)$.

As shown in Figure 8.1, if several projections are obtained using different values of the angle θ, their Fourier transform can be computed and placed along the respective radial lines in the frequency domain of the Fourier transform, $F(u, v)$, of the object function $f(x, y)$. Additional projections acquired in the space domain

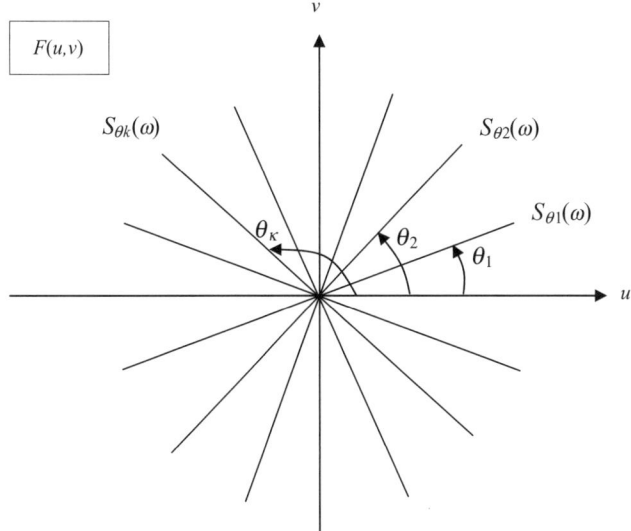

Figure 8.1 The frequency domain of the Fourier transform $F(u, v)$ with the Fourier transforms, $S_\theta(\omega)$ of individual projections $J_\theta(p)$.

provide more spectral information in the frequency domain leading to the entire frequency domain being filled up. Now the object function can be reconstructed using 2-D inverse Fourier transform of the spectrum $F(u, v)$.

8.1.2 Inverse Radon Transform

The forward Radon transform is used to obtain projections of an object function at different viewing angles. Using the central slice theorem, an object function can be reconstructed by taking the inverse Fourier transform of the spectral information in the frequency domain that is assembled with the Fourier transform of the individual projections. Thus, the reconstructed object function, $\hat{f}(x, y)$, can be obtained by taking the 2-D inverse Fourier transform of $f(u, v)$ as

$$\hat{f}(x, y) = F^{-1}\{F(u, v)\} = \int_{-\infty}^{\infty}\int_{-\infty}^{\infty} F(u, v) e^{j2\pi(xu+vy)} du\, dv \tag{8.7}$$

Representing $\hat{f}(x, y)$ in the polar coordinate system as $\hat{f}(r, \theta)$, Equation 8.7 can be rewritten with the change of variables as

$$\hat{f}(r, \theta) = \int_{0}^{\pi}\int_{-\infty}^{\infty} F(\omega, \theta) e^{j2\pi w(x\cos\theta+y\sin\theta)} |\omega|\, d\omega\, d\theta. \tag{8.8}$$

In Equation 8.8, the frequency variable ω appears because of the Jacobian due to change of variables. Replacing $F(\omega, \theta)$ with $S_\theta(\omega)$, the reconstructed image $\hat{f}(x, y)$, can be expressed as the back-projected integral (sum) of the modified projections $J_\theta^*(p')$ as

$$\hat{f}(r, \theta) = \int_{0}^{\pi}\int_{-\infty}^{\infty} |\omega| S_\theta(\omega) e^{j2\pi\omega(x\cos\theta+y\sin\theta)} d\omega\, d\theta$$

$$= \int_{0}^{\pi} J_\theta^*(p') d\theta$$

where

$$J_\theta^*(p') = \int_{-\infty}^{\infty} |\omega| S_\theta(\omega) e^{j2\pi\omega(x\cos\theta+y\sin\theta)} d\omega. \tag{8.9}$$

8.1.3 Backprojection Method

Although the object function can be reconstructed using the inverse Fourier transform of the spectral information of the frequency domain $F(u, v)$ obtained using the central slice theorem, an easier implementation of Equation 8.9 can be obtained by its realization through the modified projections, $J_\theta^*(p')$. This realization leads to the convolution–backprojection, also known as filtered backprojection method for image reconstruction from projections.

The modified projection $J_\theta^*(p')$ can be expressed in terms of a convolution of

8.1. RADON TRANSFORM AND IMAGE RECONSTRUCTION

$$J_\theta^*(p') = \int_{-\infty}^{\infty} |\omega| \, S_\theta(\omega) e^{j2\pi\omega(x\cos\theta + y\sin\theta)} \, d\omega$$

$$= \int_{-\infty}^{\infty} |\omega| \, S_\theta(\omega) e^{j2\pi\omega p} \, d\omega$$

$$= F^{-1}\{|\omega| \, S_\theta(\omega)\}$$

$$= F^{-1}\{|\omega|\} \otimes J_\theta(p) \tag{8.10}$$

where $\otimes$ represents the convolution operator.

Equation 8.10 presents some interesting challenges for implementation. The integration over the spatial frequency variable ω should be carried out from $-\infty$ to ∞. But in practice the projections are considered to be bandlimited. This means that any spectral energy beyond a spatial frequency, say Ω, must be ignored. With Equations 8.9 and 8.10, it can be shown that the reconstruction function or image, $\hat{f}(x, y)$ can be computed as

$$\hat{f}(x, y) = \frac{1}{\pi} \int_0^\pi d\theta \int_{-\infty}^\infty dp' \, J_\theta(p') h(p - p') \tag{8.11}$$

where $h(p)$ is a filter function that is convolved with the projection function.

Ramachandran and Lakshiminarayanan (7) computed the filter function $h(p)$ strictly from Equation 8.10 in the Fourier domain as

$$H_{R-L} = \begin{cases} |\omega| & \text{if } |\omega| \le \Omega \\ 0 & \text{otherwise} \end{cases} \tag{8.12}$$

where H_{R-L} is the Fourier transform of the filter kernel function $h_{R-L}(p)$ in the spatial domain and is bandlimited.

In general, $H(\omega)$, a bandlimited filter function in the frequency domain (Fig. 8.2) can be expressed as

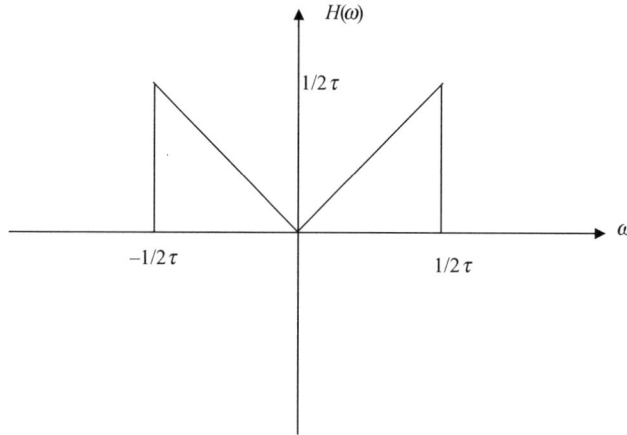

Figure 8.2 A bandlimited filter function $H(\omega)$.

$$H(\omega) = |\omega| B(\omega)$$

where $B(\omega)$ denotes the bandlimiting function

$$B(\omega) = \begin{cases} 1 & \text{if } |\omega| \leq \Omega \\ 0 & \text{otherwise} \end{cases}. \quad (8.13)$$

For the convolution operation with the projection function in the spatial domain (Eqs. 8.9 and 8.10), the filter kernel function, $H(\omega)$ can be obtained from $h(p)$ by taking the inverse Fourier transform as

$$h(p) = \int_{-\infty}^{\infty} H(\omega) e^{j2\pi\omega p} \, d\omega. \quad (8.14)$$

If the projections are sampled with a time interval of τ, the projections can be represented as $J_\theta(k\tau)$ where k is an integer. Using the sampling theorem and the bandlimited constraint, all spatial frequency components beyond Ω are ignored such that

$$\Omega = \frac{1}{2\tau}. \quad (8.15)$$

For the bandlimited projections with a sampling interval of t, Equation 8.14 can be expressed with some simplification as

$$h(p) = \frac{1}{2\tau^2} \frac{\sin(\pi p/\tau)}{\pi p/\tau} - \frac{1}{4\tau^2} \left(\frac{\sin(\pi p/2\tau)}{\pi p/2\tau} \right)^2. \quad (8.16)$$

Thus, the modified projection $J_\theta^*(p')$ and the reconstruction image can be computed as

$$J_\theta^*(p') = \int_{-\infty}^{\infty} J_\theta(p') h(p - p') \, dp'$$

$$\hat{f}(x, y) = \frac{\pi}{L} \sum_{i=1}^{L} J_{\theta_i}(p') \quad (8.17)$$

where L is the total number of projections acquired during the imaging process at viewing angles θ_i; for $i = 1, \ldots, L$.

The quality of the reconstructed image depends heavily on the number of projections and the spatial sampling interval of the acquired projection. For better quality images to be reconstructed, it is essential to acquire a large number of projections covering the entire range of viewing angles around the object. Higher resolution images with fine details can only be reconstructed if the projections are acquired with a high spatial sampling rate satisfying the basic principle of the sampling theorem. If the raw projection data is acquired at a sampling rate lower than the Nyquist sampling rate, aliasing artifacts would occur in the reconstructed image because of the overlapping spectra in the frequency domain. The fine details in the reconstructed images represent high-frequency components. The maximum frequency component that can be reconstructed in the image is thus limited by the

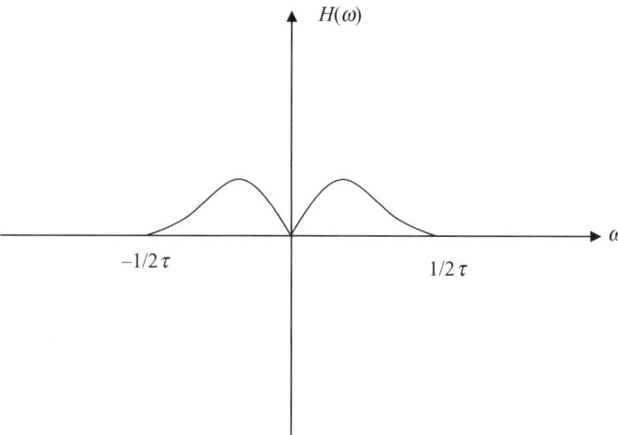

Figure 8.3 A Hamming window based filter kernel function in the frequency domain.

detector size and the scanning procedure used in the acquisition of raw projection data. To reconstruct images of higher resolution and quality, the detector size should be small. On the other hand, the projection data may suffer from poor signal-to-noise ratio (SNR) if there is not sufficient number of photons collected by the detector due to its smaller size.

There are several variations in the design of the filter function $H(\omega)$ investigated in the literature. The acquired projection data is discrete in the spatial domain. To implement the convolution–backprojection method in the spatial domain, the filter function has to be realized as discrete in the spatial domain. The major problem of the Ramachandaran–Lakshiminarayanan filter is that it has sharp cutoffs in the frequency domain at $\omega = 1/2\tau$ and $\omega = -1/2\tau$ as shown in Figure 8.2. The sharp cutoff-based function provides sinc functions for the filter in the spatial domain as shown in Equation 8.16, causing modulated ringing artifacts in the reconstructed image. To avoid such artifacts, the filter function must have smooth cutoffs such as those obtained from Hamming window function. A bandlimited generalized Hamming window can be represented as

$$H_{Hamming}(\omega) = |\omega|[\alpha + (1-\alpha)\cos(2\pi\omega\tau)]B(\omega) \quad \text{for } 0 \leq \alpha \leq 1 \quad (8.18)$$

where the parameter α can be adjusted to provide appropriate characteristic shape of the function.

The Hamming window-based filter kernel function provides smoother cutoffs as shown in Figure 8.3. The spatial domain functions for the Ramachandaran–Lakshiminarayanan and Hamming window-based filter kernels (5–7) are shown for comparison in Figure 8.4. It is apparent from Figure 8.4 that the Hamming window-based convolution function provides smoother function in the spatial domain that reduces the ringing artifacts and improves SNR in the reconstructed image. Other smoothing functions can be used to reduce ringing artifacts and improve the quality of the reconstructed image.

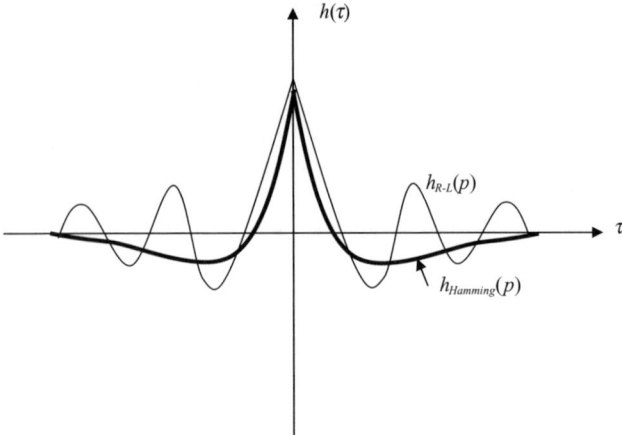

Figure 8.4 A comparison of the $h_{Ham\ min\ g}(p)$ and $h_{R-L}(p)$ convolution functions in the spatial domain.

8.2. ITERATIVE ALGEBRAIC RECONSTRUCTION METHODS

Although the filtered backprojection method is commonly used for medical image reconstruction, iterative methods are used for image reconstruction as an alternative. The iterative reconstruction methods are based on optimization strategies incorporating specific constraints about the object domain and the reconstruction process. Algebraic reconstruction techniques (ART) are popular algorithms used in iterative image reconstruction. In the algebraic reconstruction methods, the raw projection data from the scanner is distributed over a prespecified image reconstruction grid such that the error between the computed projections from the reconstructed image and the actual acquired projections is minimized. Such methods provide a mechanism to incorporate additional specific optimization criteria such as smoothing and entropy maximization in the reconstruction process to improve the image quality and SNR. The algebraic reconstruction methods are based on the series expansion representation of a function and were used by Gordon and Herman for medical image reconstruction (5, 8).

Let us assume a 2-D image reconstruction grid of N pixels as shown in Figure 8.5. Let us define p_i representing the projection data as a set of ray sums that are collected by M scanning rays passing through the image at specific angles as shown in Figure 8.5. Let f_j be the value of jth pixel of the image that is weighted by $w_{i,j}$ to meet the projection measurements. Thus, the ray sum, p_i, in the projection data can be expressed as

$$p_i = \sum_{j=1}^{N} w_{i,j} f_j \quad \text{for } i = 1, \ldots, M. \tag{8.19}$$

Equation 8.19 provides M equations of N unknown variables to be determined. The weight $w_{i,j}$ represents the contribution of the pixel value in determining the ray sum

8.2. ITERATIVE ALGEBRAIC RECONSTRUCTION METHODS

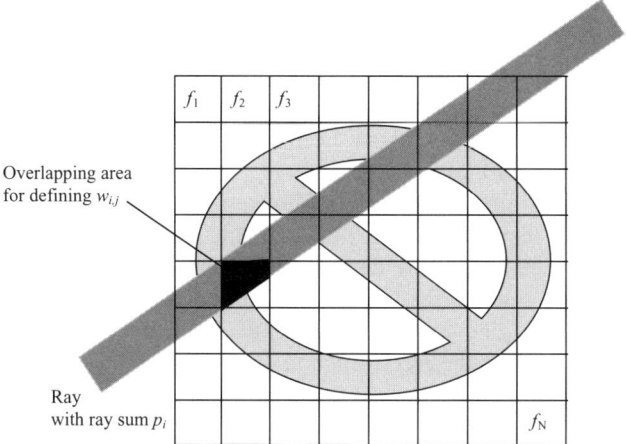

Figure 8.5 Reconstruction grid with a ray defining the ray sum for ART.

and can be determined by geometrical consideration as the ratio of the area overlapping with the scanning ray to the total area of the pixel. The problem of determining f_j for image reconstruction can be solved iteratively using the ART algorithm. Alternately, it can be solved through matrix inversion since the measured projection data p_i is known. The set of equations can also be solved using dynamic programming methods (5).

In algebraic reconstruction methods, each pixel is assigned a predetermined value such as the average of the raw projection data per pixel to start the iterative process. Any time during the reconstruction process, a computed ray sum from the image under reconstruction is obtained by passing a ray as shown in Figure 8.5. In each iteration, an error between the measured projection ray sum and the computed ray sum is evaluated and distributed on the corresponding pixels in a weighted manner. The correction to the pixel values can be obtained in an additive or multiplicative manner; that is, the correction value is either added to the current pixel value or multiplied with it to obtain the next value. The iterative process continues until the error between the measured and computed ray sums is minimized or meets a prespecified criterion. The f_j values from the last iteration provide the final reconstructed image.

Let q_j^k be the computed ray sum in the kth iteration that is projected over the reconstruction grid in the next iteration. The iterative procedure can then be expressed as

$$q_i^k = \sum_{l=1}^{N} f_l^{k-1} w_{i,l} \quad \text{for all } i = 1, \ldots, M$$

$$f_j^{k+1} = f_j^k + \left[\frac{p_i - q_i^k}{\sum_{l=1}^{N} w_{i,l}^2} \right] w_{i,j}. \tag{8.20}$$

Gordon (8) used an easier way to avoid large computation of the weight matrix by replacing the weight by 1 or 0. If the center of the pixel passes through the ray, the corresponding weight is assigned as 1, otherwise 0. This simplification provides an efficient implementation of the algorithm and is known as additive ART. Other versions of ART including multiplicative ART have been developed to improve the reconstruction efficacy and quality (5, 8).

The iterative ART methods offer an attractive alternative to the filtered backprojection method because of their abilities to deal with the noise and random fluctuations in the projection data caused by detector inefficiency and scattering. These methods are particularly suitable for limited view image reconstruction as more constraints defining the imaging geometry and prior information about the object can easily be incorporated into the reconstruction process.

8.3. ESTIMATION METHODS

Although the filtered backprojection methods are most commonly used in medical imaging, in practice, a significant number of approaches using statistical estimation methods have been investigated for image reconstruction for transmission as well as emission computed tomography (ECT). These methods assume a certain distribution of the measured photons and then find the parameters for attenuation function (in the case of transmission scans such as X-ray CT) or emitter density (in the case of emission scans such as PET).

The photon detection statistics of a detector is usually characterized by Poisson distribution. Let us define a measurement vector $\vec{J} = [J_1, J_2, \ldots, J_N]$ with J_i to be the random variable representing the number of photons collected by the detector for the ith ray such that (9)

$$E[J_i] = m_i e^{-\int_L \mu(x,y,z)dl} \quad \text{for } i = 1, 2, \ldots, N \quad (8.21)$$

where L defines the ray along which the photons with monochromatic energy have been attenuated with the attenuation coefficients denoted by μs milliseconds, and m_i is the mean number of photons collected by the detector for the ith ray position. Also, in the above formulation, the noise, scattering, and random coincidence effects are ignored.

The attenuation parameter vector $\vec{\mu}$ can be expressed in terms of a series expansion as a weighted sum of individual attenuation coefficients of corresponding pixels (for 2-D reconstruction) or voxels (for 3-D reconstruction). If the parameter vector $\vec{\mu}$ has N_p number of individual elements (pixels or voxels), it can be represented as

$$\vec{\mu} = \sum_{j=1}^{N_p} \mu_j w_j \quad (8.22)$$

where w_j is the basis function that is the weight associated with the individual μ_j belonging to the corresponding pixel or voxel.

One simple solution to obtain w_j is to assign it a value of 1 if the ray contributing to the corresponding photon measurement vector passes through the pixel (or voxel) and 0 otherwise. It can be shown that a line integral or ray sum for ith ray is given by

$$\int_{L_i} \mu(x, y, z)\, dl = \sum_{k=1}^{N_p} a_{ik} \mu_k \qquad (8.23)$$

where $a_{ik} = \int_{L_i} w_k(\vec{x})$ with $\vec{x}$ representing the position vector for (x, y, z) coordinate system.

The weight matrix $A = \{a_{ik}\}$ is defined to rewrite the measurement vector as

$$J_i(\vec{\mu}) = m_i e^{-[A\vec{\mu}]_i} \qquad (8.24)$$

where $[A\vec{\mu}]_i = \sum_{k=1}^{N_p} a_{ik} \mu_k$.

The reconstruction problem is to estimate $\vec{\mu}$ from a measured set of detector counts realizing the random variable $\vec{J}$. The maximum likelihood (ML) estimate can be expressed as (9–11)

$$\hat{\vec{\mu}} = \arg\max_{\vec{\mu} \geq \vec{0}} L(\vec{\mu})$$

$$L(\vec{\mu}) = \log P[\vec{J} = \vec{j}; \vec{\mu}] \qquad (8.25)$$

where $L(\vec{\mu})$ is the likelihood function defined as the logarithmic of the probability function $P[\vec{J} = \vec{j}; \vec{\mu}]$. The ML reconstruction methods are developed to obtain an estimate of the parameter vector $\vec{\mu}$ that maximizes the probability of observing the measured data (photon counts).

Using the Poisson distribution model for the photon counts, the measurement joint probability function $P[\vec{J} = \vec{j}; \vec{\mu}]$ can be expressed as

$$P[\vec{J} = \vec{j}; \vec{\mu}] = \prod_{i=1}^{N} P[J_i = j_i; \vec{\mu}] = \prod_{i=1}^{N} \frac{e^{-j_i(\mu)} [j_i(\mu)]^{j_i}}{j_i!}. \qquad (8.26)$$

If the measurements are obtained independently through defining ray sums, the log likelihood function can be expressed combining Equations 8.21, 8.25, and 8.26 as

$$L(\vec{\mu}) = \sum_{i=1}^{N} h_i([A\vec{\mu}]_i) \qquad (8.27)$$

where $h_i(l) = j_i \log(m_i e^{-l}) - m_i e^{-l}$.

Let us consider an additive non-negative function r_i representing the background photon count for the ith detector due to the scattering and random coincidences; the likelihood function can then be expressed as (9)

$$L(\vec{\mu}) = \sum_{i=1}^{N} h_i([A\vec{\mu}]_i) \qquad (8.28)$$

where $h_i(l) = j_i \log(m_i e^{-l} + r_i) - (m_i e^{-l} + r_i)$.

Several algorithms have been investigated in the literature to obtain an estimate of the parameter vector that maximizes the log likelihood function given in Equation 8.27. However, it is unlikely that there is a unique solution to this problem. There may be several solutions of the parameter vector that can maximize the likelihood function. All solutions may not be appropriate or even feasible for image

CHAPTER 8 IMAGE RECONSTRUCTION

reconstruction. To improve quality of reconstructed images, a number of methods imposing additional constraints such as smoothness are applied by incorporating the penalty functions in the optimization process. Several iterative optimization processes incorporating roughness penalty function for the neighborhood values of the estimated parameter vector have been investigated in the literature (9–11).

Let us represent a general roughness penalty function $R(\mu)$ (9, 10) such that

$$R(\bar{\mu}) = \sum_{k=1}^{K} \psi([\mathbf{C}\bar{\mu}]_k) \qquad (8.29)$$

where $[\mathbf{C}\bar{\mu}]_k = \sum_{l=1}^{N_p} c_{kl}\mu_l$

where ψ_k are potential functions working as a norm on the smoothness constraints $C\mu \approx 0$ and K is the number of such constraints. The matrix $\mathbf{C}$ is a $K \times N_p$ penalty matrix. It should be noted that ψ_k are convex, symmetric, non-negative, and differentiable functions (9). A potential choice for a quadratic penalty function could be by defining $\psi_k(t) = w_k t^2/2$ with non-negative weights, that is, $w_k \geq 0$. Thus, the roughness penalty function $R(\bar{\mu})$ is given by

$$R(\bar{\mu}) = \sum_{k=1}^{K} w_k \frac{1}{2}([\mathbf{C}\bar{\mu}]_k)^2. \qquad (8.30)$$

The objective function for optimization using the penalized ML approach can now be revised as

$$\widehat{\bar{\mu}} = \arg\max \Phi(\bar{\mu}) \qquad (8.31)$$

where $\Phi(\bar{\mu}) = L(\bar{\mu}) - \beta R(\bar{\mu})$.

The parameter β controls the level of smoothness in the final reconstructed image.

Several methods for obtaining the above ML estimate have been investigated in the literature. These optimization methods include expectation maximization (EM), complex conjugate gradient, gradient descent optimization, grouped coordinated ascent, fast gradient-based Bayesian reconstruction, and ordered-subsets algorithms (12–21). Such iterative algorithms have been applied to obtain a solution for the parameter vector for reconstructing an image from both transmission and emission scans.

In general, the penalized function $\Phi(\bar{\mu})$ is quite complex and difficult to optimize. De Pierro (22) used an optimization transfer method defining a surrogate function $\phi(\bar{\mu}; \bar{\mu}^{(n)})$ that is easier to optimize with an estimate of attenuation vector after the nth iteration represented by $\bar{\mu}^{(n)}$. There are many choices for surrogate functions. For example, a parabola surrogate function with an optimal curvature to ensure fast optimization process can be designed (9, 10). A quadratic surrogate function may be defined as

$$q(l; l_i^{(n)}) \equiv h(l_i^{(n)}) + \dot{h}(l_i^{(n)})(l - l_i^{(n)}) - \frac{c}{2}(l - l_i^{(n)})^2$$

$$\text{for} \quad c \geq 0 \quad \text{and} \quad l_i^{(n)} = [A\bar{\mu}]_i \qquad (8.32)$$

The variable $l_i^{(n)}$ is the ith line integral through the estimated attenuation map at the nth iteration.

The estimation problem can then be rewritten involving the surrogate function in each iteration as

$$\phi(\vec{\mu}; \vec{\mu}^{(n)}) \equiv Q(\vec{\mu}; \vec{\mu}^{(n)}) - \beta R(\vec{\mu}) \tag{8.33}$$

where $Q(\vec{\mu}; \vec{\mu}^{(n)})$ is the conditional expectation of log-likelihood function in the nth iteration.

The function $Q(\vec{\mu}; \vec{\mu}^{(n)})$ can be provided (9) as

$$Q(\vec{\mu}; \vec{\mu}^{(n)}) = \sum_{k=1}^{N_p} Q_k(\mu_k; \vec{\mu}^{(n)})$$

where

$$Q_k(\mu_k; \vec{\mu}^{(n)}) = \sum_{i=1}^{N} \overline{N}_{ik}^{(n)} \log(e^{-a_{ik}\mu_k}) + (\overline{M}_{ik}^{(n)} - \overline{N}_{ik}^{(n)}) \log(1 - e^{-a_{ik}\mu_k})$$

$$\overline{N}_{ik}^{(n)} \equiv E[J_{il}/J_i = j_i; \vec{\mu}^{(n)}]|_{l:k_i,l=j}$$

$$\overline{M}_{ik}^{(n)} \equiv E[J_{il-1}/J_i = j_i; \vec{\mu}^{(n)}]|_{l:k_i,l=j} \tag{8.34}$$

Now, the EM algorithm can be expressed as the implementation of the following steps in each iteration until convergence:

1. E-Step:

$$\text{Find } Q(\vec{\mu}; \vec{\mu}^{(n)}) \text{ and } \phi(\vec{\mu}; \vec{\mu}^{(n)})$$

2. M-Step:

$$\vec{\mu}^{(n+1)} = \arg\max_{\vec{\mu}} \phi(\vec{\mu}; \vec{\mu}^{(n)}) \tag{8.35}$$

By combining these steps with the surrogate function, it can be shown (9) that the iterative ML–EM estimate for the transmission scans can be given as

$$\mu_k^{(n+1)} = \frac{\sum_{i=1}^{N}(\overline{M}_{ik}^{(n)} - \overline{N}_{ik}^{(n)})}{\frac{1}{2}\sum_{i=1}^{N} a_{ik}(\overline{M}_{ik}^{(n)} + \overline{N}_{ik}^{(n)})} \tag{8.36}$$

8.4. FOURIER RECONSTRUCTION METHODS

As described above, the central slice theorem provides a relationship between the projection acquired in the rotated coordinate system and the Fourier domain of the object. For 2-D image reconstruction, the 1-D Fourier transform of the projection acquired at an angle θ belongs to the corresponding radial line at the same angle in the 2-D Fourier transform (represented in the polar coordinate system) of the object. If a sufficient number of projections are obtained, their respective Fourier transforms can be placed in the frequency domain as shown in Figure 8.1. This 2-D representation of the frequency information usually requires a great deal of interpolation with the change from polar to Cartesian coordinate systems. This is a necessary and computationally expensive step to fill the frequency space evenly to avoid artifacts in the reconstructed images. To reconstruct the image in the spatial domain, a 2-D inverse Fourier transform is applied to this interpolated information in the frequency domain.

The choice of interpolation function is critical in the direct Fourier reconstruction methods. Recently, sinc function-based gridding algorithms for fast Fourier reconstruction have been investigated (23, 24). The Fourier reconstruction method using the central slice theorem resamples the frequency domain information from a polar to a Cartesian grid. Walden used Shannon sampling theorem for developing sinc function-based interpolation method for the bandlimited functions in the radial direction. The interpolation in the angular direction was done with standard methods such as polynomial interpolation (25).

8.5. IMAGE RECONSTRUCTION IN MEDICAL IMAGING MODALITIES

To reconstruct images in a specific medical imaging modality, it is necessary to consider the data collection process. Filtered backprojection methods are ideal for transmission scans such as X-ray CT but do not provide a theoretically sound basis for image reconstruction for ECT. The probabilistic nature of the emission process is well suited for statistical estimation method-based image reconstruction techniques. However, the estimation-based image reconstruction methods are relatively complex and computationally expensive. Noise and detector variability cause additional problems in image reconstruction with respect to unique convergence of iterative estimation-based image reconstruction methods. Because of these difficulties, filtered backprojection methods have been modified for emission imaging and are commonly used for practical image reconstruction in single photon emission computed tomography (SPECT) and positron emission tomography (PET). However, new ML and EM approaches are attractive, provide good results, and are expected to take a more prominent role in practical image reconstruction.

Specific image reconstruction methods for medical imaging modalities are described in the following subsections.

8.5.1 Image Reconstruction in X-Ray CT

The filtered backprojection method is most commonly used in X-ray CT for image reconstruction. The method described above essentially deals with the projections obtained in parallel-beam geometry. However, recent scanners use a divergent 2-D or 3-D beam for imaging. Thus, the data obtained from the divergent beams have to be resorted before the filtered backprojection method developed for parallel projections is applied. It should be noted that each ray in the divergent beam can be reorganized in a specific projection in the parallel-beam geometry. Figure 8.6 shows a 2-D divergent beam with the angular step γ and the radial distance D between the

8.5. IMAGE RECONSTRUCTION IN MEDICAL IMAGING MODALITIES

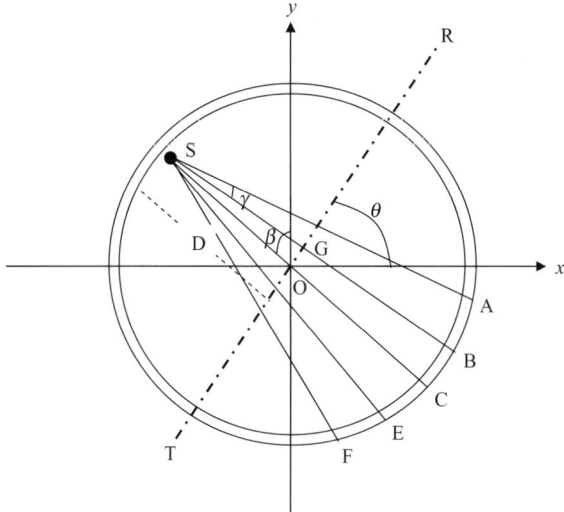

Figure 8.6 A 2-D divergent beam geometry.

source and the origin. This geometry is well suited for fourth-generation CT scanners in which the detectors are placed along circular ring(s).

Let $K_\beta(\gamma)$ represent a fan projection from the divergent beam where β is the angle that the source makes with its central reference axis and γ indicates the location of the ray as shown in Figure 8.6. The objective of the resorting algorithm is to convert fan projections $K_\beta(\gamma)$ into the parallel-beam projection representation $J_\theta(p)$ as defined earlier in this chapter. In Figure 8.6, a plane R-T is shown at an angle θ over which a parallel projection $J_\theta(p)$ is computed using the rotated coordinate system. Considering the ray SB intersecting the parallel projection plane R-T at G, it can be noted that

$$\theta = \beta + \gamma \quad \text{and} \quad OG = p = D\sin\gamma. \tag{8.37}$$

The fan projections $K_\beta(\gamma)$ can be sorted into $K'_\beta(\gamma)$ corresponding to the parallel-beam geometry suitable for implementation of the filtered backprojection method. The sorting relationship for all source positions denoted by β_i can be expressed as

$$K'_{\beta_i}(\gamma) = K_{\beta_i}(\gamma) D\cos\gamma. \tag{8.38}$$

For image reconstruction, $K'_{\beta_i}(\gamma)$ is convolved with the filter function $h(\gamma)$ to provide filtered projections $Q_{\beta_i}(\gamma)$ that are backprojected as

$$Q_{\beta_i}(\gamma) = K'_{\beta_i}(\gamma) \otimes h(\gamma)$$

$$f(x, y) = \Delta\beta \sum_{i=1}^{N} \frac{1}{L^2(x, y; \beta_i)} Q_{\beta_i}(\gamma') \tag{8.39}$$

where N is the total number of source positions, $L\gamma'$ is the angle of the divergent beam ray passing through the point (x, y), and L is the distance between the source and the point (x, y) for the source position β_i.

Recently, cone-beam geometry has been investigated for CT imaging and image reconstruction. A cone beam is a 3-D divergent beam to scan an entire or partial volume of a 3-D object. Cone-beam reconstruction method is basically derived from fan-beam geometry with the additional third dimension. However, the mathematical methods for image reconstruction from cone-beam data become complicated, requiring heuristics to deal with the uncertainties of the data mapping and interpolation issues (26). Also, a direct backprojection algorithm of 3-D Radon transform can be found in Reference (27). In this method, the 3-D Radon transform-based backprojection operation is recursively decomposed using a hierarchical approach.

8.5.2 Image Reconstruction in Nuclear Emission Computed Tomography: SPECT and PET

Although the basic principles of image reconstruction in ECT are the same as X-ray CT, there is an important difference in these two modalities regarding the parameter to be reconstructed. The objective of image reconstruction in X-ray CT is to estimate the attenuation coefficient map from the projection data while scattering is usually ignored. In case of image reconstruction in SPECT or PET, the basic objective is to reconstruct the source emission map within the object from the statistical distribution of photons that have gone through attenuation within the object but detected outside the object. In X-ray CT, the source statistics are known with a single unknown parameter of attenuation coefficients. In ECT (SPECT and PET), both source statistics and attenuation coefficient parameters are unknown. Since the distribution of the emission source is to be reconstructed, the attenuation coefficient parameter has to be assumed or estimated. Incorporation of attenuation information in the reconstruction process is called the attenuation correction. Reconstructed images without adequate attenuation corrections are noisy and poor in image quality. There are several methods for attenuation correction used in SPECT image reconstruction (28–32).

In real cases, the attenuation coefficients are nonuniformly distributed within the object. In cases where attenuation coefficients can be assumed to be constant within the object, the attenuation effect can be compensated by taking the arithmetic or geometric mean of the photon counts from a pair of detectors placed in opposite directions (30). Such methods are very efficient in preprocessing the data for attenuation compensation before the filtered backprojection algorithm is applied. However, they provide acceptable results only in low-resolution imaging applications such as full-body imaging. For specific organ imaging, a transmission scan is done to estimate the attenuation coefficient parameter, which is then used in the reconstruction process.

The transmission scans in SPECT for computing the attenuation coefficient parameter usually suffer from low photon statistics and scattering effects. Although filtered backprojection methods are applied with some modification to reconstruct transmission images in SPECT because of computational efficiency, the iterative ML estimation-based algorithms have provided better results (17–19). These algorithms can be used to estimate the attenuation coefficient parameter from the transmission scan separately or in conjunction with the iterative statistical algorithms for estimation of source distribution for image reconstruction (19).

The current practice in SPECT and PET imaging is to obtain separate transmission scans to compute attenuation maps. However, attenuation maps could be obtained directly from the emission scans by applying the consistency conditions using the projection operator (31, 32).

8.5.2.1 A General Approach to ML–EM Algorithms

The ML-based reconstruction algorithms such as ML–EM find an estimate of the photon emission distribution such that its projections are as close as possible to the measured projection data. A general ML–EM algorithm for ECT is described below (12–14).

Let us assume that the object to be reconstructed has an emission density function $\lambda(x, y, z) = \bar{\lambda} = [\lambda_1, \lambda_2, \ldots, \lambda_B]^t$ with a Poisson process over a matrix of B spatially distributed boxes in the object space or pixels in the reconstruction space. The emitted photons (in case of SPECT) or photon pairs (in case of PET) are detected by the detectors with the measurement vector $\bar{J} = [J_1, J_2, \ldots, J_D]^t$ with D measurements. The problem is then to estimate $\lambda(b)$; $b = 1, \ldots, B$ from the measurement vector.

Each emission in box b is detected by the detector d (SPECT) or the detector tube d (PET) with a probability $p(b, d) = P(\text{detection in } d \text{ for a photon emitted in } b)$. The transition matrix $p(b, d)$ is derived from the geometry of the detector array and the object or reconstruction space.

Let $j(b, d)$ denote the number of emissions in box b detected in the detector or detector tube d. These are independent Poisson variables with the expected value $E[j(b, d)] = \bar{\lambda}(b, d) = \lambda(b)p(b, d)$.

The likelihood function (13) is defined as

$$L(\lambda) = P(\bar{j} \mid \bar{\lambda}) = \sum_A \prod_{\substack{b=1,\ldots,B \\ d=1,\ldots,D}} e^{-\bar{\lambda}(b,d)} \frac{\bar{\lambda}(b, d)^{j(b,d)}}{j(b, d)!} \qquad (8.40)$$

where the sum is over all possible detector arrays A of $j(b, d)$.

It can be shown that $L(\lambda)$ is concave (13). An iterative scheme based on the EM algorithm can be used to maximize $L(\lambda)$. The algorithm starts with an initial guess $\lambda^0(b)$ and then, in each iteration, a new estimate $\hat{\lambda}^{new}(b)$ is computed from $\hat{\lambda}^{old}(b)$, the current estimate of $\lambda(b)$ by

$$\hat{\lambda}^{new}(b) = \hat{\lambda}^{old}(b) \sum_{d=1}^{D} \frac{j(d)p(b, d)}{\sum_{b'=1}^{B} \hat{\lambda}^{old}(b')p(b', d)}; \quad b = 1, \ldots, B. \qquad (8.41)$$

The general convergence of the above ML–EM algorithm is quite slow and sensitive to the noise in the iteration process. As described above, the ML reconstruction process in emission imaging is an ill-posed problem and can provide a number of solutions fitting the projection data. Some of these solutions are not appropriate and cause large variations when the iteration process continues. Regularization methods such as penalized likelihood estimation, weighted least squares, ordered subsets, and Bayesian estimation algorithms have been applied to obtain a better reconstruction

(19–21). A multigrid EM reconstruction algorithm to improve the efficiency and quality of image reconstruction was investigated with the multiresolution approach using the standard interpolation functions and wavelets (33, 34).

8.5.2.2 A Multigrid EM Algorithm A multigrid expectation maximization (MGEM) algorithm has been applied to the problem of image reconstruction in PET (33). The MGEM algorithm uses the ML–EM method on a set of reconstruction grids with different resolutions. The wavelet-based multiresolution EM algorithm uses wavelet transform for the transition criterion for switching the resolution level. A wavelet spline interpolation method is used to project intermediate reconstructions from a specific grid level to the next finer grid (34).

Let us assume there are a number of grids, G^k, where $k = 1, \ldots, K$ represents the same reconstruction space at different resolutions. G^0 is the coarsest grid while G^K is the finest resolution grid. The reconstruction pyramid consists of square grids of size S^k, $k = 1, \ldots, K$, such that the ratio, $S^{k+1}:S^k = 1:2$. The maximum frequency, f^k, of the image on grid G^k is given by $1/2S^k$, which is twice the maximum frequency that can be represented by G^{k-1}. By using the hierarchical structure of the reconstruction pyramid, the low-frequency components of the finest resolution are recovered quickly at the coarser grids. The problem of slow convergence of the single-grid EM algorithm can then be solved by appropriate utilization of different grid sizes. The low-frequency components are recovered first, using the coarser grids, and then the high-frequency components are recovered by projecting the solutions onto finer grids and reconstructing using the single-grid EM algorithm. Since coarser grid solutions can be found much faster, the MGEM algorithm is computationally much more efficient. Also, some a priori information can be incorporated into the initialization step to reduce the pattern dependency of the EM algorithm. A flow diagram of the MGEM algorithm is shown in Figure 8.7.

The wavelet based multiresolution expected maximization (WMREM) algorithm performs a wavelet based-decomposition of the reconstructed image at each iteration and the energy of the high-high-frequency band of the wavelet decomposition provides the transition criterion to switch to the next grid level. The energy in the high-high-frequency band represents the high-frequency content of the image at that grid level. The grid level is switched when the energy in this band ceases to increase. The switching of the grid levels is continued until a grid level finer than the desired resolution is reached. This is done in order to retrieve the high-frequency components of the desired grid resolution, which are the low frequency components of a grid level finer than the desired grid resolution. The low-low-frequency component of the wavelet decomposition of the reconstructed image is the final image at the desired grid level.

Wavelet-based interpolation methods have been used for several applications (35–39). For the class of smooth functions used in regularization, the ideal basis for transformation would be both spatially and spectrally localized and fast to compute. The desire for spectral localization stems from the fact that the projection of a system onto a spectrally localized basis tends to produce a well-conditioned system. The spatial localization requirement stems from the requirement that the basis vectors must compactly describe the available data. Figure 8.8 shows a wavelet-based interpolation method. Figure 8.9 shows a Shepp and Logan phantom and reconstructed

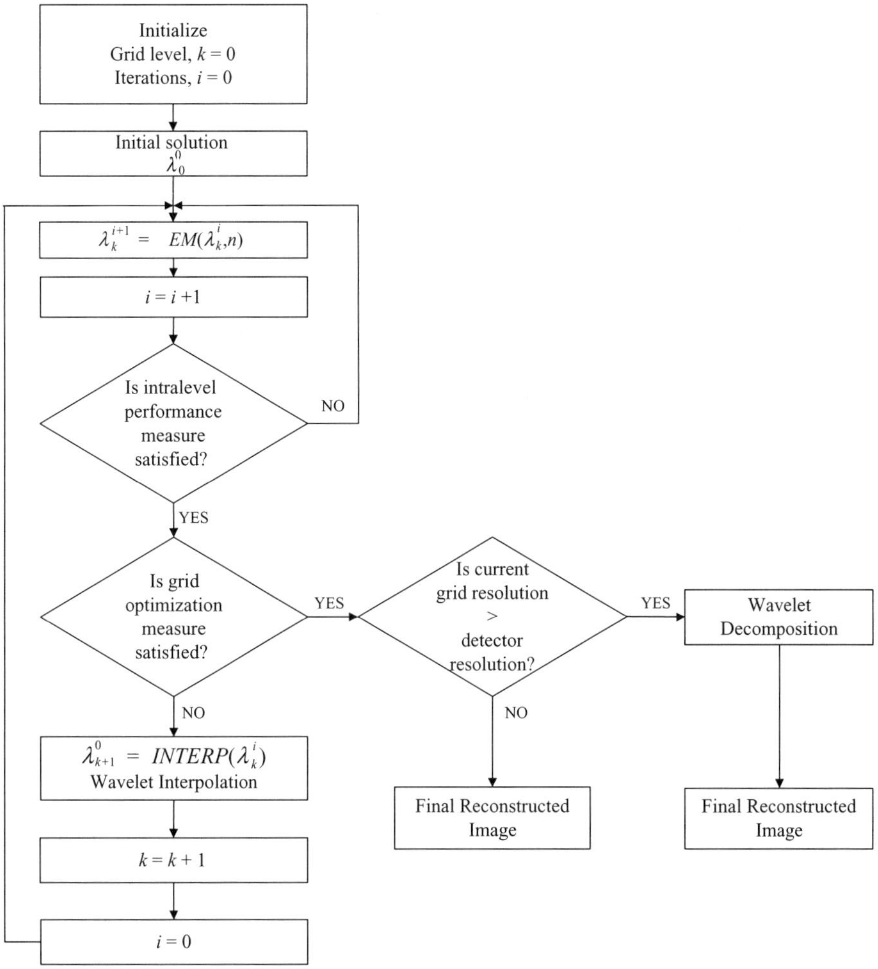

8.5. IMAGE RECONSTRUCTION IN MEDICAL IMAGING MODALITIES

Figure 8.7 A flowchart of the MGEM algorithm for PET image reconstruction.

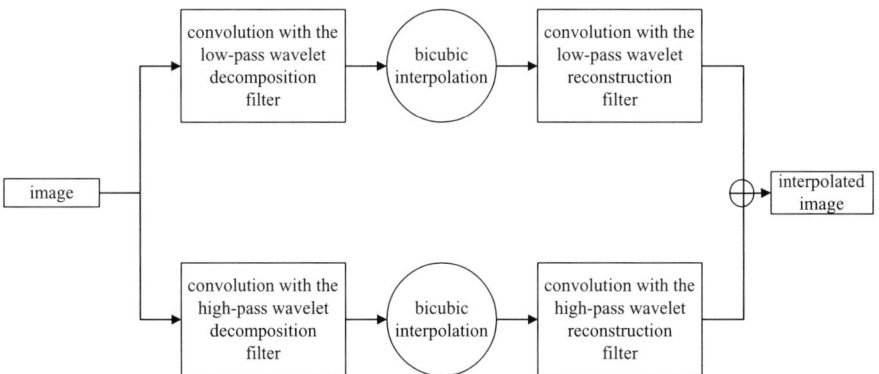

Figure 8.8 A wavelet-based interpolation method.

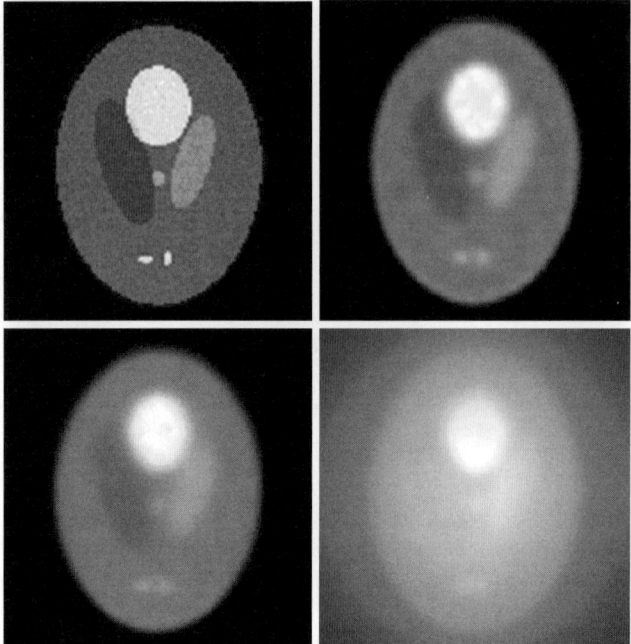

Figure 8.9 Shepp and Logan phantom (top left) and reconstructed phantom images using WMREM algorithm (top right), ML–EM algorithm (bottom left), and filtered backprojection method (bottom right).

images from the ML–EM algorithm (13), WMREM algorithm (35), and the filtered backprojection method. Figure 8.10 shows reconstructed brain images from a PET scan of a patient with a tumor, using a generalized EM algorithm, the backprojection method, and the WMREM algorithm for comparison.

8.5.3 Image Reconstruction in Magnetic Resonance Imaging

The Fourier reconstruction method is commonly applied in magnetic resonance imaging (MRI) for image reconstruction. The electromagnetic free induction decay (FID) signal acquired in MRI image is in the frequency domain. As presented in Equation 5.19 in Chapter 5, the signal $S(\vec{\omega}) = S(\omega_x, \omega_y, \omega_z)$ can be expressed as

$$S(\vec{\omega}) = \bar{M}_0 \iiint f(x, y, z) e^{-i(\omega_x x + \omega_y y + \omega_z z)} dx\, dy\, dz \tag{8.42}$$

where $f(x, y, z)$ is the image to be reconstructed. For 2-D image reconstruction, the image function is reduced to $f(x, y)$.

Inverse Fourier transform of the signal $S(\vec{\omega})$ provides the reconstructed image. However, this is implemented using discrete fast Fourier transform (FFT) algorithms that may require interpolation of data points depending on the resolution of the reconstructed image and data samples in the k-space. Gridding interpolation algorithms may be used for this purpose (23–25). Specific parameter-based images (such as proton-density, T_1-weighted, and T_2-weighted images) are reconstructed using

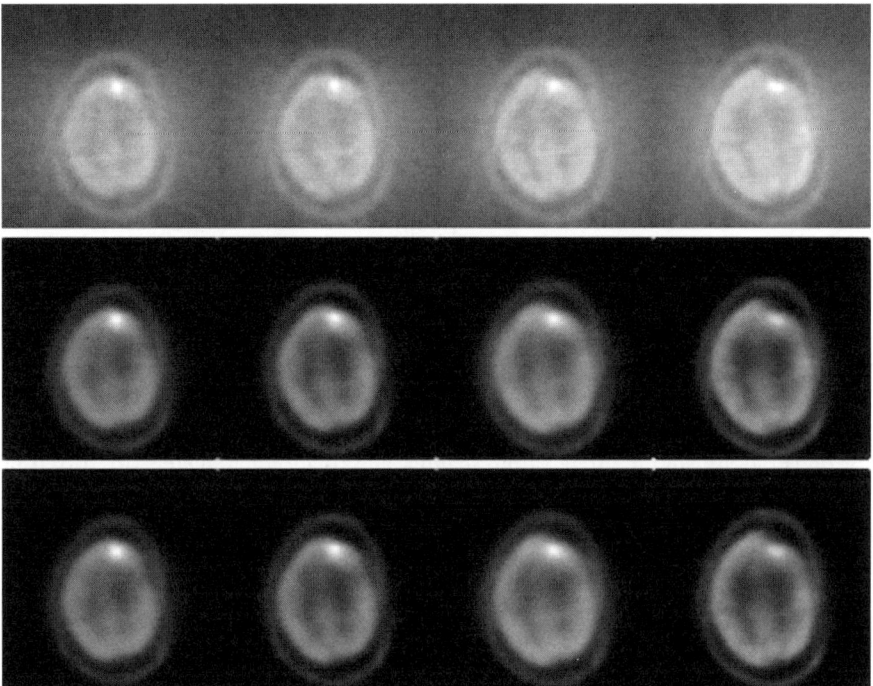

Figure 8.10 Four PET-reconstructed axial brain images of a patient with a tumor. Images in the top row are reconstructed using filtered backprojection method; images in the middle row are reconstructed using WMREM algorithm; and images in the bottom row are reconstructed using a generalized ML–EM algorithm for the same axial cross-sections.

appropriate pulse sequences to acquire the desired signal as explained in Chapter 5, but the image reconstruction method remains the same. Special preprocessing and correlation methods are used in blood flow imaging or functional MRI (fMRI) using the snapshot pulse sequencing, such as spiral echo planar imaging (SEPI), for fast imaging (40, 41). A signal estimation-based analysis in fMRI is discussed in Reference (42).

An important aspect of blood flow imaging or fMRI is that the snapshot pulse sequence (SEPI) has to acquire the entire signal in the k-space in a very short time. The k-space is filled in a spiral geometry by a SEPI sequence as discussed in Chapter 5. Acquisition of all data samples in the k-space in a short time causes other off-resonance effects such as chemical shift and field inhomogeneities to be accumulated, degrading the MR signal. To compensate for these effects, an iterative reconstruction method using ART is presented in Reference (43).

8.5.4 Image Reconstruction in Ultrasound Imaging

Ultrasound imaging is primarily based on the point measurements as described in Chapter 7. The point-by-point measurements lead to a line scan. A collection of line scans can provide a 2-D ultrasound image. Ultrasound arrays can be used to obtain line measurements more efficiently. To improve the quality of ultrasound image, the most important issue is the reduction of speckle noise. Ultrasound speckle-reduction methods can be characterized into two categories: image averaging and image filtering. In the first approach, several images of a target object are averaged to improve the SNR. It is apparent that such methods suffer from the loss of spatial resolution. Various filters such as weighted median and Wiener filters are used in the second approach to reduce speckle noise (44–46).

Three-dimensional image reconstruction in ultrasound imaging is usually obtained by stacking up 2-D images in the third dimension (47, 48). The difficulty of this approach is the localization of 2-D images in the desired plan to accurately register and interpolate 2-D images for visualization of 3-D structures. In addition, the optimal 2-D image plane may be restricted by the patient's anatomy such that the acquisition of 2-D images along the desired axis may not be feasible. The acquired 2-D images are tagged with some visual landmarks, which are then used for registration using the translation, scaling, and rotation parameters, discussed in Chapter 2. However, the 3-D image reconstruction in ultrasound imaging from 2-D tomographic images suffer from uncertainties in imaging geometry and variability of the structures in the imaging medium. Geometrical distortions and signal variances in 3-D ultrasound image reconstruction from stacking of parallel 2-D images are discussed in Reference (49).

8.6. EXERCISES

8.1. Assume an object $f(x, y)$ in x–y coordinate system with parallel rays passing through the object at an angle θ. Define a projection $J_\theta(p)$ graphically and express it in mathematical terms using the Radon transform.

8.2. How does a set of projections $J_\theta(p)$ with different viewing angles (with rotated coordinates) relate to the Fourier transform of the object $f(x, y)$?

8.3. Describe a direct Fourier reconstruction method using the central slice theorem.

8.4. Write and describe the mathematical expression of image reconstruction using the backprojection method. Why is there a need for filtering operation in the backprojection reconstruction method?

8.5. What should be the properties of an ideal filter function for the filtered backprojection method? Describe a filter function of your choice and explain the reasons for your selection.

8.6. Implement the filtered backprojection method selected in Exercise 8.5 in the MATLAB environment. Use the Shepp and Logan phantom as an object for image reconstruction. Compute projections every 20 degrees from the Shepp and Logan phantom.

8.7. Repeat Exercise 8.6 with the R-L filter defined in Equation 8.12 to reconstruct Shepp and Logan phantom. Compare and comment on the quality of the reconstructed image with the image obtained in Exercise 8.6.

8.8. Repeat Exercise 8.6 with projections computed every 5 degrees. Compare the reconstructions to those obtained in Exercise 8.6. Comment on the aliasing artifacts, if any.

8.9. What is the significance of interpolation in rebinning algorithm for divergent beam-based projection data to implement parallel-beam based filtered backprojection method?

8.10. What is the basis for iterative algebraic reconstruction methods? What are the advantages and disadvantages of ART compared with the filtered backprojection method?

8.11. Derive an expression for the correction factor for multiplicative ART. Is it a better algorithm than the additive ART? Explain your answer.

8.12. Repeat Exercise 8.6 with the additive ART and compare the reconstructed images with those obtained using the filtered backprojection method. Also, compare the reconstruction error and computation time for ART and filtered backprojection methods.

8.13. Why is attenuation correction important in image reconstruction for SPECT imaging?

8.14. Define an objective function for the penalized ML–EM algorithm for PET. What is the significance of the penalty function? What are the required mathematical properties of the penalty function?

8.15. What is the optimization transfer principle? How does it help in the optimization of the objective function in Exercise 8.11?

8.16. Implement the image reconstruction method for the optimization of the objective function in Exercise 8.11 in the MATLAB environment using a Shepp and Logan phantom for 1 million events of photon emission for 720 detectors and a reconstruction grid of 512×512. Comment on the reconstructed image quality and error in reconstruction by comparing intensity profiles for three oblique cross-sections of the phantom.

8.17. Obtain three multiresolution reconstructions on 64×64, 128×128, and 256×256 separately and compare the reconstruction errors for three reconstruction interpolated to the 512×512 resolution. Use a wavelet-based interpolation method in the MATLAB environment as described in Figure 8.7.

8.7. REFERENCES

1. J. Radon, "Uber die Bestimmung von Funktionen durch ihre Integralwerte langs gewisser Mannigfaltigkeiten," *Ber. Verb. Saechs. AKAD. Wiss., Leipzig, Match Phys.*, Kl 69, pp. 262–277, 1917.
2. G.N. Hounsfield, "A method and apparatus for examination of a body by radiation such as X or gamma radiation," Patent 1283915, The Patent Office, London, England, 1972.
3. G.N. Hounsfield, "Computerized transverse axial scanning tomography: Part-1, description of the system," *Br. J. Radiol.*, Vol. 46, pp. 1016–1022, 1973.
4. A.M. Cormack, "Representation of a function by its line integrals with some radiological applications," *J. Appl. Phys.*, Vol. 34, pp. 2722–2727, 1963.

5. G.T. Herman, *Image Reconstruction from Projections*, Academic Press, New York, 1980.
6. A. Rosenfeld and A.C. Kak, *Digital Picture Processing:* Volume 1, Academic Press, Orlando, FL, 1982.
7. G.N. Ramachandran and A.V. Lakshminaryanan, "Three-dimensional reconstruction from radiographs and electron micrographs," *Proc. Nat. Acad. Sci. USA*, Vol. 68, pp. 2236–2240, 1971.
8. R. Gordon, "A tutorial on ART (algebraic reconstruction techniques)," *IEEE Trans. Nucl. Sci.*, Vol. 21, pp. 78–93, 1974.
9. J.A. Fessler, "Statistical image reconstruction methods for transmission tomography," in M. Sonka and J.M. Fitzpatrick (Eds), *Handbook of Medical Imaging:* Volume 2, *Medical Image Processing and Analysis*, SPIE Press, Bellingham, WA, pp. 1–70, 2000.
10. H. Erdogen and J. Fessler, "Monotonic algorithms for transmission tomography," *IEEE Trans. Med. Imaging*, Vol. 18, pp. 801–814, 1999.
11. D.F. Yu, J.A. Fessler, and E.P. Ficaro, "Maximum likelihood transmission image reconstruction for overlapping transmission beams," *IEEE Trans. Med. Imaging*, Vol. 19, pp. 1094–1105, 2000.
12. A.P. Dempster, N.M. Laird, and D.B. Rubin, "Maximum likelihood from incomplete data via the EM algorithm," *J. R. Stat. Soc. Ser. B*, Vol. 39, pp. 1–38, 1977.
13. L.A. Shepp and Y. Vardi, "Maximum likelihood reconstruction for emission tomography," *IEEE Trans. Med. Imaging*, Vol. 1, pp. 113–121, 1982.
14. K. Lange and R. Carson, "EM reconstruction algorithms for emission and transmission tomography," *J. Comput. Assist. Tomogr.*, Vol. 8, pp. 306–316, 1984.
15. J.M. Olinger, "Maximum likelihood reconstruction of transmission images in emission computed tomography via the EM algorithm," *IEEE Trans. Med. Imaging*, Vol. 13, pp. 89–101, 1994.
16. C.A. Bouman and K. Saur, "A unified approach to statistical tomography using coordinate descent optimization," *IEEE Trans. Image Process.*, Vol. 5, pp. 480–492, 1996.
17. J. Fessler, E. Ficaro, N.H. Climhome, and K. Lange, "Grouped coordinate ascent algorithms for penalized likelihood transmission image reconstruction," *IEEE Trans. Med. Imaging*, Vol. 16, pp. 166–175, 1997.
18. H. Erdogen, G. Gualtiere, and J.A. Fessler, "Ordered subsets algorithms for transmission tomography," *Phys. Med. Biol.*, Vol. 44, pp. 2835–2851, 1999.
19. E.U. Mumcuoglu, R. Leahy, S.R. Cherry, and Z. Zhou, "Fast gradient-based methods for Bayesian reconstruction of transmission and emission PET images," *IEEE Trans. Med. Imaging*, Vol. 13, pp. 687–701, 1994.
20. T. Hebert and R. Leahy, "A generalized EM algorithm for 3-D Bayesian reconstruction from Poisson data using Gibbs priors," *IEEE Trans. Med. Imaging*, Vol. 8, pp. 194–202, 1989.
21. P.J. Green, "Bayesian reconstructions from emission tomography data using a modified EM algorithm," *IEEE Trans. Med. Imaging*, Vol. 9, pp. 84–93, 1990.
22. A.R. De Pierro, "A modified expectation maximization algorithm for penalized likelihood estimation in emission tomography," *IEEE Trans. Med. Imaging*, Vol. 14, pp. 132–137, 1995.
23. J.D. O'Sullivan, "A fast sinc function gridding algorithm for Fourier inversion in computed tomography," *IEEE Trans. Med. Imaging*, Vol. 4, pp. 200–207, 1985.
24. H. Schomberg and J. Timmer, "The gridding method for image reconstruction by Fourier transformation," *IEEE Trans. Med. Imaging*, Vol. 14, pp. 595–607, 1995.
25. J. Walden, "Analysis of the direct Fourier method for computed tomography," *IEEE Trans. Med. Imaging*, Vol. 19, pp. 211–222, 2000.
26. B. Smith and C. Peck, "Implementation, comparison and investigation of heuristic techniques for cone beam tomography," *IEEE Trans. Med. Imaging*, Vol. 15, pp. 519–531, 1996.
27. S. Basu and Y. Bresler, "$O(N^3 \log N)$Backprojection algorithm for the 3-D Radon transform," *IEEE Trans. Med. Imaging*, Vol. 21, pp. 76–88, 2002.
28. A.V. Bronnikov, "Approximate reconstruction of attenuation map in SPECT imaging," *IEEE Trans. Nucl. Sci.*, Vol. 42, pp. 1483–1488, 1995.
29. B.M.W. Tsui, G.T. Gulberg, E.R. Edgerton, J.G. Ballard, J.R. Perry, W.H. McCartney, and J. Berg, "Correction of non-uniform attuentaion in cardiac SPECT imaging," *J. Nuc. Med.*, Vol. 30, pp. 497–507, 1989.
30. J.A. Sorenson, "Quantitative measurement of radioactivity in vivo by whole body counting," *Instrum. Nucl. Med.*, Vol. 2, pp. 311–347, 1974.
31. A.V. Bronnikov, "Reconstruction of attenuation map using discrete consistency conditions," *IEEE Trans. Med. Imaging*, Vol. 19, pp. 451–462, 2000.

32. A. Welch, R. Clack, F. Natterer, and G. Gullberg, "Toward accurate attenuation correction in SPECT without transmission measurements," *IEEE Trans. Med. Imaging*, Vol. 16, pp. 532–541, 1997.
33. M.V. Ranganath, A.P. Dhawan, and N. Mullani, "A multigrid expectation maximization reconstruction algorithm for positron emission tomography," *IEEE Trans. Med. Imaging*, Vol. 7, pp. 273–278, 1988.
34. A. Raheja and A.P. Dhawan, "Wavelet based multiresolution expectation maximization reconstruction algorithm for emission tomography," *Comput. Med. Imaging Graph.*, Vol. 24, pp. 87–98, 2000.
35. S.K. Mitra and J.F. Kasier (Eds), *Handbook of Digital Signal Processing*, John Wiley and Sons, Inc., 1993.
36. A.P. Pentland, "Interpolation using wavelet bases," *IEEE Trans. Pattern Anal. Mach. Intell.*, Vol. 16, No. 4, pp. 410–414, 1994.
37. M.-H. Yaou and W.-T. Chang, "Fast surface interpolation using multiresolution wavelet transform," *IEEE Trans. Pattern Anal. Mach. Intell.*, Vol. 16, No. 7, pp. 673–688, 1994.
38. C.K. Chui, "On compactly supported spline wavelets and a duality priciple," *Trans. Am. Math. Soc.*, Vol. 330, No. 2, pp. 903–915, 1992.
39. A. Cohen, I. Daubechies, and J.-C. Feauveau, "Biorthogonal bases of compactly supported wavelets," *Comm. Pure Appl. Math.*, Vol. 45, No. 5, pp. 485–560, 1992.
40. S. Ogawa, D.W. Tank, R. Menon, J.M. Eillermann, S.G. Kim, H. Merkle, and K. Ugurbil, "Intrinsic signal changes accompanying sensory simulation," *Proc. Nat. Acad. Sci. USA*, Vol. 89, pp. 5951–5955, 1992.
41. M.S. Cohen and S.Y. Bookheimer, "Localization of brain function using MRI," *Trends Neurosci.*, Vol. 17, pp. 208–276, 1994.
42. V. Solo, P. Purdon, R. Weisskoff, and E. Brown, "A signal estimation approach to functional MRI," *IEEE Trans. Med. Imaging*, Vol. 20, pp. 26–35, 2001.
43. T.B. Harshbarger and D.B. Tweig, "Iterative reconstruction of single-shot spiral MRI with off resonance," *IEEE Trans. Med. Imaging*, Vol. 18, pp. 196–205, 1999.
44. J.U. Quistguard, "Signal acquisition and processing in medical diagnostic ultrasound," *IEEE Signal Process. Mag.*, pp. 67–74, 1997.
45. M. Karaman, M.A. Kutay, and G. Bozdagi, "An adaptive speckle suppression filter for medical ultrasound imaging," *IEEE Trans. Med. Imaging*, Vol. 14, pp. 283–292, 1995.
46. X. Hao, S. Gao, and X. Gao, "A novel multiscale nonlinear thesholding method for ultrasonic speckle suppressing," *IEEE Trans. Med. Imaging*, Vol. 18, pp. 787–794, 1999.
47. T.R. Nelson, D.B. Downey, D.H. Pretorius, and A. Fenster, *Three-Dimensional Ultrasound*, Lippincott Williams and Wilkins, Philadelphia, 1999.
48. E.O. Ofili and N.C. Nanda, "Three-dimensional and four-dimensional echocardiography," *Ultrasound Med. Biol.*, Vol. 20, pp. 669–675, 1994.
49. H.N. Cardinal, J.D. Gill, and A. Fenster, "Analysis of geometrical distortion and statistical variance in length, area and volume in a linearly scanned ultrasound image," *IEEE Trans. Med. Imaging*, Vol. 19, pp. 632–651, 2000.

CHAPTER 9

IMAGE PROCESSING AND ENHANCEMENT

Medical images acquired in most radiological applications are visually examined by a physician. The purpose of image enhancement methods is to process an acquired image for better contrast and visibility of features of interest for visual examination as well as subsequent computer-aided analysis and diagnosis. As described in Chapters 4–7, different medical imaging modalities provide specific information about internal organs or biological tissues. Image contrast and visibility of the features of interest depend on the imaging modality as well as the anatomical regions.

There is no unique general theory or method for processing all kinds of medical images for feature enhancement. Specific medical imaging applications (such as cardiac, neurological, and mammography) present different challenges in image processing for feature enhancement and analysis. Medical images show characteristic information about the physiological properties of the structures and tissues. However, the quality and visibility of information depends on the imaging modality and the response functions (such as the point spread function [PSF]) of the imaging scanner. Medical images from specific modalities need to be processed using a method that is suitable to enhance the features of interest. For example, a chest X-ray radiographic image shows the anatomical structure of the chest based on the total attenuation coefficients. If the radiograph is being examined for a possible fracture in the ribs, the image enhancement method is required to improve the visibility of hard bony structures. But if an X-ray mammogram is obtained for examination of potential breast cancer, an image processing method is required to enhance visibility of microcalcifications, speculated masses, and soft-tissue structures such as parenchyma. A single image enhancement method may not serve both of these applications. Image enhancement methods for improving the soft tissue contrast in magnetic resonance (MR) brain images may be entirely different from those used for positron emission tomography (PET) brain images. Thus, image enhancement tasks and methods are very much application-dependent.

Image enhancement methods may also include image restoration methods, which are generally based on minimum mean-squared error operations, such as Wiener filtering and other constrained deconvolution methods incorporating some a priori knowledge of degradation (1–5). Since the main objective is to enhance

---

Medical Image Analysis, Second Edition, by Atam P. Dhawan
Copyright © 2011 by the Institute of Electrical and Electronics Engineers, Inc.

features of interest, a suitable combination of both restoration and contrast enhancement algorithms is the integral part of preprocessing in image analysis. The selection of a specific restoration algorithm for noise removal is highly dependent on the image acquisition system. For example, in the filtered-backprojection method for reconstructing images in computed tomography (CT), the raw data obtained from the scanner is first deconvolved with a specific filter. Filter functions such as Hamming window, as described in Chapter 8, may also be used to reduce noise in the projection data. On the other hand, several image enhancement methods, such as neighborhood-based operations and frequency filtering operations, implicitly de-emphasize noise for feature enhancement.

Image enhancement tasks are usually characterized in two categories (1–5):

1. **Spatial Domain Methods:** These methods manipulate image pixel values in the spatial domain based on the distribution statistics of the entire image or local regions. Histogram transformation, spatial filtering, region-growing, morphological image processing, and model-based image estimation methods are some examples in this category of image and feature enhancement.
2. **Frequency Domain Methods:** These methods manipulate information in the frequency domain based on the frequency characteristics of the image. Frequency filtering, homomorphic filtering, and wavelet processing methods are some examples in this category of frequency representation-based image and feature enhancement.

In addition to the above general approaches for image and feature enhancement, model-based techniques such as Hough transform, matched filtering, neural networks, and knowledge-based systems are also used to extract specific features for pattern recognition and classification. These methods are discussed in detail in the next chapter.

9.1. SPATIAL DOMAIN METHODS

Spatial domain methods process an image with pixel-by-pixel transformation based on the histogram statistics or neighborhood operations. These methods are usually faster in computer implementation as compared to frequency filtering methods that require computation of Fourier transform for frequency domain representation. However, frequency filtering methods may provide better results in some applications if a priori information about the characteristic frequency components of the noise and features of interest is available. For example, specific spike degradations due to mechanical stress and vibration on the gradient coils in the raw signal often cause striation artifacts in fast MR imaging techniques. The spike degradation-based noise in the MR signal can be modeled with their characteristic frequency components and can be removed by selective filtering and wavelet processing methods (7). Wiener filtering methods have been applied for signal enhancement to remove frequency components related to the undesired resonance effects of the nuclei and noise suppression in MR imaging (8–10).

9.1.1 Histogram Transformation and Equalization

A histogram of an image provides information about the intensity distribution of pixels in the image. The simplest form of a histogram is the plot of occurrence of specific gray-level values of the pixels in the image. For example, there are 256 gray levels ranging from 0 to 255 in an image with 8-bit gray-level resolution. The occurrence of gray levels can be provided in terms of the absolute values, that is, the number of times a specific gray level has occurred in the image, or the probability values, that is, the probability of occurrence of a specific gray level in the image. In mathematical terms, a histogram $h(r_i)$ is expressed as

$$h(r_i) = n_i \quad \text{for } i = 0, 1, \ldots, L-1 \tag{9.1}$$

where r_i is the ith gray level in the image for a total of L gray values and n_i is the number of occurrences of gray-level r_i in the image.

If a histogram is expressed in terms of the probability of occurrence of gray levels, it can be expressed as

$$p_r(r_i) = \frac{n_i}{n} \tag{9.2}$$

where n is the total number of pixels in the image.

Thus, a histogram is a plot of $h(r_i)$ or $p_r(r_i)$ versus r_i. Figure 9.1 shows X-ray CT and T_2-weighted proton density MR images of brain with their respected histogram $h(r_i)$.

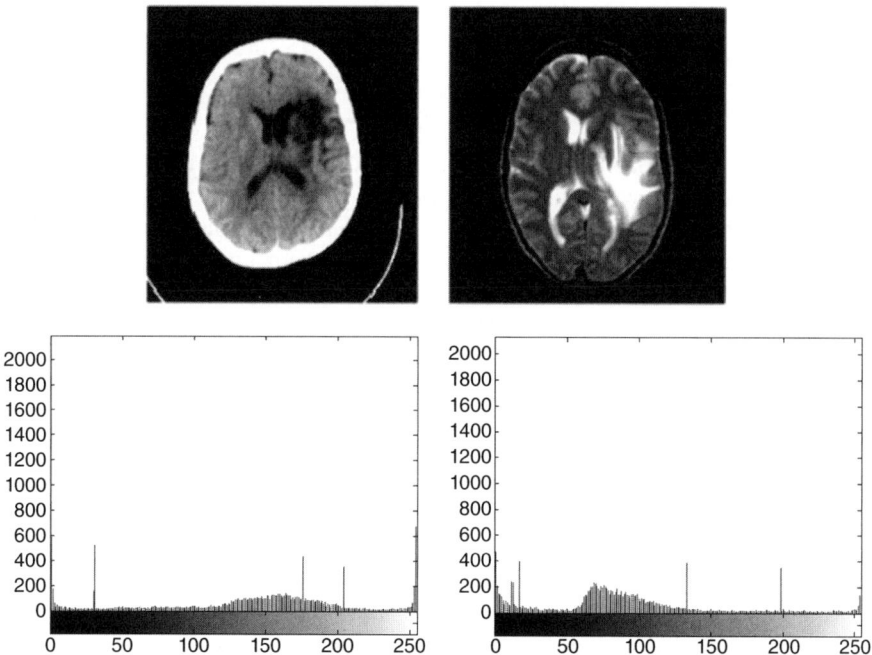

Figure 9.1 An X-ray CT image (top left) and T_2-weighted proton density image (top right) of human brain cross-sections with their respective histograms at the bottom.

A histogram can be scaled linearly to change the dynamic range of gray levels in the image. Let us assume that an image has all of its gray levels in the range [a, b] where the minimum gray level is represented by a and the maximum gray level value is given by b. The utilization of dynamic range of gray levels in the image can be seen in the histogram. Using a histogram scaling method, the gray level range of [a, b] can be changed to a new gray level range of [c, d] by a linear transformation as

$$z_{new} = \frac{d-c}{b-a}(z-a) + c \tag{9.3}$$

where z and z_{new} are, respectively, the original and new gray-level values of a pixel in the image.

If an image is not using the full dynamic range of gray levels (e.g., 256 gray levels from 0 to 255 for an image with 8-bit gray level resolution), a histogram scaling method can be used to expand the dynamic range to its full possible range to improve the contrast and brightness in general. An example of image histogram scaling is shown in Figure 1.8 in Chapter 1.

A popular general-purpose method of image enhancement is histogram equalization. In this method, a monotonically increasing transformation function, $T(r)$, is used to map the original gray values, r_i of the input image, into new gray values, s_i of the output image, such that

$$s_i = T(r_i) = \sum_{j=0}^{i} p_r(r_j)$$

$$= \sum_{j=0}^{i} \frac{n_j}{n} \quad for \quad i = 0, 1, \ldots, L-1 \tag{9.4}$$

where $p_r(r_i)$ is the probability-based histogram of the input image that is transformed into the output image with the histogram $p_s(s_i)$.

The transformation function $T(r_i)$ in Equation 9.4 stretches the histogram of the input image such that the gray values occur in the output image with equal probability of occurrence. It should be noted that the uniform distribution of the histogram of the output image is limited by discrete computation of the gray-level transformation. The histogram equalization method forces image intensity levels to be redistributed with an equal probability of occurrence.

Figure 9.2 shows the enhanced images of the brain images shown in Figure 9.1 as obtained by the histogram equalization method. The respective histograms of the enhanced images are shown at the bottom.

The histogram equalization method stretches the contrast of an image by redistributing the gray values to achieve a uniform distribution. This general method may not provide good results in many applications. The histogram equalization method may cause saturation in some regions of the image resulting in loss of details and high-frequency information that may be necessary for interpretation. Sometimes, local histogram equalization is applied separately on predefined local neighborhood regions, such as 7 × 7 pixels, to provide better results (1).

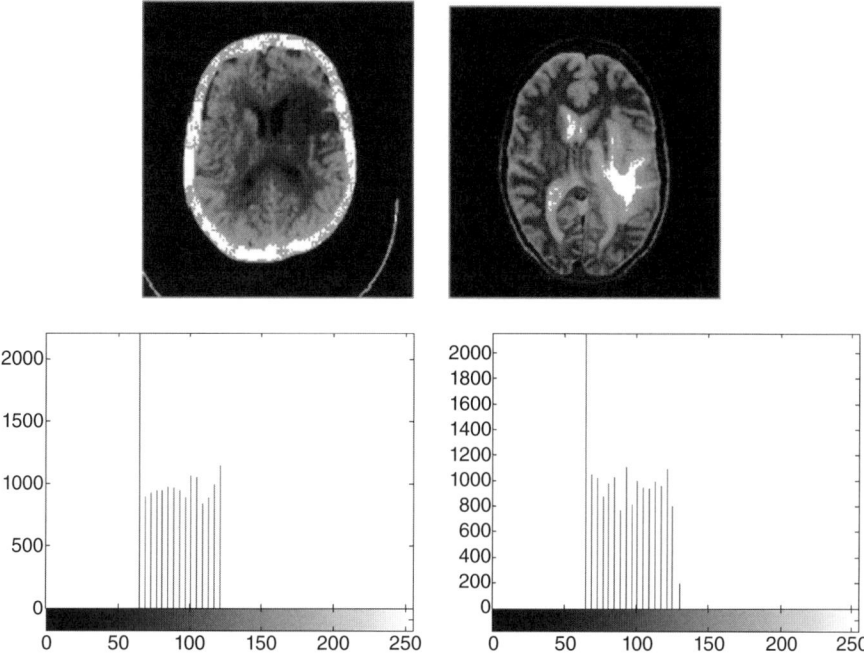

Figure 9.2 Histogram equalized images of the CT and MR brain images shown in Figure 9.1 (top) and their respective histograms (bottom).

9.1.2 Histogram Modification

If a desired distribution of gray values is known a priori, a histogram modification method is used to apply a transformation that changes the gray values to match the desired distribution. The target distribution can be obtained from a good contrast image that is obtained under similar imaging conditions. Alternatively, an original image from a scanner can be interactively modified through regional scaling of gray values to achieve the desired contrast. This image can now provide a target distribution to the rest of the images, obtained under similar imaging conditions, for automatic enhancement using the histogram modification method.

Let us assume that $p_z(z_i)$ is the target histogram expressed, and $p_r(r_i)$ and $p_s(s_i)$ are, respectively, the histograms of the input and output image. A transformation is needed such that the output image $p_s(s_i)$ should have the desired histogram of $p_z(z_i)$. The first step in this process is to equalize $p_r(r_i)$ using the Equation 9.3 such that (1, 6)

$$u_i = T(r_i) = \sum_{j=0}^{i} p_r(r_j) \quad \text{for} \quad i = 0, 1, \ldots, L-1 \tag{9.5}$$

where is u_i represents the equalized gray values of the input image.

A new transformation V is defined to equalize the target histogram such that

$$u_i = V(z_i) = \sum_{k=0}^{i} p_z(z_k) \quad \text{for} \quad i = 0, 1, \ldots, L-1. \tag{9.6}$$

Putting $V(z_i) = T(r_i) = u_i$ to achieve the target distribution, new gray values s_i for the output image are computed from the inverse transformation V^{-1} as

$$s_i = z_i = V^{-1}[T(r_i)] = V^{-1}(u_i). \tag{9.7}$$

With the transformation defined in Equation 9.7, the histogram distribution of the output image $p_s(s_i)$ would become similar to the target histogram $p_z(z_i)$.

9.1.3 Image Averaging

Signal averaging is a well-known method for enhancing signal-to-noise ratio (SNR). In medical imaging, data from the detector is often averaged over time or space for signal enhancement. However, such signal enhancement is achieved at the cost of some loss of temporal or spatial resolution. Sequence images, if properly registered and acquired in nondynamic applications, can be averaged for noise reduction leading to smoothing effects. Selective weighted averaging can also be performed over a specified neighborhood of pixels in the image.

Let us assume that an ideal image $f(x, y)$ is degraded by the presence of additive noise $n(x, y)$. The acquired image $g(x, y)$ then can be represented as

$$g(x, y) = f(x, y) + n(x, y). \tag{9.8}$$

In a general imaging process, the noise is assumed to be uncorrelated and random with a zero average value. If a sequence of K images is acquired for the same object under the same imaging conditions, the average image $\bar{g}(x, y)$ can be obtained as

$$\bar{g}(x, y) = \frac{1}{K}\sum_{i=1}^{K} g_i(x, y) \tag{9.9}$$

where $g_i(x, y); i = 1, 2, \ldots, K$ represents the sequence of images to be averaged.

As the number of images K increases, the expected value of the average image $\bar{g}(x, y)$ approaches to $f(x, y)$, reducing the noise per pixel in the averaged image as

$$E\{\bar{g}(x, y)\} = f(x, y)$$

$$\sigma_{\bar{g}(x, y)} = \frac{1}{\sqrt{K}}\sigma_{n(x,y)} \tag{9.10}$$

where σ represents the standard deviation of the respective random field.

9.1.4 Image Subtraction

If two properly registered images of the same object are obtained with different imaging conditions, a subtraction operation on the acquired image can enhance the information about the changes in imaging conditions. This simple enhancement method is applied in angiography where an image of the anatomy with vascular structure is obtained first. An appropriate dye or tracer drug is then administered in the body and flows through the vascular structure. A second image is acquired of the same anatomy at the peak of the tracer flow. The subtraction of these two images then produces an image with good contrast and visibility of the vascular structure. Figure 9.3 shows an MR angiographic image obtained using the subtraction method.

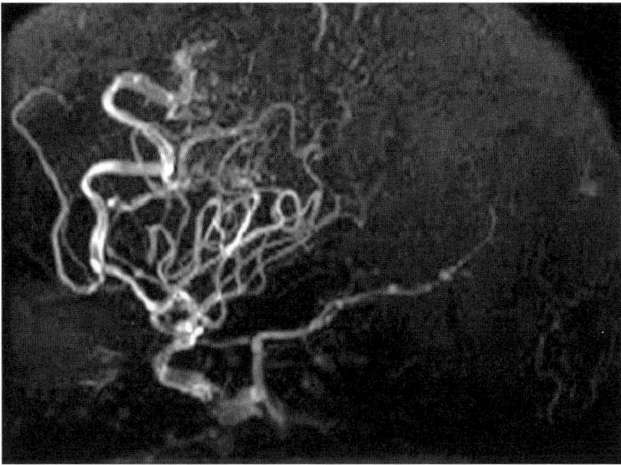

Figure 9.3 An MR angiography image obtained through image subtraction method.

	$f(x-1,y)$	
$f(x,y-1)$	$f(x,y)$	$f(x,y+1)$
	$f(x+1,y)$	

$f(x-1,y-1)$	$f(x-1,y)$	$f(x-1,y+1)$
$f(x,y-1)$	$f(x,y)$	$f(x,y+1)$
$f(x+1,y-1)$	$f(x+1,y)$	$f(x+1,y+1)$

Figure 9.4 A 4-connected (left) and 8-connected neighborhood of a pixel $f(x, y)$.

9.1.5 Neighborhood Operations

The spatial filtering methods using neighborhood operations involve the convolution of the input image with a specific mask (such as Laplacian-based high-frequency emphasis filtering mask) to enhance an image. The gray value of each pixel is replaced by the new value computed according to the mask applied in the neighborhood of the pixel. The neighborhood of a pixel may be defined in any appropriate manner based on a simple connectedness or any other adaptive criterion (13). Figure 9.4 shows 4- and 8-connected neighborhoods of a central pixel in 3×3 pixel regions.

A weight mask is first created by assigning weights for each pixel location in the selected type of neighborhood. The weight mask is then convolved with the image. With an appropriate design of the mask, specific operations including image smoothing and enhancement can be performed. For example, using a Laplacian weight mask, edge features can be emphasized in the enhanced image.

Let us assume a general weight mask of $(2p + 1) \times (2p + 1)$ pixels where p can take integer values, such as 1, 2, ... , depending on the size of the mask. For $p = 1$, the size of the weight mask is 3×3 pixels. A discrete convolution of an image $f(x, y)$ with a spatial filter represented by a weight mask $w(x, y)$ is given by

1	2	1
2	4	2
1	2	1

Figure 9.5 A weighted averaging mask for image smoothing. The mask is used with a scaling factor of 1/16 that is multiplied to the values obtained by convolution of the mask with the image (Eq. 9.11).

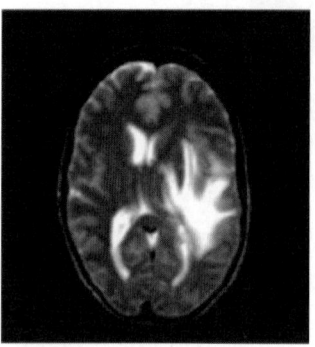

Figure 9.6 Smoothed image of the MR brain image shown in Figure 9.1 as a result of the spatial filtering using the weighted averaging mask shown in Figure 9.5.

$$g(x, y) = \frac{1}{\sum_{x'=-p}^{p}\sum_{y'=-p}^{p} w(x', y')} \sum_{x'=-p}^{p}\sum_{y'=-p}^{p} w(x', y') f(x+x', y+y'). \quad (9.11)$$

The convolution in Equation 9.11 is performed for all values of x and y in the image. In other words, the weight mask of the filter is translated and convolved over the entire extent of the input image to provide the output image.

The values of the weight mask are derived from a discrete representation of the selected filter. Based on the filter, the characteristics of the input image are changed in the output image. For example, Figure 9.5 shows a weighted averaging mask that can be used for image smoothing and noise reduction. In this mask, the locations of pixels in the 4-connected neighborhood are weighted two times more than other pixels. The reason is that pixels in the 4-connected neighborhood are closer than others to the central pixel. Figure 9.6 shows the MR brain image smoothed by spatial filtering using the weighted averaging mask shown in Figure 9.5 on the image shown in Figure 9.1. Some loss of details can be noted in the smoothed image because of the averaging operation. To minimize the loss of details, an adaptive median filtering may be applied (1–4).

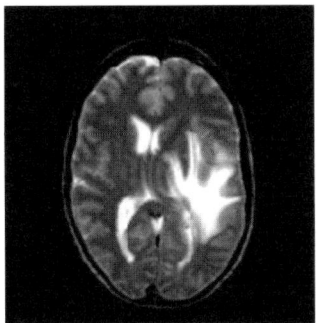

Figure 9.7 A smoothed MR brain image obtained by spatial filtering using the median filter method over a fixed neighborhood of 3 × 3 pixels.

9.1.5.1 Median Filter Median filter is a well-known order-statistics filter that replaces the original gray value of a pixel by the median of gray values of pixels in the specified neighborhood. For example, for 3 × 3 pixels-based fixed neighborhood (Fig. 9.4), the gray value of the central pixel $f(x, y)$ is replaced by the median of gray values of all 9 pixels in the neighborhood. Instead of replacing the gray value of the central pixel by the median operation of the neighborhood pixels, other operations such as midpoint, arithmetic mean, and geometric mean can also be used in order-statistics filtering methods (1–5). A median filter operation for a smoothed image $\hat{f}(x, y)$, computed from the acquired image $g(x, y)$, is defined as

$$\hat{f}(x, y) = \underset{(i, j) \in N}{\operatorname{median}} \{g(i, j)\} \tag{9.12}$$

where N is the prespecified neighborhood of the pixel (x, y).

Figure 9.7 shows the smoothed MR brain image as obtained by median filtering over the neighborhoods of 3 × 3 pixels. Adaptive neighborhoods can be used for median filtering to preserve the edges better. Several methods of adaptive neighborhoods are used in the literature including fixed shape and feature adaptive neighborhoods (1, 13). In adaptive neighborhood processing, a region centered at a pixel is grown until a prespecified criterion of region growing is satisfied. One simple method of region growing is to grow a neighborhood around the central pixel from 3 × 3 pixels to 5 × 5 pixels and so on, until the difference between the gray value of the central pixel and the average of all other pixels in the neighborhood is within a preselected threshold. Thus, local neighborhoods with different sizes can be used for median filtering for preserving edge details in the smoothed image.

9.1.5.2 Adaptive Arithmetic Mean Filter Adaptive local noise-reduction filtering can be applied using the variance information of the selected neighborhood and an estimate of the overall variance of noise in the image. If the noise variance of the image is similar to the variance of gray values in the specified neighborhood of pixels, the filter provides an arithmetic mean value of the neighborhood. Let σ_n^2 be an estimate of the variance of the noise in the image and σ_s^2 be the variance of gray values of pixels in the specified neighborhood. An adaptive local noise-reduction filtering can be implemented as

$$\hat{f}(x, y) = g(x, y) - \frac{\sigma_n^2}{\sigma_s^2}[g(x, y) - \bar{g}_{ms}(x, y)] \tag{9.13}$$

where $\bar{g}_{ms}(x, y)$ is the mean of the gray values of pixels in the specified neighborhood.

It should be noted that if the noise variance is zero in the image, the resultant image is the same as the input image. If an edge were present in the neighborhood, the local variance would be higher than the noise variance of the image. In such cases, the above estimate in Equation 9.13 would return the value close to the original gray value of the central pixel.

9.1.5.3 Image Sharpening and Edge Enhancement
Edges in an image are basically defined by the change in gray values of pixels in the neighborhood. The change of gray values of adjacent pixels in the image can be expressed by a derivative (in continuous domain) or a difference (in discrete domain) operation.

A first-order derivative operator, such as Sobel, computes the gradient information in a specific direction. The derivative operator can be encoded into a weight mask. Figure 9.8 shows two Sobel weight masks that are used, respectively, in computing the first-order gradient in x- and y-directions (defined by $\frac{\partial f(x, y)}{\partial x}$ and $\frac{\partial f(x, y)}{\partial y}$). These weight masks of 3×3 pixels each are used for convolution to compute respective gradient images. For spatial image enhancement based on the first-order gradient information, the resultant gradient image can simply be added to the original image and rescaled using the full dynamic range of gray values. Four weight masks to compute directional first-order gradients are shown in Figure 9.9. These masks compute gradient in, respectively, horizontal, 45-degree vertical, and 135-degree directions. The gradient information thus obtained can be further used for specific directional feature enhancement and extraction for image segmentation (discussed in the next chapter).

A second-order derivative operator, known as Laplacian, can be defined as

$$\nabla^2 f(x, y) = \frac{\partial^2 f(x, y)}{\partial x^2} + \frac{\partial^2 f(x, y)}{\partial y^2}$$
$$= [f(x+1, y) + f(x-1, y) + f(x, y+1) + f(x, y-1) - 4f(x, y)] \tag{9.14}$$

-1	-2	-1
0	0	0
1	2	1

-1	0	1
-2	0	2
-1	0	1

Figure 9.8 Weight masks for first-order derivative-based Sobel operator. The mask at the left is for computing gradient in the x-direction while the mask at the right computes the gradient in the y-direction.

−1	−1	−1
0	0	0
1	1	1

−1	0	1
−1	0	1
−1	0	1

−1	−1	0
−1	0	1
−0	1	1

0	1	1
−1	0	1
−1	−1	0

Figure 9.9 Weight masks for computing first-order gradient in (clockwise from top left) in horizontal, 45-degree, vertical, and 135-degree directions.

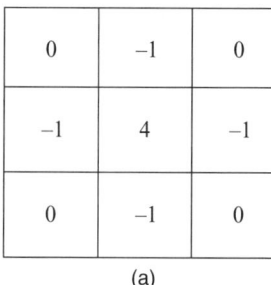
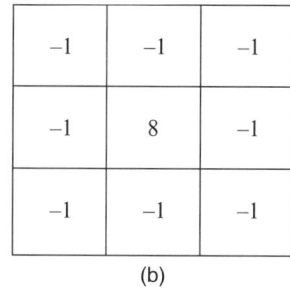
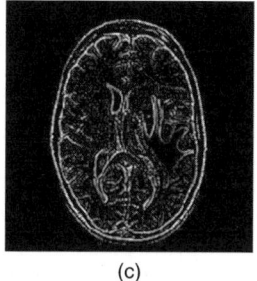

(a)   (b)   (c)

Figure 9.10 (a) A Laplacian weight mask using 4-connected neighborhood pixels only; (b) a Laplacian weight mask with all neighbors in a window of 3 × 3 pixels; and (c) the resultant second-order gradient image obtained using the mask in (a).

where $\nabla^2 f(x, y)$ represents the second-order derivative or Laplacian of the image $f(x, y)$.

A Laplacian mask with diagonal neighbors is shown in Figure 9.10 with the resultant MR brain image showing edge as obtained by spatial filtering convolving the MR brain image shown in Figure 9.1 with this mask. Adding the Laplacian (edge information) to the image provides a simple method of edge-based image enhancement. This can be accomplished by changing the weight value of the central location in the mask from 8 to 9. A different value can be assigned to this location to change the relative emphasis of edges to the image. Figure 9.11 shows the weight mask- and edge-based image enhancement of the same image.

9.1.5.4 Feature Enhancement Using Adaptive Neighborhood Processing

An automated gray-level remapping method for enhancement of details in chest

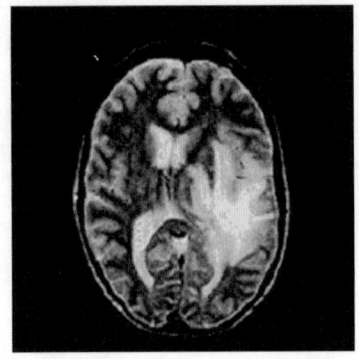

Figure 9.11 Laplacian-based image-enhancement weight mask with diagonal neighbors and the resultant enhanced image with emphasis on second-order gradient information.

region CT images was used by Davis and Wallenslager (11). The objective of this enhancement is to reduce dark line artifacts in CT chest images and to provide an aid to the automatic detection of the lung region. Pizer et al. (12) developed an adaptive gray-level assignment method for CT image enhancement. Dhawan et al. (13) used an adaptive neighborhood-based image processing technique that utilizes a low-level analysis and knowledge about desired features in designing a contrast enhancement function. The contrast enhancement function (CEF) is then used to enhance mammographic features while suppressing the noise. In this method, an adaptive neighborhood structure is defined as a set of two neighborhoods: inner and outer. Three types of adaptive neighborhoods can be defined: constant ratio, constant difference, and feature adaptive. A constant ratio adaptive neighborhood criterion is one that maintains the ratio of the inner to outer neighborhood size at 1:3, that is, each adaptive neighborhood around a pixel had an inner neighborhood of size $c \times c$ and an outer neighborhood of size $3c \times 3c$, where c is an odd number. A constant difference neighborhood criterion is the one that allows the size of the outer neighborhood to be $(c + n) \times (c + n)$, where n is a positive even integer. Note that both of the above mentioned neighborhoods are of fixed shape, that is, square. These neighborhoods can only provide the closest possible approximation of the local features into square regions. However, mammographic features are of arbitrary shape and are highly variable in shape and size. The approximation of local features into square regions may cause loss of fine details about these features.

A variable shaped feature adaptive neighborhood criterion that adapts the arbitrary shape and size of the local features to obtain the "center" (consisting of pixels forming the feature) and the "surround" (consisting of pixels forming the background for that feature) regions is defined using the predefined similarity and distance criteria. These regions are used to compute the local contrast for the centered pixel. The procedure to obtain the center and the surround regions is as follows.

1. The inner and outer neighborhoods around a pixel are grown using the constant difference adaptive neighborhood criterion. To define the similarity criterion, gray-level and percentage thresholds are defined. For example, a gray level

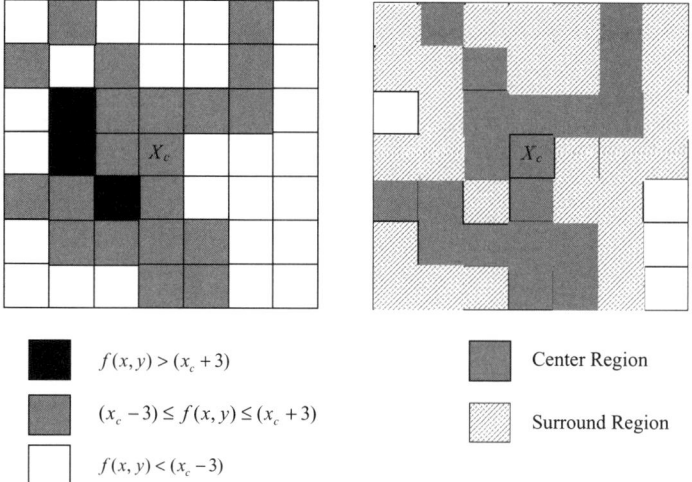

Figure 9.12 Region growing for a feature adaptive neighborhood: image pixel values in a 7 × 7 neighborhood (left) and central and surround regions for the feature-adaptive neighborhood.

threshold of 3 and a percentage threshold of 60 are used in Figure 9.12. Using these thresholds, the region around each pixel in the image is grown in all the directions until the similarity criterion is violated. At the point of violation, the region forming all pixels, which have been included in the neighborhood of the centered pixel satisfying the similarity criterion, are designated as the center region. The surround region is then computed using the distance criterion, which may be a unit distance in all directions (Fig. 9.12). Thus, the surround region is comprised of all pixels contiguous to the center region. The local contrast $C(x, y)$ for the centered pixel is then computed as

$$C(x, y) = \frac{|P_c(x, y) - P_s(x, y)|}{\max\{P_c(x, y), P_s(x, y)\}} \quad (9.15)$$

where $P_c(x, y)$ and $P_s(x, y)$ are the average gray-level values of the pixels corresponding to the center and the surround regions, respectively, centered on the pixel.

2. The CEF is used as a function to modify the contrast distribution in the contrast domain of the image. A contrast histogram is computed as a tool for controlling the efficiency and the performance of the algorithm. The contrast histogram is the plot of occurrence of contrast levels (discretized with a suitable degree of resolution) in the contrast domain. The contrast histogram is analyzed and correlated to the requirements of feature enhancement, such as microcalcification enhancement. Using the CEF, a new contrast value, $C'(x, y)$, is computed.

3. The new contrast value $C'(x, y)$ is used to compute a new pixel value for the enhanced image $g(x, y)$ as

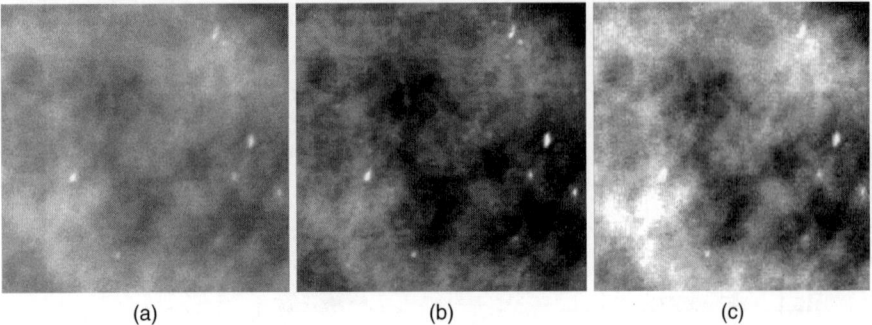

(a) (b) (c)

Figure 9.13 (a) A part of a digitized breast film-mammogram with microcalcification areas. (b) Enhanced image through feature adaptive contrast enhancement algorithm. (c) Enhanced image through histograph equalization method.

$$g(x, y) = \frac{P_s(x, y)}{1 - C'(x, y)} \quad \text{if } P_c(x, y) \geq P_s(x, y)$$

$$g(x, y) = P_s(x, y)(1 - C'(x, y)) \quad \text{if } P_c(x, y) < P_s(x, y). \quad (9.16)$$

Figure 9.13 shows a selected region for microcalcification feature enhancement from a digitized film-mammogram along with the enhanced image using feature-adaptive neighborhood processing. The microcalcification details can be seen more clearly in the enhanced image. The enhanced image using the histogram equalization method is also shown in Figure 9.13 for comparison. A loss of resolution resulting from the saturated regions can be seen in the enhanced image provided by the histogram equalization method.

An adaptive image enhancement method using the first-order derivative information has been used for enhancing specific mammographic features such as stellate lesions, circumscribed masses, and microcalcification (14).

9.2. FREQUENCY DOMAIN FILTERING

Frequency domain filtering methods process an acquired image in the Fourier domain to emphasize or de-emphasize specified frequency components. In general, the frequency components can be expressed in low and high ranges. The low-frequency range components usually represent shapes and blurred structures in the image, while high-frequency information belongs to sharp details, edges, and noise. Thus a low-pass filter with attenuation to high-frequency components would provide image smoothing and noise removal. A high-pass filtering with attenuation to low-frequency extracts edges and sharp details for image enhancement and sharpening effects.

As presented in Chapter 2, an acquired image $g(x, y)$ can be expressed as a convolution of the object $g(x, y)$ with a PSF $h(x, y)$ of a linear spatially invariant imaging system with additive noise $n(x, y)$ as

$$g(x, y) = h(x, y) \otimes f(x, y) + n(x, y) \quad (9.17)$$

9.2. FREQUENCY DOMAIN FILTERING

The Fourier transform of Equation 9.17 provides a multiplicative relationship of $F(u, v)$, the Fourier transform of the object, and $H(u, v)$, the Fourier transform of the PSF.

$$G(u, v) = H(u, v)F(u, v) + N(u, v) \tag{9.18}$$

where u and v represent frequency domain along x- and y-directions, and $G(u, v)$ and $N(u, v)$ are, respectively, the Fourier transforms of the acquired image $g(x, y)$ and the noise $n(x, y)$.

The object information in the Fourier domain can be recovered by inverse filtering as

$$\hat{F}(u, v) = \frac{G(u, v)}{H(u, v)} - \frac{N(u, v)}{H(u, v)} \tag{9.19}$$

where $\hat{F}(u, v)$ is the restored image in the frequency domain.

The inverse filtering operation represented in Equation 9.19 provides a basis for image restoration in the frequency domain. The inverse Fourier transform of $F(u, v)$ provides the restored image in the spatial domain. The PSF of the imaging system can be experimentally determined or statistically estimated (1).

9.2.1 Wiener Filtering

The image restoration approach presented in Equation 9.19 appears to be simple but poses a number of challenges in practical implementation. Besides the difficulties associated with the determination of the PSF, low values or zeros in $H(u, v)$ cause computational problems. Constrained deconvolution approaches and weighted filtering have been used to avoid the "division by zero" problem in Equation 9.19 (1–3). Wiener filtering is a well-known and effective method for image restoration to perform weighted inverse filtering as

$$\hat{F}(u, v) = \left[\left(\frac{1}{H(u, v)} \right) \left(\frac{|H(u, v)|^2}{|H(u, v)|^2 + \frac{S_n(u, v)}{S_f(u, v)}} \right) \right] G(u, v) \tag{9.20}$$

where $S_f(u, v)$ and $S_n(u, v)$ are, respectively, the power spectrum of the signal and noise.

The Wiener filter, also known as the minimum square error filter, provides an estimate determined by exact inverse filtering if the noise spectrum is zero. In cases of nonzero signal-to-noise spectrum ratio, the division is appropriately weighted. If the noise can be assumed to be spectrally white, Equation 9.20 reduces to a simple parametric filter with a constant K as

$$\hat{F}(u, v) = \left[\left(\frac{1}{H(u, v)} \right) \left(\frac{|H(u, v)|^2}{|H(u, v)|^2 + K} \right) \right] G(u, v). \tag{9.21}$$

In implementing inverse filtering-based methods for image restoration, the major issue is the estimation of the PSF and noise spectra. The estimation of PSF is dependent on the instrumentation and parameters of the imaging modality. For example, in the echo planar imaging (EPI) sequence method of MR imaging, an image formation process can be described in a discrete representation by (15, 16)

$$g(x, y) = \sum_{x'=0}^{M-1} \sum_{y'=0}^{N-1} f(x', y') H(x', y'; x, y) \qquad (9.22)$$

where $g(x, y)$ is the reconstructed image of $M \times N$ pixels, $f(x, y)$ is the ideal image of the object, and $H(x', y'; x, y)$ is the PSF of the image formation process in EPI. The MR signal $s(k, l)$ at a location (k, l) in the k-space for the EPI method can be represented as

$$s(k, l) = \sum_{x=0}^{M-1} \sum_{y=0}^{N-1} f(x, y) A(x, y; k, l) \qquad (9.23)$$

where

$$A(x, y; k, l) = e^{-2\pi j((kx/M)+(ly/N)-(\gamma/2\pi)\Delta B_{x,y} t_{k,l})} \qquad (9.24)$$

where $\Delta B_{x,y}$ is spatially variant field inhomogeneity and $t_{k,l}$ is the time between the sampling of the k-space location (k, l) and the RF excitation.

With the above representation, the PSF $H(x', y'; x, y)$ can be obtained from the two-dimensional (2-D) inverse FFT of the function $A(x, y; k, l)$ as

$$\begin{aligned} H(x', y'; x, y) &= \sum_{k=0}^{M-1} \sum_{l=0}^{N-1} A(x, y; k, l) e^{2\pi j((kx/M)+ly/N))} \\ &= \sum \sum e^{2\pi j((k(x'-x)/M)+(l(y'-y)/N)-(\gamma/2\pi)\Delta B_{x,y} t_{k,l})}. \end{aligned} \qquad (9.25)$$

9.2.2 Constrained Least Square Filtering

The constrained least square filtering method uses optimization techniques on a set of equations representing the image formation process. Equation 9.18 can be rewritten in matrix form as

$$\mathbf{g} = \mathbf{H}\mathbf{f} + \mathbf{n} \qquad (9.26)$$

where $\mathbf{g}$ is a column vector representing the reconstructed image $g(x, y)$, $\mathbf{f}$ is a column vector of $MN \times 1$ dimension, representing the ideal image $f(x, y)$, and $\mathbf{n}$ represents the noise vector. The PSF is represented by the matrix $\mathbf{H}$ of $MN \times MN$ elements.

For image restoration using the above equation, an estimate $\hat{\mathbf{f}}$ needs to be computed such that the mean-square error between the ideal image and the estimated image is minimized. The overall problem may not have a unique solution. Also, small variations in the matrix $\mathbf{H}$ may have significant impact on the noise content of the restored image. To overcome these problems, regularization methods involving constrained optimization techniques are used. Thus, the optimization process is subjected to specific constraints such as smoothness to avoid noisy solutions for the vector $\hat{\mathbf{f}}$. The smoothness constraint can be derived from the Laplacian for the estimated image. Using the theory of random variables, the optimization process is defined to estimate $\hat{\mathbf{f}}$ such that the mean-square error, e^2 given by

$$e^2 = \text{Trace } E\left\{\left(\mathbf{f} - \hat{\mathbf{f}}\right)\mathbf{f}^t\right\}$$

is minimized subject to the smoothness constraint involving the minimization of the roughness or Laplacian of the estimated image as

$$\min \{\hat{\mathbf{f}}^t [\mathbf{C}]^t [\mathbf{C}] \hat{\mathbf{f}}\}$$

where

$$[\mathbf{C}] = \begin{bmatrix} 1 & & & & & & \\ -2 & 1 & & & & & \\ 1 & -2 & 1 & & & & \\ & 1 & -2 & & & & \\ & & 1 & \cdot & & & \\ & & & \cdot & 1 & & \\ & & & & \cdot & -2 & \\ & & & & & 1 & \end{bmatrix}. \quad (9.27)$$

It can be shown that the estimated image $\hat{\mathbf{f}}$ can be expressed as (4)

$$\hat{\mathbf{f}} = \left([\mathbf{H}]^t [\mathbf{H}] + \frac{1}{\lambda} [\mathbf{C}]^t [\mathbf{C}] \right)^{-1} [\mathbf{H}]^t \mathbf{g} \quad (9.28)$$

where λ is a Lagrange multiplier.

9.2.3 Low-Pass Filtering

The ideal low-pass filter suppresses noise and high-frequency information providing a smoothing effect to the image. A 2-D low-pass filter function $H(u, v)$ is multiplied with the Fourier transform $G(u, v)$ of the image to provide a smoothed image as

$$\hat{F}(u, v) = H(u, v) G(u, v) \quad (9.29)$$

where $\hat{F}(u, v)$ is the Fourier transform of the filtered image $\hat{f}(x, y)$ that can be obtained by taking an inverse Fourier transform.

An ideal low-pass filter can be designed by assigning a frequency cutoff value, ω_0. The frequency cutoff value can also be expressed as the distance D_0 from the origin in the Fourier (frequency) domain.

$$H(u, v) = \begin{cases} 1 & \text{if } D(u, v) \leq D_0 \\ 0 & \text{otherwise} \end{cases} \quad (9.30)$$

where $D(u, v)$ is the distance of a point in the Fourier domain from the origin representing the dc value.

An ideal low-pass filter has sharp cutoff characteristics in the Fourier domain, causing a rectangular window for the pass band. From Chapter 2, it can be shown that a rectangular function in the frequency domain provides a sinc function in the spatial domain. Also, the multiplicative relationship of the filter model in Equation 9.29 causes a convolution operation in the spatial domain. The rectangular pass-band window in the ideal low-pass filter causes ringing artifacts in the spatial domain. To reduce ringing artifacts, the pass band should have a smooth fall-off characteristic.

A Butterworth low-pass filter of nth order can be used to provide smoother fall-off characteristics and is defined as

$$H(u, v) = \frac{1}{1+[D(u, v)/D_0]^{2n}}. \quad (9.31)$$

As the order n increases, the fall-off characteristics of the pass band become sharper. Thus, a first-order Butterworth filter provides the least amount of ringing artifacts in the filtered image.

A Gaussian function is also commonly used for low-pass filtering to provide smoother fall-off characteristics of the pass band and is defined by

$$H(u, v) = e^{-D^2(u,v)/2\sigma^2} \quad (9.32)$$

where $D(u, v)$ is the distance from the origin in the frequency domain and σ represents the standard deviation of the Gaussian function that can be set to the cutoff distance D_0 in the frequency domain.

In the above case, the gain of the filter is down to 0.607 of its maximum value at the cutoff frequency. Figure 9.14 shows a low-pass filter function with Gaussian window-based roll-off characteristics and the results of low-pass filtering of the MR brain image shown in Figure 9.1.

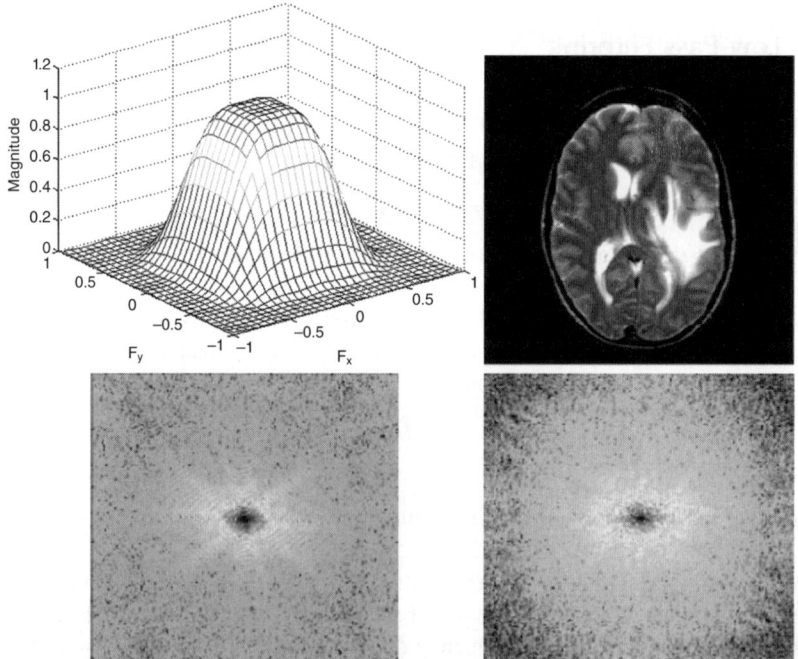

Figure 9.14 From top left clockwise: A low-pass filter function $H(u, v)$ in the Fourier domain, the low-pass filtered MR brain image, the Fourier transform of the original MR brain image shown in Figure 9.1, and the Fourier transform of the low-pass filtered MR brain image.

9.2.4 High-Pass Filtering

High-pass filtering is used for image sharpening and extraction of high-frequency information such as edges. The low-frequency information is attenuated or blocked depending on the design of the filter. An ideal high-pass filter has a rectangular window function for the high-frequency pass band. Since the noise in the image usually carries high-frequency components, high-pass filtering shows the noise along with edge information. An ideal 2-D high-pass filter with a cutoff frequency at a distance D_0 from the origin in the frequency domain is defined as

$$H(u, v) = \begin{cases} 0 & \text{if } D(u, v) \geq D_0 \\ 1 & \text{otherwise} \end{cases}. \quad (9.33)$$

As described above for an ideal low-pass filter, the sharp cutoff characteristic of the rectangular window function in the frequency domain as defined in Equation 9.33 causes the ringing artifacts in the filtered image in the spatial domain. To avoid ringing artifacts, filter functions with smoother fall-off characteristics such as Butterworth and Gaussian are used. A Butterworth high-pass filter of nth order is defined in the frequency domain as

$$H(u, v) = \frac{1}{1 + [D_0 / D(u, v)]^{2n}}. \quad (9.34)$$

A Gaussian high-pass filter is defined in the frequency domain as

$$H(u, v) = 1 - e^{-D^2(u, v)/2\sigma^2}. \quad (9.35)$$

Figure 9.15 shows a Gaussian high-pass filter function and the results of high-pass filtering of the MR brain image shown in Figure 9.1.

9.2.5 Homomorphic Filtering

The filtering model described above utilizes a single function or property (such as brightness) of the image. However, in homomorphic systems, the image formation can be described as a multiplication of two or more functions. For example, an image acquired by a photographic camera can be expressed as

$$f(x, y) = i(x, y)r(x, y) \quad (9.36)$$

where $i(x, y)$ and $r(x, y)$, respectively, represent the illumination and reflectance for a spatial point (x, y) in the image. In general, a two-function-based homomorphic system can be described as

$$f(x, y) = f_1(x, y)f_2(x, y) \quad (9.37)$$

where $f_1(x, y)$ and $f_2(x, y)$, respectively, represent two properties of the image.

The multiplicative relationship of two functions in Equation 9.37 can be converted into an additive relationship by applying a logarithmic operator as

$$g(x, y) = \ln f(x, y) = \ln f_1(x, y) + \ln f_2(x, y). \quad (9.38)$$

Homomorphic filtering is a method to perform frequency filtering in the logarithmic transform domain. Since the filtering is done in the frequency domain of the log of

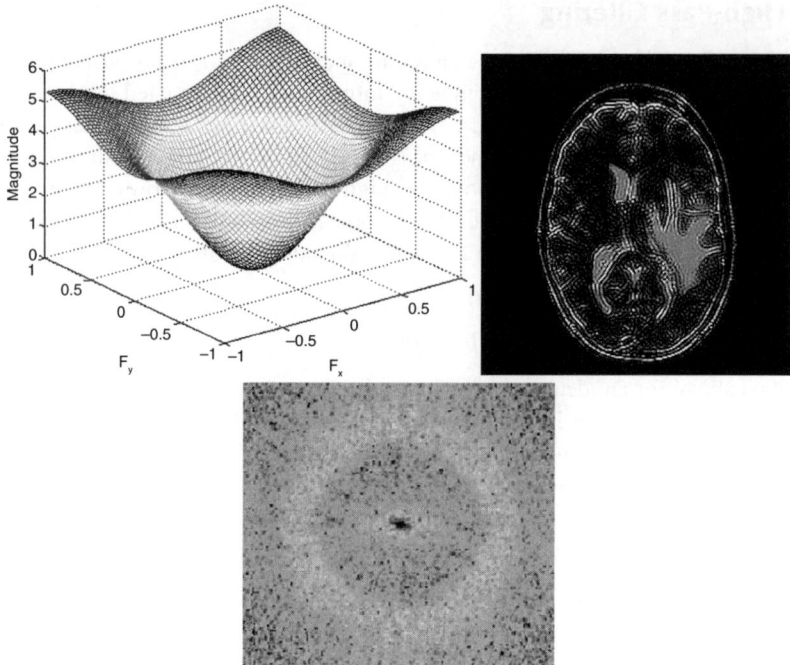

Figure 9.15   From top left clockwise: A high-pass filter function $H(u, v)$ in the Fourier domain, the high-pass filtered MR brain image, and the Fourier transform of the high-pass filtered MR brain image.

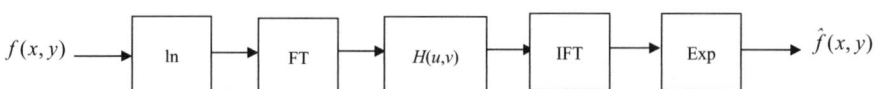

Figure 9.16   A schematic block diagram of homomorphic filtering method.

the image, after the filtering operation, an exponential operation has to be performed to get back to the spatial image domain. A block diagram of the homomorphic filtering method is shown in Figure 9.16.

The Fourier transform of Equation 9.38 provides

$$G(u, v) = F_1(u, v) + F_2(u, v). \tag{9.39}$$

With the application of a filter function $H(u, v)$ in the frequency domain, the filtered version can be expressed as

$$S(u, v) = H(u, v)G(u, v) = H(u, v)F_1(u, v) + H(u, v)F_2(u, v). \tag{9.40}$$

Taking inverse Fourier transform on Equation 9.40 provides

$$\begin{aligned} s(x, y) &= F^{-1}\{H(u, v)F_1(u, v)\} + F^{-1}\{H(u, v)F_2(u, v)\} \\ &= f_1'(x, y) + f_2'(x, y). \end{aligned} \tag{9.41}$$

Finally, an exponential operation is applied to obtain the filtered image $\hat{f}(x, y)$ in the spatial image domain as

$$\hat{f}(x, y) = e^{s(x,y)} = \hat{f}_1(x, y)\hat{f}_2(x, y). \tag{9.42}$$

If a model for the identification of functions, $f_1(x, y)$ and $f_2(x, y)$, is available, two different filter functions can be applied separately on the corresponding representation of each function. Typical filter functions such as Butterworh or Gaussian can be applied to implement homomorphic filter function $H(u, v)$ in the Fourier transform of the log domain of the image. In the absence of an imaging model, heuristic knowledge can be used to implement homomorphic filtering. For example, $f_1(x, y)$ and $f_2(x, y)$ components can represent, respectively, low- and high-frequency components in the image. A circularly symmetric homomorphic filter function can then be designed, as shown in Figure 9.17 (1).

A Gaussian high-pass filter function can then be used with some modification for implementation in the homomorphic filtering scheme for image sharpening as (1)

$$H(u, v) = (\gamma_H - \gamma_L)[1 - e^{c(D^2(u,v)/\sigma^2)}] + \gamma_L \tag{9.43}$$

where c is the parameter to control the sharpness effect in the filtered image. The MR brain image sharpened by homomorphic filtering using a circularly symmetric function obtained from the function shown in Figure 9.17 is shown in Figure 9.18.

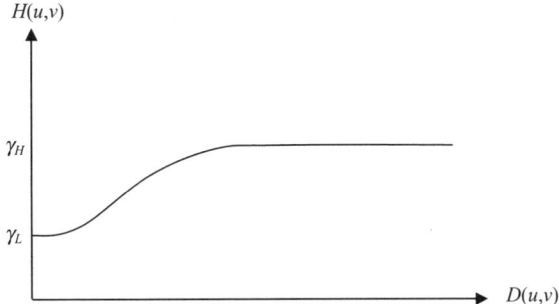

Figure 9.17 A circularly symmetric filter function for homomorphic filtering.

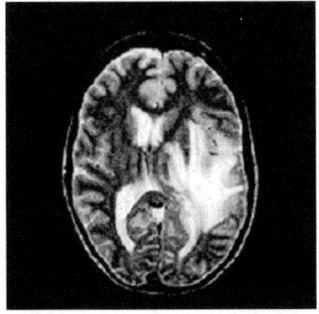

Figure 9.18 The enhanced MR brain image obtained by homomorphic filtering using a circularly symmetric function shown in Equation 9.43.

9.3. WAVELET TRANSFORM FOR IMAGE PROCESSING

As described in Chapter 2, wavelet transform provides a complete localization of spatio-frequency features in the image. Wavelet transform decomposes an image into a set of linearly weighted orthonormal basis functions through scaling and shifting operations. For wavelet transform analysis, a set of orthonormal basis functions is generated by scaling and translation of the mother wavelet $\psi(t)$ and the scaling function $\phi(t)$. Using the scaling operations, the multiresolution approach of the wavelet transform provides localization and representation of different frequencies in the image at different scales.

The wavelet functions with scaling and translations form an orthonormal basis in $L^2(R)$. The wavelet-spanned multiresolution subspace satisfies the relation

$$V_{j+1} = V_j \oplus W_j$$
$$= V_{j-1} \oplus W_{j-1} \oplus W_j$$
$$= V_{j-2} \oplus W_{j-2} \oplus W_{j-1} \oplus W_j$$

where $\oplus$ denotes the union operation of subspaces, and

$$L^2(R) = \ldots \oplus W_{-2} \oplus W_{-1} \oplus W_0 \oplus W_1 \oplus W_2 \oplus \ldots \quad (9.44)$$

where the original space V_{j+1} is divided into V_j and W_j spectral subspaces as the output of the low-pass and high-pass filters, respectively. These subspaces are then further decomposed into smaller spectral bands.

The wavelet functions span the orthogonal complement spaces with scaling and wavelet filter coefficients that are related as

$$h_\psi(n) = (-1)^n h_\phi(1-n). \quad (9.45)$$

As described in Chapter 2, an arbitrary square summable sequence $x[n]$ representing a signal in the time or space domain is expressed as

$$x[n] \in L^2(R). \quad (9.46)$$

The discrete signal $x[n]$ is decomposed into wavelet transform domain to obtain coefficients $X[k]$ as

$$x[n] = \sum_{k \in Z} \langle \varphi_k[l] x[l] \rangle \varphi_k[n] = \sum_{k \in Z} X[k] \varphi_k[n]$$

where

$$\varphi_{2k}[n] = h_0[2k-n] = g_0[n-2k]$$
$$\varphi_{2k+1}[n] = h_1[2k-n] = g_1[n-2k]$$

and

$$X[2k] = \langle h_0[2k-l], x[l] \rangle$$
$$X[2k+1] = \langle h_1[2k-l], x[l] \rangle. \quad (9.47)$$

In Equation 9.47, the orthonormal bases $\phi_k[n]$ are expressed as low-pass and high-pass filters for decomposition and reconstruction of a signal using the quadrature-mirror filter theory. The low-pass and high-pass filters for signal decomposition or analysis are expressed, respectively, as h_0 and h_1, while g_0 and g_1 are, respectively, the low-pass and high-pass filters for signal reconstruction or synthesis. A perfect reconstruction of the signal can be obtained from the wavelet coefficients as

$$\begin{aligned} x[n] &= \sum_{k \in Z} X[2k]\phi_{2k}[n] + \sum_{k \in Z} X[2k+1]\phi_{2k+1}[n] \\ &= \sum_{k \in Z} X[2k]g_0[n-2k] + \sum_{k \in Z} X[2k+1]g_1[n-2k]. \end{aligned} \quad (9.48)$$

Figure 9.19a (reproduced from Chapter 2) shows a schematic diagram of multiresolution signal decomposition using low-pass (H_0) and high-pass (H_1) decomposition filters to obtain wavelet coefficients. Figure 9.19b shows a schematic diagram of signal reconstruction from wavelet coefficients using low-pass (G_0) and high-pass (G_1) reconstruction filters. As described in Chapter 2, an image can be analyzed using one-dimensional (1-D) wavelet transform with low-pass and high-pass decomposition filters in multiresolution space for image processing applications. The image is first sampled along the rows and then along the columns for analysis using 1-D low-pass and high-pass filters. The image, at resolution 2^{j+1}, represented by A_{j+1}, is first low-pass and then high-pass filtered along the rows. The result of each filtering process is subsampled. Next, the subsampled results are low-pass and high-pass filtered along each column. The results of these filtering processes are again subsampled. The frequency band denoted by A_j in Figure 9.20 is referred to as the low-low-frequency band. It contains the scaled low-frequency information. The frequency bands labeled D_j^1, D_j^2, and D_j^3 denote the detail information. They are referred to as low-high, high-low, and high-high-frequency bands, respectively. This analysis can be iteratively applied to an image for further decompose into narrower frequency bands, that is, each frequency band can be further decomposed into four

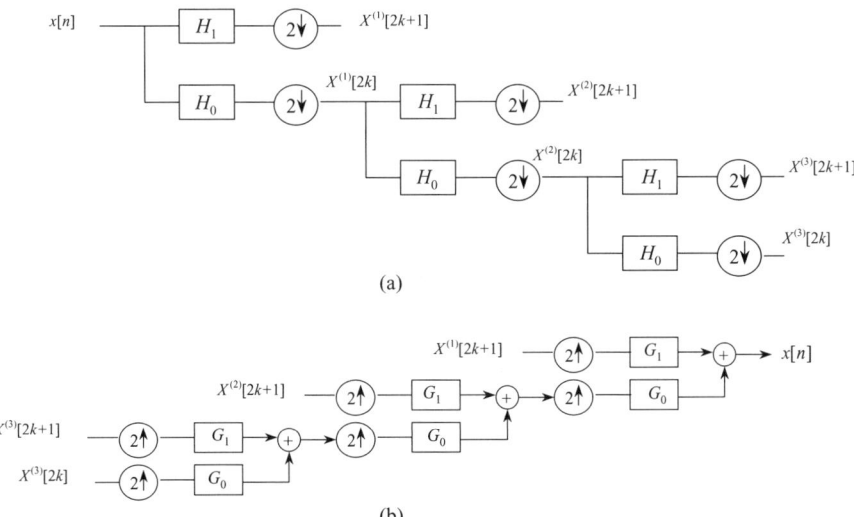

Figure 9.19 (a) A multiresolution signal decomposition using wavelet transform and (b) the reconstruction of the signal from wavelet transform coefficients.

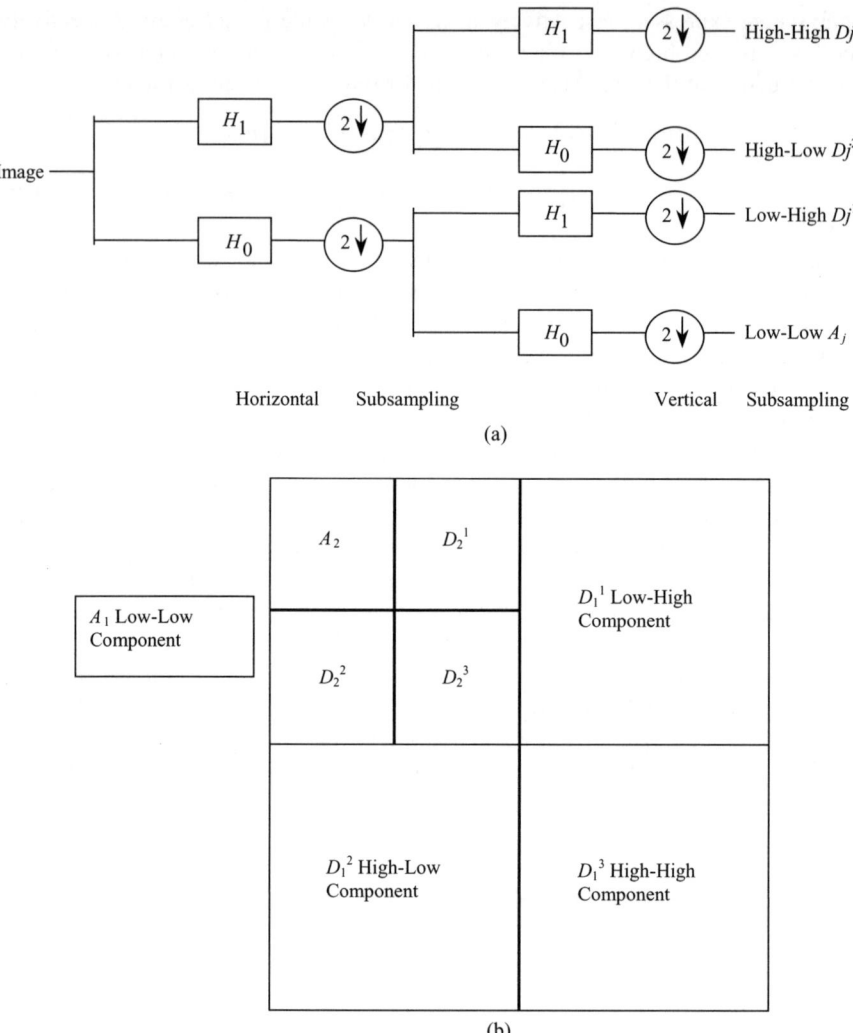

Figure 9.20 (a) Multiresolution decomposition of an image using the wavelet transform. (b) Wavelet transform-based image decomposition: the original resolution image ($N \times N$) is decomposed into four low-low A_1, low-high D_1^1, high-low D_1^2, and high-high D_1^3 images each of which is subsampled to resolution $[(N/2) \times (N/2)]$. The low-low image is further decomposed into four images of $[(N/4) \times (N/4)]$ resolution each in the second level of decomposition. For a full decomposition, each of the "Detail" component can also be decomposed into four sub-images with $[(N/4) \times (N/4)]$ resolution each.

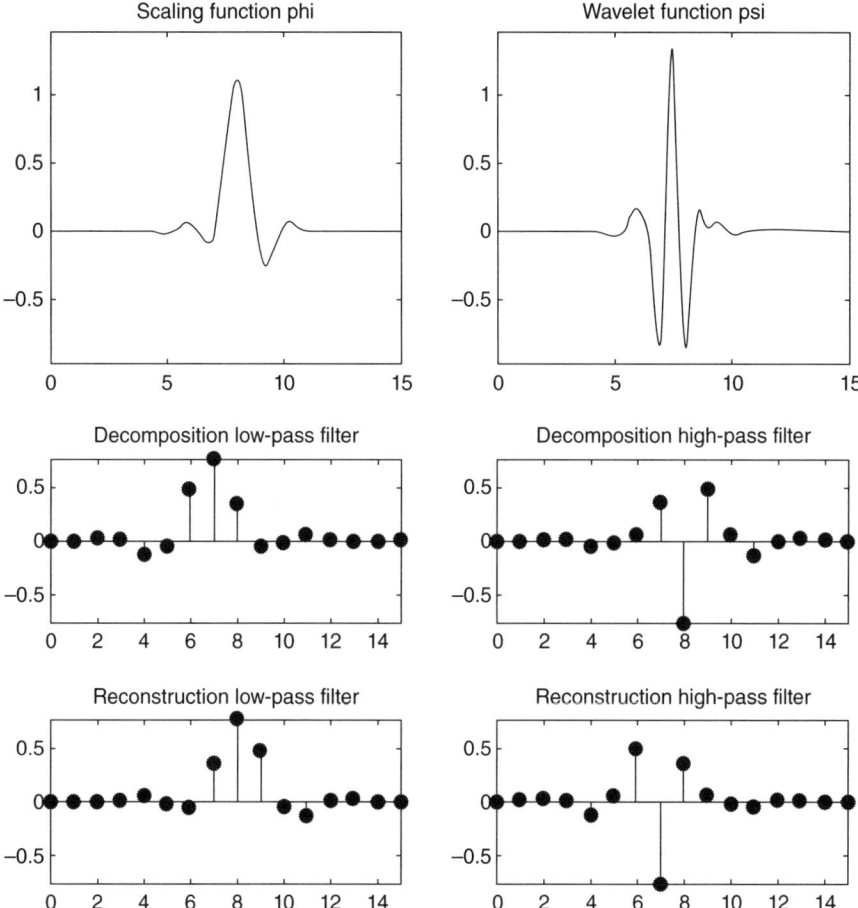
Figure 9.21 A least asymmetric wavelet with eight coefficients.

narrower bands. Each level of decomposition reduces the resolution by a factor of two. The multiscale framework of signal decomposition into narrower frequency bands is also called wavelet packet analysis.

The "least asymmetric" wavelets were designed by Daubechies (17) for applications in signal and image processing. A least asymmetric wavelet is shown in Figure 9.21 with the coefficients of the corresponding low-pass and high-pass filters given in Table 9.1.

9.3.1 Image Smoothing and Enhancement Using Wavelet Transform

The wavelet transform provides a set of coefficients representing the localized information in a number of frequency bands. A popular method for denoising and smoothing is to threshold the coefficients in those bands that have high probability

TABLE 9.1 The Coefficients for the Corresponding Low-Pass and High-Pass Filters for the Least Asymmetric Wavelet

N	High-pass	Low-pass
0	−0.107148901418	0.045570345896
1	−0.041910965125	0.017824701442
2	0.703739068656	−0.140317624179
3	1.136658243408	−0.421234534204
4	0.421234534204	1.136658243408
5	−0.140317624179	−0.703739068656
6	−0.017824701442	−0.041910965125
7	0.045570345896	0.107148901418

of noise and then reconstruct the image using reconstruction filters. Reconstruction filters, as described in Equation 9.48, can be derived from the decomposition filters using the quadrature-mirror theory (17–20). The reconstruction process integrates information from specific bands with successive upscaling of resolution to provide the final reconstructed image at the same resolution as the input image. If certain coefficients related to the noise or noise-like information are not included in the reconstruction process, the reconstructed image shows a reduction of noise and smoothing effects.

Wavelet coefficients are correlated with specific spatio-frequency features in the image (21, 22). A specific feature can be eliminated if the respective wavelet coefficient(s) in the wavelet transform domain are thresholded and then the image is reconstructed using nonthresholded coefficients. Similarly, a specific feature can be enhanced if the corresponding wavelet coefficients are strengthened (multiplied by appropriate gain factor while others may be threshold and normalized) in the wavelet transform domain, and then the image is reconstructed from using modified wavelet coefficients with an appropriate interpolation method (23, 24). For image denoising or smoothing, hard or soft thresholding methods may be applied in the wavelet transform domain. With the hard thresholding method, all coefficients below the predetermined threshold are set to zero as

$$\omega_T(X) = \begin{cases} X & \text{if } |X| > T \\ 0 & \text{if } |X| \leq T \end{cases} \quad (9.49)$$

where $\omega_T(X)$ represents modified coefficient value for thresholding the wavelet coefficient X at the threshold T.

In the soft thresholding method, the nonthresholded coefficients are rearranged to the range of 0 to maximum value as

$$\omega_T(X) = \begin{cases} X - T & \text{if } |X| \geq T \\ X + T & \text{if } |X| \leq -T \\ 0 & \text{if } |X| < T \end{cases}. \quad (9.50)$$

Monotonically increasing or piecewise linear enhancement functions can be used in rescaling and thresholding wavelet coefficients in the wavelet transform domain for specific feature enhancement (25–27). Laine et al. (26) used a simple piecewise linear enhancement function to modify wavelet coefficients for feature enhancement as

$$E(X) = \begin{cases} X - (K-1)T & \text{if } X < -T \\ KX & \text{if } |X| \leq T \\ X + (K-1)T & \text{if } X > T \end{cases}$$
(9.51)

where $E(X)$ represents enhanced coefficient value for the wavelet coefficient X at the threshold T.

As can be seen in Figure 9.22, the coefficients available in the low-high, high-low, and high-high-frequency bands in the decomposition process provide edge-related information that can be emphasized in the reconstruction process for image sharpening (10, 22). Figure 9.23 shows a smoothed version of the MR brain image reconstructed using all bands, except the high-high-frequency band. Figure 9.24 shows an image that is reconstructed using the high-high-frequency band information only.

It is difficult to discriminate image features from noise based on the spatial distribution of gray values. The noise, which is usually of a high-frequency nature, should be de-emphasized when other high-frequency features of interest, such as edges, are enhanced. A useful distinction between the noise and image features may be made, if some knowledge about the processed image features and their behavior is known a priori. This points out the need for some partial image analysis that must be performed before the image enhancement operations are performed. Thus, an intelligent or knowledge-based feature enhancement may provide better

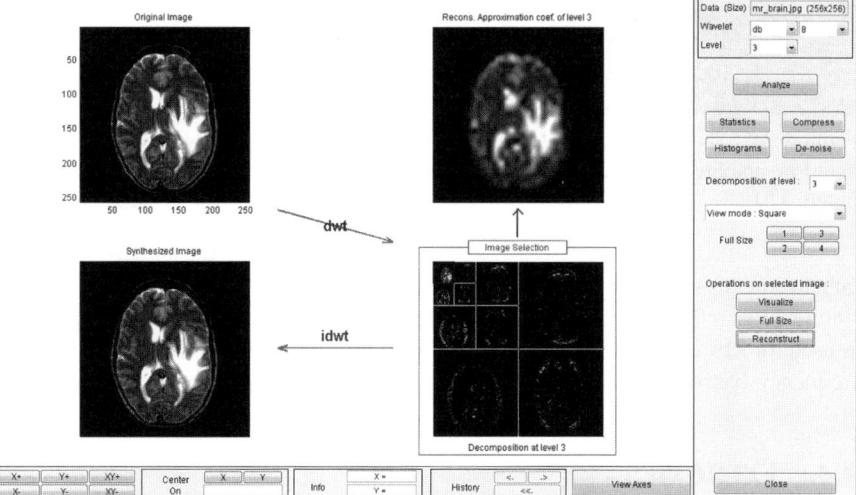

Figure 9.22 Three-level wavelet decomposition of the MR brain image (top left) is shown at the bottom right with inverse discrete wavelet transform shown at bottom left. A reconstruction from low-low pass-band decomposition at the third level is shown at the top right.

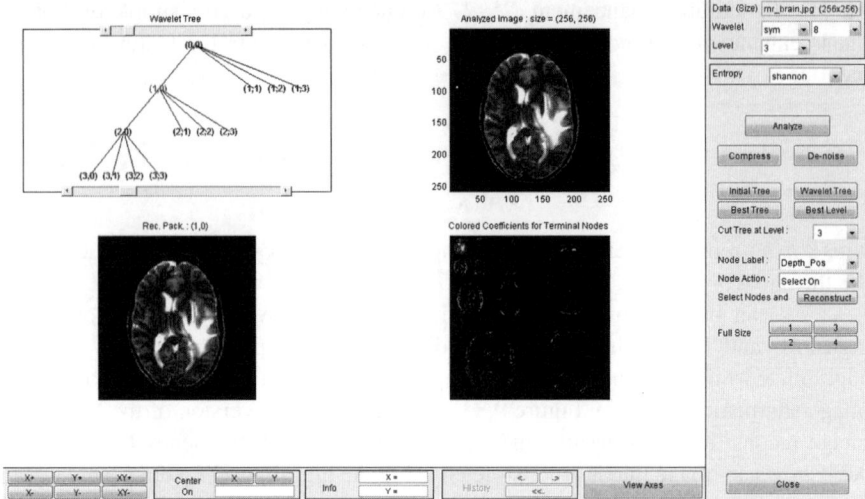

Figure 9.23 The MR brain image of Figure 9.1 (top right) reconstructed from the low-low-frequency band at the first decomposition level (node [1, 0] in the wavelet tree) is shown at the bottom left with three levels of wavelet decomposition (bottom right).

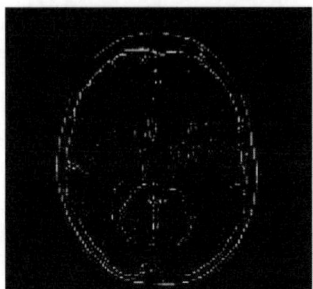

Figure 9.24 The MR brain image of Figure 9.1 reconstructed from the low-high, high-low, and high-high-frequency bands using the wavelet decomposition shown in Figure 9.21.

enhancement. An example is provided above for the enhancement of microcalcification features in X-ray mammography. A scale-based diffusive image filtering method is used for MR images for image enhancement and denoising while preserving high-frequency-based fine structures (25–27).

9.4. EXERCISES

9.1. **a.** Why are image smoothing and image sharpening operations important in medical image processing and analysis?

  b. What is the difference between image smoothing and image sharpening?

9.2. What is the difference between spatial and frequency filtering methods? Compare the advantages of both types of methods.

9.3. Does median filtering provide better image smoothing and denoising than weighted averaging? Apply both methods in MATLAB on a CT brain image and compare their results.

9.4. Use the following image enhancement methods in MATLAB on a T_1-weighted MR brain image and comment on the contrast of features in enhanced images:

  a. Histogram equalization

  b. Sobel gradient masks

  c. Laplacian gradient mask

  d. Local histogram equalization

9.5. Repeat Exercise 9.4 for an X-ray mammography image and comment on the results on contrast enhancement for each method. Do you observe similar effects of feature enhancement on the mammography image as you observed for the MR brain image in Exercise 9.4?

9.6. Use the image selected in Exercise 9.4 for Gaussian high-pass filtering for image sharpening. Compare the filtered image with the enhanced image obtained using Laplacian mask.

9.7. Apply a parametric Weiner filtering method on the image selected in Exercise 9.5 and compare the results for three choices of the parameter K. Assume a Gaussian blur function with a variance of 9 pixels to compute a PSF. What is the effect of using different values of the parameter K on the output image?

9.8. Add Gaussian noise to the mammography image used in Exercise 9.5 using the "noise" function in MATLAB. Repeat Exercise 9.5 on the noisy image and compare restored images with those obtained in Exercise 9.5.

9.9. Use a brain image for wavelet-based three-level decomposition using the following wavelets (level 4) in the MATLAB environment:

  a. HAAR

  b. db6

  c. db8

  d. sym4

9.10. Using the decomposition tree in the MATLAB environment, reconstruct the image using the following subbands and compare the results with respect to visible features:

  a. Low-low-low

  b. High-high-high

  c. All bands except low-low-low

9.11. Repeat Exercise 9.13 for the X-ray mammography image selected in Exercise 9.5. Compare wavelet-based image enhancement results with those obtained from Gaussian low-pass and high-pass frequency filtering in Exercise 9.5.

9.5. REFERENCES

1. R.C. Gonzalez and R.E. Woods, *Digital Image Processing*, Prentice Hall, Englewood Cliffs, NJ, 2002.
2. A.K. Jain, *Fundamentals of Digital Image Processing*, Prentice Hall, Englewood Cliffs, NJ, 1989.
3. R. Jain, R. Kasturi, and B.G. Schunck, *Machine Vision*, McGraw-Hill, New York, 1995.
4. A. Rosenfeld and A.V. Kak, *Digital Picture Processing*, Volumes 1 and 2, 2nd Edition, Academic Press, Orlando, FL, 1982.
5. J.C. Russ, *The Image Processing Handbook*, 2nd Edition, CRC Press, Boca Raton, FL, 1995.
6. R.J. Schalkoff, *Digital Image Processing and Computer Vision*, John Wiley & Sons, New York, 1989.
7. Y.H. Kao and J.R. MacFall, "Correction of MR-k space data corrupted by spike noise," *IEEE Trans. Med. Imaging*, Vol. 19, pp. 671–680, 2000.
8. O.A. Ahmed and M.M. Fahmy, "NMR signal enhancement via a new time-frequency transform," *IEEE Trans. Med. Imaging*, Vol. 20, pp. 1018–1025, 2001.
9. C. Goutte, F.A. Nielson, and L.K. Hansen, "Modeling of hemodynamic response in fMRI using smooth FIR filters," *IEEE Trans. Med. Imaging*, Vol. 19, pp. 1188–1201, 2000.
10. S. Zaroubi and G. Goelman, "Complex denoising of MR data via wavelet analysis: Applications for functional MRI," *Magn. Reson. Imaging*, Vol. 18, pp. 59–68, 2000.
11. G.W. Davis and S.T. Wallenslager, "Improvement of chest region CT images through automated gray-level remapping," *IEEE Trans. Med. Imaging*, Vol. MI-5, pp. 30–35, 1986.
12. S.M. Pizer, J.B. Zimmerman, and E.V. Staab, "Adaptive gray-level assignment in CT scan display," *J. Comput. Assist. Tomog.*, Vol. 8, pp. 300–306, 1984.
13. A.P. Dhawan and E. LeRoyer, "Mammographic feature enhancement by computerized image processing," *Comput. Methods Programs Biomed.*, Vol. 27, pp. 23–29, 1988.
14. J.K. Kim, J.M. Park, K.S. Song, and H.W. Park, "Adaptive mammographic image enhancement using first derivative and local statistics," *IEEE Trans. Med. Imaging*, Vol. 16, pp. 495–502, 1997.
15. G. Chen, H. Avram, L. Kaufman, J. Hale, and D. Kramer, "T2 restoration and noise suppression of hybrid MR images using Wiener and linear prediction techniques," *IEEE Trans. Med. Imaging*, Vol. 13, pp. 667–676, 1994.
16. P. Munger, G.R. Crelier, T.M. Peters, and G.B. Pike, "An inverse problem approach to the correction of distortion in EPI images," *IEEE Trans. Med. Imaging*, Vol. 19, pp. 681–689, 2000.
17. I. Daubechies, *Ten Lectures on Wavelets*, Society for Applied Mathematics, Philadelphia, 1992.
18. S. Mallat, "A theory for multiresolution signal decomposition: The wavelet representation," *IEEE Trans. Pattern Anal. Mach. Intell.*, Vol. 11, No. 7, pp. 674–693, 1989.
19. S. Mallat, "Wavelets for a vision," *Proc. IEEE*, Vol. 84, No. 4, pp. 604–614, 1996.
20. M. Vetterli and J. Kovacevic, *Wavelets and Subband Coding*, Prentice Hall, Englewood Cliffs, 1995.
21. A. Bovik, M. Clark, and W. Geisler, "Multichannel texture analysis using localized spatial filters," *IEEE Trans. Pattern Anal. Mach. Intell.*, Vol. 12, pp. 55–73, 1990.
22. J.B. Weaver, X. Yansun, D.M. Healy Jr., and L.D. Cromwell, "Filtering noise from images with wavelet transforms," *Mag. Reson. Med.*, Vol. 21, No. 2, pp. 288–295, 1991.
23. A.P. Pentland, "Interpolation using wavelet bases," *IEEE Trans. Pattern Anal. Mach. Intell.*, Vol. 16, No. 4, pp. 410–414, 1994.
24. M-H. Yaou and W-T. Chang, "Fast surface interpolation using multiresolution wavelet transform," *IEEE Trans. Pattern Anal. Mach. Intell.*, Vol. 16, No. 7, pp. 673–688, 1994.
25. P.K. Saha and J.K. Udupa, "Scale-based diffusive image filtering preserving boundary sharpness and fine structures," *IEEE Trans. Med. Imaging*, Vol. 20, pp. 1140–1155, 2001.
26. A. Laine, "Wavelets in spatial processing of biomedical images," *Annu. Rev. Biomed. Eng.*, Vol. 2, pp. 511–550, 2000.
27. M. Unser, A. Aldroubi, and A. Laine, "IEEE transactions on medical imaging," Special Issue on Wavelet s in Medical Imaging, 2003.

CHAPTER 10

IMAGE SEGMENTATION

Segmentation is an important step in medical image analysis and classification for radiological evaluation or computer-aided diagnosis. Image segmentation refers to the process of partitioning an image into distinct regions by grouping together neighborhood pixels based on some predefined similarity criterion. The similarity criterion can be determined using specific properties or features of pixels representing objects in the image. In other words, segmentation is a pixel classification technique that allows the formation of regions of similarities in the image.

Image segmentation methods can be broadly classified into three categories:

1. Edge-based methods in which the edge information is used to determine boundaries of objects. The boundaries are then analyzed and modified as needed to form closed regions belonging to the objects in the image.

2. Pixel-based methods in which heuristics or estimation methods derived from the histogram statistics of the image are used to form closed regions belonging to the objects in the image.

3. Region-based methods in which pixels are analyzed directly for a region-expansion process based on a predefined similarity criterion to form closed regions belonging to the objects in the image.

Once the regions are defined, features can be computed to represent regions for characterization, analysis, and classification. These features may include shape and texture information of the regions as well as statistical properties, such as variance and mean of gray values.

This chapter describes major image segmentation methods for medical image analysis and classification.

10.1. EDGE-BASED IMAGE SEGMENTATION

Edge-based approaches use a spatial filtering method to compute the first-order or second-order gradient information of the image. As described in Chapter 9, Sobel or other directional derivative masks can be used to compute gradient information. The Laplacian mask can be used to compute second-order gradient information of the image. For segmentation purposes, edges need to be linked to form closed regions. Gradient information of the image is used to track and link relevant edges.

Medical Image Analysis, Second Edition, by Atam P. Dhawan
Copyright © 2011 by the Institute of Electrical and Electronics Engineers, Inc.

The second step is usually very tedious. In addition, it has to deal with the uncertainties in the gradient information due to noise and artifacts in the image.

10.1.1 Edge Detection Operations

The gradient magnitude and directional information from the Sobel horizontal and vertical direction masks can be obtained by convolving the respective G_x and G_y masks with the image as (1, 2)

$$G_x = \begin{bmatrix} -1 & 0 & 1 \\ -2 & 0 & 2 \\ -1 & 0 & 1 \end{bmatrix}$$

$$G_y = \begin{bmatrix} 1 & 2 & 1 \\ 0 & 0 & 0 \\ -1 & -2 & -1 \end{bmatrix}$$

$$M = \sqrt{G_x^2 + G_y^2} \approx |G_x| + |G_y| \qquad (10.1)$$

where M represents the magnitude of the gradient that can be approximated as the sum of the absolute values of the horizontal and vertical gradient images obtained by convolving the image with the horizontal and vertical masks G_x and G_y.

The second-order gradient operator Laplacian can be computed by convolving one of the following masks, $G_{L(4)}$ and $G_{L(8)}$, which, respectively, use a 4- and 8-connected neighborhood.

$$G_{L(4)} = \begin{bmatrix} 0 & -1 & 0 \\ -1 & 4 & -1 \\ 0 & -1 & 0 \end{bmatrix}$$

$$G_{L(8)} = \begin{bmatrix} -1 & -1 & -1 \\ -1 & 8 & -1 \\ -1 & -1 & -1 \end{bmatrix}. \qquad (10.2)$$

The second-order derivative, Laplacian, is very sensitive to noise as can be seen from the distribution of weights in the masks in Equation 10.2. The Laplacian mask provides a nonzero output even for a single pixel-based speckle noise in the image. Therefore, it is usually beneficial to apply a smoothing filter first before taking a Laplacian of the image. The image can be smoothed using a Gaussian weighted spatial averaging as the first step. The second step then uses a Laplacian mask to determine edge information. Marr and Hildreth (3) combined these two steps into a single Laplacian of Gaussian (LOG) function as

$$h(x, y) = \nabla^2[g(x, y) \otimes f(x, y)]$$
$$= \nabla^2[g(x, y)] \otimes f(x, y) \qquad (10.3)$$

where $\nabla^2[g(x, y)]$ is the LOG function that is used for spatial averaging and is commonly expressed as the Mexican hat operator:

$$\nabla^2[g(x,y)] = \left(\frac{x^2 + y^2 - 2\sigma^2}{\sigma^4}\right) e^{-\frac{(x^2+y^2)}{2\sigma^2}} \quad (10.4)$$

where σ^2 is the variance of the Gaussian function.

A LOG mask for computing the second-order gradient information of the smoothed image can be computed from Equation 10.4. With $\sigma = 2$, the LOG mask G_{LOG} of 5×5 pixels is given by

$$G_{LOG} = \begin{bmatrix} 0 & 0 & -1 & 0 & 0 \\ 0 & -1 & -2 & -1 & 0 \\ -1 & -2 & 16 & -2 & -1 \\ 0 & -1 & -2 & -1 & 0 \\ 0 & 0 & -1 & 0 & 0 \end{bmatrix}. \quad (10.5)$$

The image obtained by convolving the LOG mask with the original image is analyzed for zero crossing to detect edges since the output image provides values from negative to positive. One simple method to detect zero crossing is to threshold the output image for zero value. This operation provides a new binary image such that a "0" gray value is assigned to the binary image if the output image has a negative or zero value for the corresponding pixel. Otherwise, a high gray value (such as "255" for an 8 bit image) is assigned to the binary image. The zero crossing of the output image can now be easily determined by tracking the pixels with a transition from black ("0" gray value) to white ("255" gray value) on an 8-bit gray-level scale.

10.1.2 Boundary Tracking

Edge detection operations are usually followed up by the edge-linking procedures to assemble meaningful edges to form closed regions. Edge-linking procedures are based on pixel-by-pixel search to find connectivity among the edge segments. The connectivity can be defined using a similarity criterion among edge pixels. In addition, geometrical proximity or topographical properties are used to improve edge-linking operations for pixels that are affected by noise, artifacts, or geometrical occlusion. Estimation methods based on probabilistic approaches, graphs, and rule-based methods for model-based segmentation have also been used (4–27).

In neighborhood search methods, the simplest method is to follow the edge detection operation by a boundary-tracking algorithm. Let us assume that the edge detection operation produces edge magnitude $e(x, y)$ and edge orientation $\phi(x, y)$ information. The edge orientation information can be directly obtained from the directional masks, as described in Chapter 9, or computed from the horizontal and vertical gradient masks. Let us start with a list of edge pixels that can be selected by scanning the gradient image obtained from the edge detection operation. Assuming the first edge pixel as a boundary pixel b_j, a successor boundary pixel b_{j+1} can be found in the 4- or 8-connected neighborhood if the following conditions are satisfied:

$$|e(b_j)| > T_1$$
$$|e(b_{j+1})| > T_1$$
$$|e(b_j) - e(b_{j+1})| < T_2$$
$$|\phi(b_j) - \phi(b_{j+1})| \bmod 2\pi < T_3 \qquad (10.6)$$

where T_1, T_2, and T_3 are predetermined thresholds.

If there is more than one neighboring pixel that satisfies these conditions, the pixel that minimizes the differences is selected as the next boundary pixel. The algorithm is recursively applied until all neighbors are searched. If no neighbor is found satisfying these conditions, the boundary search for the striating edge pixel is stopped and a new edge pixel is selected. It can be noted that such a boundary-tracking algorithm may leave many edge pixels and partial boundaries unconnected. Some a priori knowledge about the object's boundaries is often needed to form regions with closed boundaries. Relational tree structures or graphs can also be used to help form the closed regions (28, 29).

A graph-based search method attempts to find paths between the start and end nodes minimizing a cost function that may be established based on the distance and transition probabilities. The start and end nodes are determined by scanning the edge pixels based on some heuristic criterion. For example, an initial search may label the first edge pixel in the image as the start node and all the other edge pixels in the image or a part of the image as potential end nodes. Among several graph-based search algorithms, the A* algorithm is widely used (28, 29).

The A* search algorithm can be implemented using the following steps (29):

1. Select an edge pixel as the start node of the boundary and put all of the successor boundary pixels in a list, OPEN.

2. If there is no node in the OPEN list, stop; otherwise continue.

3. For all nodes in the OPEN list, compute the cost function $t(z_k)$ and select the node z_k with the smallest cost. Remove the node z_k from the OPEN list and label it as CLOSED. The cost function $t(z)$ may be computed as

$$t(z_k) = c(z_k) + h(z_k)$$
$$c(z_k) = \sum_{i=2}^{k} s(z_{i-1}, z_i) + \sum_{j=1}^{k} d(z_j) \qquad (10.7)$$

where $s(z_{i-1}, z_i)$ and $d(z_i)$ are the transition and local costs, and $h(z_k)$ is the lower bound estimate of the cost function.

4. If z_k is the end node, exit with the solution path by backtracking the pointers; otherwise continue.

5. Expand the node z_k by finding all successors of z_i. If there is no successor, go to step 2; otherwise continue.

6. If a successor z_i is not labeled yet in any list, put it in the list OPEN with updated cost as $c(z_i) = c(z_k) + s(z_k, z_i) + d(z_i)$ and a pointer to its predecessor z_k.

10.1. EDGE-BASED IMAGE SEGMENTATION

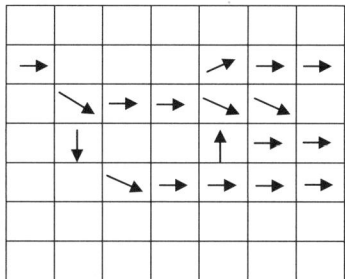

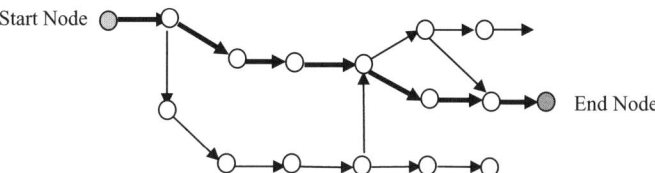

Figure 10.1 Top: An edge map with magnitude and direction information. Bottom: A graph derived from the edge map with a minimum cost path (dark arrows) between the start and end nodes.

7. If a successor z_i is already labeled as CLOSED or OPEN, update its value by $c'(z_i) = \min[c(z_i), c(z_k) + s(z_k, z_i)]$. Put those CLOSED successors, whose cost functions $c'(z_i)$ were lowered, in the OPEN list and redirect to z_k the pointers from all nodes whose costs were lowered.

8. Go to step 2.

The A* algorithm may not always find the optimal solution with minimum cost path a suboptimal solution can be found with the use of some a priori or heuristic information (29). Figure 10.1 shows a schematic representation of an example edge map and a graph of edge nodes with a probable minimum cost path. It can be seen that the path marked with bold arrows may not necessarily be the optimal path.

10.1.3 Hough Transform

The Hough transform is used to detect straight lines and other parametric curves such as circles and ellipses (14). It can also be used to detect boundaries of an arbitrarily shaped object if the parameters of the object are known. The basic concept of the generalized Hough transform is that an analytical function such as a straight line, a circle, or a closed shape, represented in the image space (spatial domain), has a dual representation in the parameter space. For example, the general equation of a straight line can be given as

$$y = mx + c \qquad (10.8)$$

where m is the slope and c is the y-intercept.

As can be seen from Equation 10.8, the locus of points is described by two parameters, slope and y-intercept. Therefore, a line in the image space forms a point

(m, c) in the parameter space. Likewise, a point in the image space forms a line in the parameter space. Therefore, a locus of points forming a line in the image space will form a set of lines in the parameter space, whose intersection represents the parameters of the line in the image space. If a gradient image is thresholded to provide edge pixels, each edge pixel can be mapped to the parameter space. The mapping can be implemented using the bins of points in the parameter space. For each edge pixel of the straight line in the image space, the corresponding bin in the parameter space is updated. At the end, the bin with the maximum count represents the parameters of the straight line detected in the image. The concept can be extended to map and detect boundaries of a predefined curve. In general, the points in the image space become hyperplanes in the N-dimensional parameter space and the parameters of the object function in the image space can be found by searching the peaks in the parameter space caused by the intersection of the hyperplanes.

To detect object boundaries using the Hough transform, it is necessary to create a parameter model of the object. The object model is transferred into a table called an R-table. The R-table can be considered as a one-dimensional array where each entry of the array is a list of vectors. For each point in the model description (MD), a gradient along with the corresponding vector extending from the boundary point to the centroid (Fig. 10.2) is computed. The gradient acts as an index for the R-table.

For object recognition, a two-dimensional (2-D) parameter space of possible x–y coordinate centers is initialized, with the accumulator values associated with each location set to zero. An edge pixel from the gradient image is selected. The gradient information is indexed into the R-table. Each vector in the corresponding list is added to the location of the edge pixel. The endpoint of the vector should now point to a new edge pixel in the gradient image. The accumulator of the corresponding location in the parameter space is then increased by one. As each edge pixel is examined, the accumulator for the corresponding location receives the highest count. If the model object is considered to be translated in the image, the accumulator for the correct translation location would receive the highest count. To deal with rotation and scaling, the process must be repeated for all possible rotations and scales. Thus, the complete process could become very tedious if a large number of rotations and

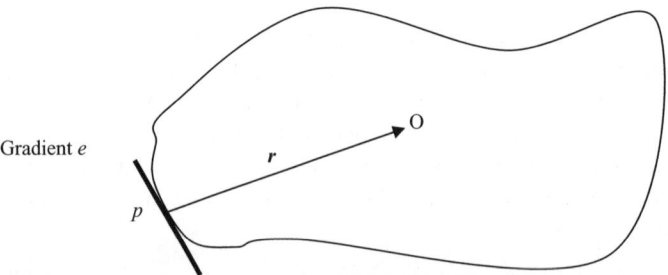

Figure 10.2 A model of an object shape to be detected in the image using Hough transform. The vector r connects the centroid and a tangent point p. The magnitude and angle of the vector r are stored in the R-table at a location indexed by the gradient of the tangent point p.

scales are examined. To avoid this complication, simple transformations can be made in the *R*-table of the transformation (14).

10.2. PIXEL-BASED DIRECT CLASSIFICATION METHODS

The pixel-based direct classification methods use histogram statistics to define single or multiple thresholds to classify an image pixel by pixel. The threshold for classifying pixels is obtained from the analysis of the histogram of the image. A simple approach is to examine the histogram for bimodal distribution. If the histogram is bimodal, the threshold can be set to the gray value corresponding to the deepest point in the histogram valley. If not, the image can be partitioned into two or more regions using some heuristics about the properties of the image. The histogram of each partition can then be used for determining thresholds. By comparing the gray value of each pixel to the selected threshold, a pixel can be classified into one of two classes.

Let us assume that an image or a part of an image has a bimodal histogram of gray values as shown in Figure 10.3. The image $f(x, y)$ can be segmented into two classes using a gray value threshold T such that

$$g(x, y) = \begin{cases} 1 & \text{if } f(x, y) > T \\ 0 & \text{if } f(x, y) \leq T \end{cases} \tag{10.9}$$

where $g(x, y)$ is the segmented image with two classes of binary gray values, "1" and "0", and T is the threshold selected at the valley point from the histogram.

A simple approach to determine the gray-value threshold T is by analyzing the histogram for the peak values and then finding the deepest valley point between the two consecutive major peaks. If a histogram is clearly bimodal, this method gives good results. However, medical images may have multiple peaks with specific requirements of regions to be segmented. For example, the magnetic resonance (MR) brain image shown in Figure 10.3 has two major peaks in the histogram. The first major peak is at the gray value 0, representing the black background. The second major peak is at the gray value 71, with a distribution of gray values corresponding to the brain tissue regions within the skull. The first requirement of the MR brain image segmentation may be to extract the overall brain area under the skull. This can be accomplished by finding out the deepest valley point between the two major peaks. The threshold T of gray value 12 is thus selected to separate the brain area from the background as shown in Figure 10.3. It can be noted that there are some holes within the segmented brain region using the gray-value threshold. These holes may be filled to quantify the overall brain area under the skull in the image.

To segment specific brain regions such as ventricles (the large structure in the middle of the image), additional thresholds can be determined from the histogram. These thresholds can be determined by finding out additional peaks in the remaining distribution of the histogram belonging to the second major peak, that is, around or after the gray value 12. A close examination of the histogram in Figure 10.3 shows a third peak around the gray value 254, representing the brightest pixels in the image.

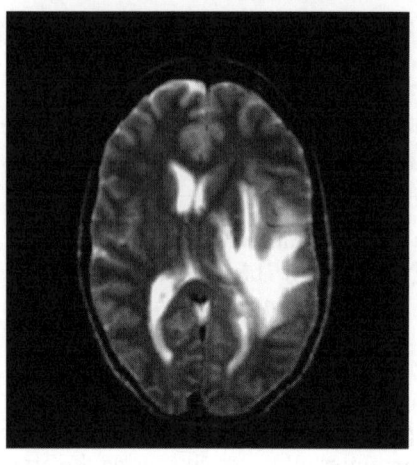

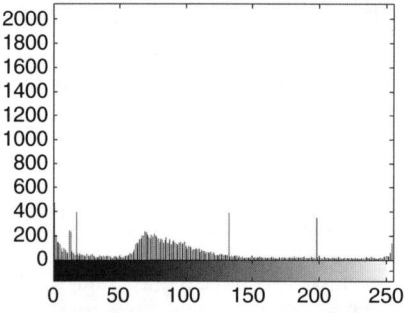

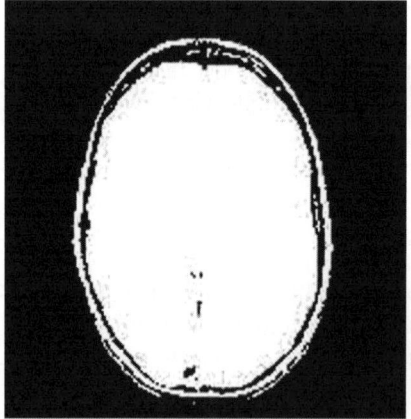

Figure 10.3 The original MR brain image (top), its gray-level histogram (middle), and the segmented image (bottom) using a gray-value threshold $T = 12$ at the first major valley point in the histogram.

A threshold between the values 12 and 254 can be determined interactively to segment the regions of interest. An alternative approach is to recompute another histogram for the gray values between 12 and 255 (corresponding to the segmented brain area only) and then to analyze this histogram for peaks and values to determine

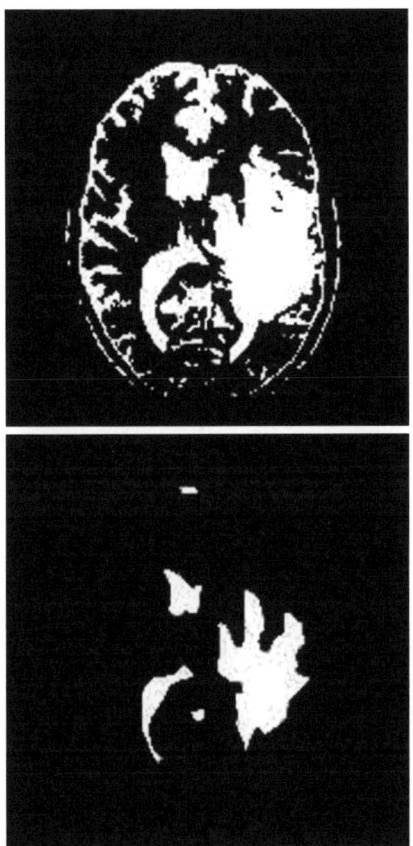

Figure 10.4 Two segmented MR brain images using a gray-value threshold $T = 166$ (top) and $T = 225$ (bottom).

additional thresholds recursively (5, 7). Figure 10.4 shows two segmentations obtained using the thresholds at, respectively, gray values 166 and 225. These thresholds were determined by analyzing the peaks and valleys of the remaining histograms in a recursive manner. The brain regions related to the white matter, cerebrospinal fluid in the sulci, ventricles, and a lesion (in the right half of the image) can be seen in the segmented image obtained using the gray-value threshold of 166. The segmented image using the gray-value threshold of 255 shows only the ventricles and lesion. The higher gray values of the ventricle and lesion regions are due to higher proton density and T_2 relaxation times of MR imaging parameters.

10.2.1 Optimal Global Thresholding

To determine an optimal global gray-value threshold for image segmentation, parametric distribution-based methods can be applied to the histogram of an image (2, 13). Let us assume that the histogram of an image to be segmented has two Gaussian distributions belonging to two respective classes, such as background and object. Thus, the histogram can be represented by a mixture probability density function $p(z)$ as

$$p(z) = P_1 p_1(z) + P_2 p_2(z) \tag{10.10}$$

where $p_1(z)$ and $p_2(z)$ are the Gaussian distributions of classes 1 and 2, respectively, with the class probabilities of P_1 and P_2 such that

$$P_1 + P_2 = 1. \tag{10.11}$$

Using a gray-value threshold T, a pixel in the image $f(x, y)$ can be sorted into class 1 or class 2 in the segmented image $g(x, y)$ as

$$g(x, y) = \begin{cases} \text{Class 1} & \text{if } f(x,y) > T \\ \text{Class 2} & \text{if } f(x,y) \leq T \end{cases}. \tag{10.12}$$

Let us define the error probabilities of misclassifying a pixel as

$$E_1(T) = \int_{-\infty}^{T} p_2(z) dz$$

and

$$E_2(T) = \int_{-\infty}^{T} p_1(z) dz \tag{10.13}$$

where $E_1(T)$ and $E_2(T)$ are, respectively, the probability of erroneously classifying a class 1 pixel to class 2 and a class 2 pixel to class 1.

The overall probability of error in pixel classification using the threshold T is then expressed as

$$E(T) = P_2(T) E_1(T) + P_1(T) E_2(T). \tag{10.14}$$

For image segmentation, the objective is to find an optimal threshold T that minimizes the overall probability of error in pixel classification. The optimization process requires the parameterization of the probability density distributions and likelihood of both classes. These parameters can be determined from a model or set of training images (10, 13).

Let us assume σ_i and μ_i to be the standard deviation and mean of the Gaussian probability density function of the class i ($i = 1, 2$ for two classes) such that

$$p(z) = \frac{P_1}{\sqrt{2\pi}\sigma_1} e^{-(z-\mu_1)^2/2\sigma_1^2} + \frac{P_2}{\sqrt{2\pi}\sigma_2} e^{-(z-\mu_2)^2/2\sigma_2^2}. \tag{10.15}$$

The optimal global threshold T can be determined by finding a general solution that minimizes Equation 10.14 with the mixture distribution in Equation 10.15 and thus satisfies the following quadratic expression (2)

$$AT^2 + BT + C = 0$$

where

$$A = \sigma_1^2 - \sigma_2^2$$
$$B = 2(\mu_1 \sigma_2^2 - \mu_2 \sigma_1^2)$$
$$C = \sigma_1^2 \mu_2^2 - \sigma_2^2 \mu_1^2 + 2\sigma_1^2 \sigma_2^2 \ln(\sigma_2 P_1 / \sigma_1 P_2). \tag{10.16}$$

If the variances of both classes can be assumed to ¾ equal to σ^2, the optimal threshold T can be determined as

$$T = \frac{\mu_1 + \mu_2}{2} + \frac{\sigma^2}{\mu_1 - \mu_2} \ln\left(\frac{P_2}{P_1}\right). \tag{10.17}$$

It should be noted that in case of equal likelihood of classes, the above expression for determining the optimal threshold is simply reduced to the average of the mean values of two classes.

10.2.2 Pixel Classification Through Clustering

In the histogram-based pixel classification method for image segmentation, the gray values are partitioned into two or more clusters, depending on the peaks in the histogram to obtain thresholds. The basic concept of segmentation by pixel classification can be extended to clustering the gray values or feature vectors of pixels in the image. This approach is particularly useful when images with pixels representing a feature vector consisting of multiple parameters of interest are to be segmented. For example, a feature vector may consist of gray value, contrast, and local texture measures for each pixel in the image. A color image may have additional color components in a specific representation such as red, green, and blue components in the RGB color coordinate system that can be added to the feature vector. MR or multimodality medical images may also require segmentation using a multidimensional feature space with multiple parameters of interest.

Images can be segmented by pixel classification through clustering of all features of interest. The number of clusters in the multidimensional feature space thus represents the number of classes in the image. As the image is sorted into cluster classes, segmented regions are obtained by checking the neighborhood pixels for the same class label. However, clustering may produce disjointed regions with holes or regions with a single pixel. After the image data are clustered and pixels are classified, a postprocessing algorithm such as region growing, pixel connectivity, or a rule-based algorithm is usually applied to obtain the final segmented regions (19). In the literature there are a number of algorithms for clustering used for a wide range of applications (13, 18, 21, 23–27).

10.2.2.1 Data Clustering Clustering is the process of grouping data points with similar feature vectors together in a single cluster while data points with dissimilar feature vectors are placed in different clusters. Thus, the data points that are close to each other in the feature space are clustered together. The similarity of feature vectors can be represented by an appropriate distance measure such as Euclidean or Mahalanobis distance (30). Each cluster is represented by its mean (centroid) and variance (spread) associated with the distribution of the corresponding feature vectors of the data points in the cluster. The formation of clusters is optimized with respect to an objective function involving prespecified distance and similarity measures, along with additional constraints such as smoothness.

Since similarity is fundamental to the formation of a cluster, a measure of the similarity between two patterns drawn from the same feature space is essential (30).

For image segmentation, the feature space can simply be represented by gray levels of pixels. However, other features such as contrast can be added to the feature space. It is common to compute dissimilarity between two patterns using a distance measure defined in a feature space.

The Minkowski distance $d_p(\mathbf{x}, \mathbf{y})$ of order p (also known as p-norm distance) defines a distance between two vectors $\mathbf{x} = (x_1, x_2, \ldots, x_n)$ and $\mathbf{y} = (y_1, y_2, \ldots, y_n)$ as

$$d_p(\mathbf{x}, \mathbf{y}) = \left(\sum_{i=1}^{n} |x_i - y_i|^p\right)^{1/p}. \tag{10.18}$$

Euclidean distance $d_2(\mathbf{x}, \mathbf{y})$ is the most popular metric; it is defined as the 2-norm distance measure as:

$$d_2(\mathbf{x}, \mathbf{y}) = \left(\sum_{i=1}^{n} |x_i - y_i|^2\right)^{1/2} = \|\mathbf{x} - \mathbf{y}\|_2. \tag{10.19}$$

The Euclidean distance has an intuitive appeal as it is commonly used to evaluate the proximity of objects in 2- or 3-D space. It works well when a data set has "compact" or "isolated" clusters (30, 31). The Minkowski metric favors the largest scaled feature, which dominates others. The problem can be addressed by proper normalization or other weighting schemes applied in the feature space. Linear correlation among features can also distort distance measures. This distortion can be alleviated by applying a whitening transformation to the data by using the Mahalanobis distance measure $d_M(\mathbf{x}, \mathbf{y})$ as

$$d_M(\mathbf{x}, \mathbf{y}) = \left((\mathbf{x} - \mathbf{y})A^{-1}(\mathbf{x} - \mathbf{y})^T\right)^{1/2} \tag{10.20}$$

where A is the covariance matrix.

In this process, $d_M(\mathbf{x}, \mathbf{y})$ assigns different weights to different features based on their variances and correlations. It is implicitly assumed here that both vectors have the same statistical distributions.

Conventional data clustering methods can be classified into two broad categories: hierarchical and partitional. In hierarchical clustering, the number of clusters need not be specified a priori. Hierarchical clustering methods consider only local neighbors in each step. For this reason, it is difficult to handle overlapping clusters through the hierarchical clustering method. In addition, hierarchical clustering is static in the sense that data points allocated to a cluster in the early stages may not be moved to a different cluster.

Partitional clustering methods develop a clustering structure by optimizing a criterion function defined either locally (on a subset of the patterns) or globally (defined over all of the data). Partitional clustering can be further divided into two classes: crisp clustering and fuzzy clustering. In crisp clustering, a data point belongs to only one cluster and clusters are separated by crisp boundaries among them. In fuzzy clustering methods, data points belong to all clusters through a degree determined by the membership function (32, 33). Partitional algorithms are dynamic in the sense that data points can be efficiently moved from one cluster to another. They can incorporate knowledge about the shape or size of clusters by using appropriate prototypes and constraints.

A popular hierarchical clustering algorithm is the agglomerative method, which is simply based on the distance between clusters. From a representation of single-point-based clusters, two clusters that are nearest and satisfy a similarity criterion are progressively merged to form a reduced number of clusters. This is repeated until just one cluster is obtained, containing the entire data set. Let us suppose that there are n points in the data vector $\mathbf{x} = (x_1, x_2, \ldots, x_n)$; the initial number of clusters will then be equal to n. An agglomerative algorithm for clustering can be defined as follows.

algorithm (agglomerative hierarchical clustering):

Step 1: for $i = 1, \ldots, n$ define cluster $C_i = \{x_i\}$

Step 2: Loop: While there is more than one cluster left compute distance between any two clusters find cluster C_j with minimum distance to C_i
$C_i = C_i \cup C_j$;
Remove cluster C_j;

End

In the above algorithm, a distance measure should be carefully chosen. Euclidean distance measure is commonly used but other measures can also be used depending on the data. It can be noted from the above algorithm that the agglomerative clustering method yields a hierarchical structure of clusters that can be shown graphically in a dendrogram showing the merging links among the data points. A dendrogram shows all data points as individual clusters at the bottom with progressively merging links and reducing number of clusters until all data points form one single cluster at the top.

A nonhierarchical or partitional clustering algorithm provides clusters as a result of the optimization of data partitioning in the feature space. Clusters can be obtained with crisp partitions (as done in k-means clustering method) or fuzzy partitions (as done in fuzzy c-means clustering method). It should be noted that these algorithms are described here for use in image segmentation but are also used for feature analysis and classification as described in Chapter 11.

10.2.2.2 k-Means Clustering

The k-means clustering method is a popular approach to partition d-dimensional data into k clusters such that an objective function providing the desired properties of the distribution of feature vectors of clusters in terms of similarity and distance measures is optimized (31). A generalized k-means clustering algorithm initially places k clusters at arbitrarily selected cluster centroids $\mathbf{v}_i$; $i = 1, \ldots, 2, k$ and modifies centroids for the formation of new cluster shapes, optimizing the objective function. The k-means clustering algorithm includes the following steps:

1. Select the number of clusters k with initial cluster centroids $\mathbf{v}_i$; $i = 1, \ldots 2, k$.

2. Partition the input data points into k clusters by assigning each data point $\mathbf{x}_j$ to the closest cluster centroid $\mathbf{v}_i$ using the selected distance measure, e.g., Euclidean distance, defined as

$$d_{ij} = \|\mathbf{x}_j - \mathbf{v}_i\| \qquad (10.21)$$

where $\mathbf{X} = \{\mathbf{x}_1, \mathbf{x}_2, \ldots, \mathbf{x}_n\}$ is the input data set.

3. Compute a cluster assignment matrix **U** representing the partition of the data points with the binary membership value of the jth data point to the ith cluster such that

$$\mathbf{U} = [u_{ij}] \qquad (10.22)$$

where $u_{ij} \in \{0, 1\}$ for all i, j

$$\sum_{i=1}^{k} u_{ij} = 1 \quad \text{for all } j \quad \text{and} \quad 0 < \sum_{j=1}^{n} u_{ij} < n \quad \text{for all } i$$

4. Recompute the centroids using the membership values as

$$\mathbf{v_i} = \frac{\sum_{j=1}^{n} u_{ij} \mathbf{x_j}}{\sum_{j=1}^{n} u_{ij}} \quad \text{for all } i \qquad (10.23)$$

5. If cluster centroids or the assignment matrix does not change from the previous iteration, stop; otherwise go to step 2.

The k-means clustering method optimizes the sum-of-squared-error-based objective function $J_w(\mathbf{U}, \mathbf{v})$ such that

$$J_w(\mathbf{U}, \mathbf{v}) = \sum_{i=1}^{k} \sum_{j=1}^{n} \|\mathbf{x}_j - \mathbf{v}_i\|^2 \qquad (10.24)$$

It can be noted from the above algorithm that the k-means clustering method is quite sensitive to the initial cluster assignment and the choice of the distance measure. Additional criterion such as within-cluster and between-cluster variances can be included in the objective function as constraints to force the algorithm to adapt the number of clusters k (as needed for optimization of the objective function). Figure 10.5 shows the results of k-means clustering on a T_2-weighted MR brain image with $k = 9$. Regions segmented from different clusters are shown in Figure 10.5b.

10.2.2.3 Fuzzy c-Means Clustering

The k-means clustering method utilizes hard binary values for the membership of a data point to the cluster. The fuzzy c-means (FCM) clustering method utilizes an adaptable membership value that can be updated based on the distribution statistics of the data points assigned to the cluster minimizing the following objective function $J_m(\mathbf{U}, \mathbf{v})$

$$J_m(\mathbf{U}, \mathbf{v}) = \sum_{i=1}^{c} \sum_{j=1}^{n} u_{ij}^m d_{ij}^2 = \sum_{i=1}^{c} \sum_{j=1}^{n} u_{ij}^m \|\mathbf{x_j} - \mathbf{v_i}\|^2 \qquad (10.25)$$

where c is the number of clusters, n is the number of data vectors, u_{ij} is the fuzzy membership, and m is the fuzziness index.

Based on the constraints defined in the distribution statistics of the data points in the clusters, the fuzziness index can be defined between 1 and a very large value for the highest level of fuzziness (maximum allowable variance within a cluster). The membership values in the FCM algorithm can be defined as (33):

10.2. PIXEL-BASED DIRECT CLASSIFICATION METHODS

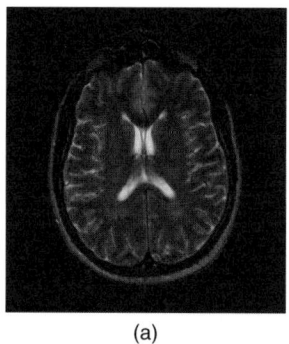

(a)

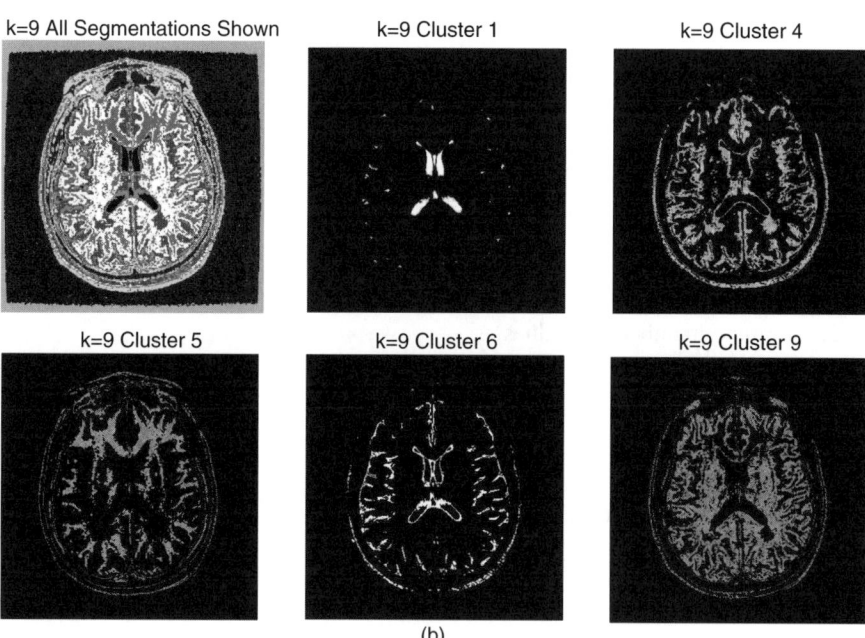

(b)

Figure 10.5 (a) A T_2-weighted MR brain image used for segmentation. (b) Results of segmentation of the image shown in Figure 2a using k-means clustering algorithm with $k = 9$: Top left: all segmented regions belonging to all nine clusters. Top middle: regions segmented from cluster $k = 1$. Top right: regions segmented from cluster $k = 4$. Bottom left: regions segmented from cluster $k = 5$. Bottom middle: regions segmented from cluster $k = 6$. Bottom right: regions segmented from cluster $k = 9$. (Courtesy of Don Adams, Arwa Gheith, and Valerie Rafalko from their class project).

$$0 \le u_{ij} \le 1 \quad \text{for all } i, j$$
$$\sum_{i=1}^{c} u_{ij} = 1 \quad \text{for all } j \quad \text{and} \quad 0 < \sum_{j=1}^{n} u_{ij} < n \quad \text{for all } i. \qquad (10.26)$$

The algorithm described for k-means clustering can be used for fuzzy c-means clustering with the update of the fuzzy membership values as defined in Equation 10.26, minimizing the objective function as defined in Equation 10.25.

10.2.2.4 An Adaptive FCM Algorithm

Additional constraints such as smoothness can be included in the objective function for clustering for better results. An adaptive version of the fuzzy c-means (FCM) clustering algorithm using a weighted derivative information is described by Pham and Prince (34). As the objective function is minimized for clustering, the minimization of the derivative information provides smooth homogenous clusters. The objective function $J_{AFCM}(\mathbf{U}, \mathbf{v})$ to be minimized for an adaptive fuzzy c-means clustering algorithm can be given as

$$J_{ACFM}(\mathbf{U}, \mathbf{v}) = \sum_{i=1}^{c}\sum_{j=1}^{n} u_{ij}^m \|\mathbf{x_j} - g_j\mathbf{v_i}\|^2 + \lambda_1 \sum_{j=1}^{n}\sum_{r=1}^{R}(D_r \otimes g)_j^2 + \lambda_2 \sum_{j=1}^{n}\sum_{r=1}^{R}\sum_{s=1}^{R}(D_r \otimes D_s \otimes g)_j^2 \tag{10.27}$$

where g_j is the unknown gain field to be estimated during the iterative clustering process, m is the fuzziness index ($m > 1$), R is the dimension of the image, D_r is the derivative operator along the rth dimension of the image, and λ_1 and λ_2 are, respectively, the weights for the first-order and second-order derivative terms.

Thus, the second and third terms in the objective function provide the smoothness constraints on clustering.

The adaptive fuzzy c-means algorithm involves the following steps (34):

1. Start with initial centroids $\mathbf{v_i}$; $i = 1, \ldots 2, c$ for c clusters and set the initial gain field $g_j = 1$ for all values of j belonging to the image data.

2. Compute membership values as

$$u_{ij} = \frac{\|\mathbf{x_j} - g_j\mathbf{v_i}\|^{-2/(m-1)}}{\sum_{i=1}^{c}\|\mathbf{x_j} - g_j\mathbf{v_i}\|^{-2/(m-1)}}. \tag{10.28}$$

3. Compute new centorids as

$$\mathbf{v_i} = \frac{\sum_{j=1}^{n} u_{ij}^m g_j \mathbf{x_j}}{\sum_{j=1}^{n} u_{ij}^m g_j^2}, \quad \text{for all } i = 1, 2, \ldots, c. \tag{10.29}$$

4. Compute a new gain field by solving the following equation for g_j

$$\sum_{i=1}^{c} u_{ij}^m (\mathbf{x_j}, \mathbf{v_i}) = g_j \sum_{i=1}^{c} u_{ij}^m (\mathbf{v_i}, \mathbf{v_i}) + \lambda_1 (H_1 \otimes g)_j + \lambda_2 (H_2 \otimes g)_j$$

with

$$H_1 = \sum_{r=1}^{R}(D_r \otimes \bar{D}_r)_j$$

$$H_2 = \sum_{r=1}^{R}((D_r \otimes D_r) \otimes (\bar{D}_s \otimes \bar{D}_s))_j \tag{10.30}$$

where $\bar{D}_r$ is the mirror reflection of D_r derivative operator.

5. If there is no difference in the centroids from the previous iteration, or if there is not a significant difference in the membership values, the algorithm has converged. Stop. Otherwise, go to step 2.

The adaptive FCM algorithm provides good regularization in the clustering process through the first- and second-order derivative terms that force the bias field to be smooth. For large values of weights, λ_1 and λ_2, the algorithm yields a constant bias field leading to the standard FCM method.

10.3. REGION-BASED SEGMENTATION

Region-growing based segmentation algorithms examine pixels in the neighborhood based on a predefined similarity criterion. The neighborhood pixels with similar properties are merged to form closed regions for segmentation. The region-growing approach can be extended to merging regions instead of merging pixels to form larger meaningful regions with similar properties. Such a region-merging approach is quite effective when the original image is segmented into a large number of regions in the preprocessing phase. Large meaningful regions may provide better correspondence and matching to the object models for recognition and interpretation. An alternate approach is region splitting, in which either the entire image or large regions of the image are split into two or more regions based on a heterogeneity or dissimilarity criterion. For example, if a region has a bimodal distribution of gray-value histogram, it can be split into two regions of connected pixels with gray values falling into their respective distributions. The basic difference between region- and thresholding-based segmentation approaches is that region-growing methods guarantee the segmented regions of connected pixels. On the other hand, pixel thresholding-based segmentation methods as defined in the previous section may yield regions with holes and disconnected pixels.

10.3.1 Region-Growing

Region-growing methods merge pixels of similar properties by examining the neighborhood pixels. The process of merging pixels continues, with the region adapting a new shape and size, until there are no eligible neighborhood pixels to be added to the current region. Thus, the region-growing process requires two criteria: a similarity criterion that defines the basis for inclusion of pixels in the growth of the region, and a stopping criterion that stops the growth of the region. The stopping criterion is usually based on the minimum number or percentage of neighborhood pixels required to satisfy the similarity criterion for inclusion in the growth of the region.

An example of a region-growing process is shown in Figure 10.6. Let us assume that a pixel at the center, as shown in Figure 10.6, is the origin of the region-growing process. In the first iteration, there are 8 pixels in the 3×3 neighborhood of the center pixel satisfying the similarity criterion. All of these pixels are grouped tighter in the region, which has now grown to a 3×3 size with a square shape. In the second iteration, the pixels in the 5×5 neighborhood are examined for similarity

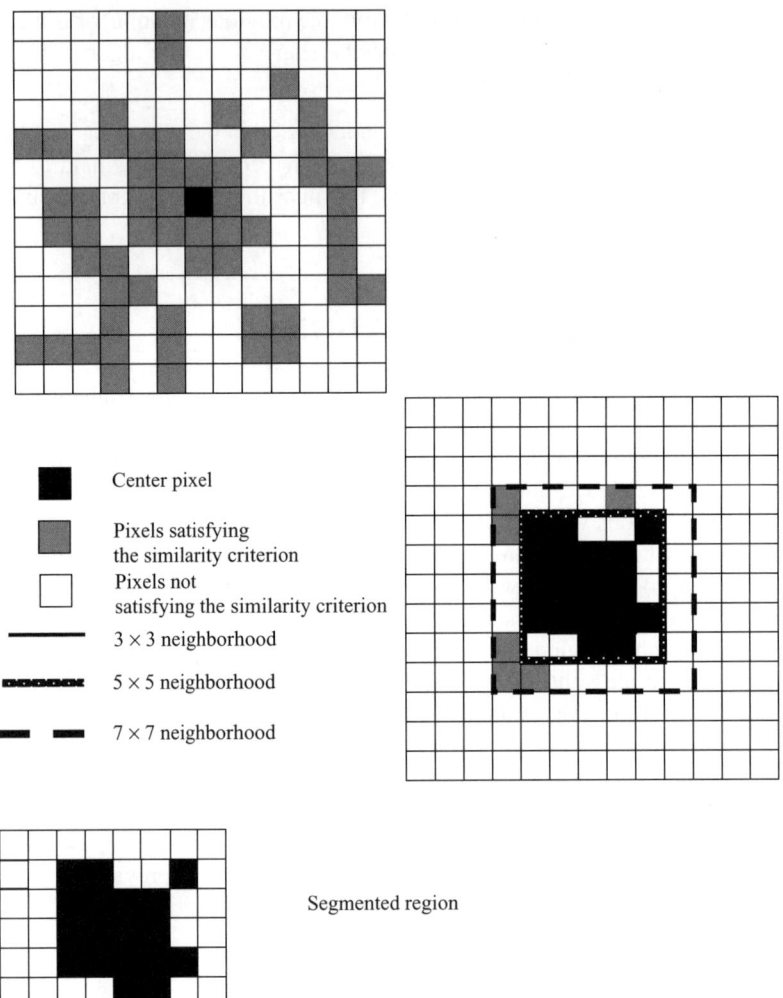

Figure 10.6 A pixel map of an image (top) with the region-growing process (middle) and the segmented region (bottom).

criterion. There are 16 new pixels in the 5 × 5 neighborhood, out of which 9 spixels satisfy the similarity criterion. These pixels are now included in the region. Let us assume that the stopping criterion is defined as the minimum percentage of pixels to be included in the growth of the region to be 30%. Therefore, in the second iteration, 56% of neighborhood pixels (9/16) are included in the growth of the region. In the third iteration, only 25% of the new neighborhood pixels satisfy the similarity criterion. The region-growing process stops when the stopping criterion is met. The region thus grown is shown in Figure 10.6. In this example, the neighborhoods are grown in a fixed shape, that is, 3 × 3 to 5 × 5 to 7 × 7, and so on. A feature-adaptive region-growing method is described in Chapter 9 for feature enhancement, which can be used to grow regions that are adaptive to the size and shape of the growing region by examining the neighborhood (9, 10).

In the region-merging algorithms, an image may be partitioned into a large number of potential homogeneous regions. For example, an image of 1024 × 1024 pixels can be portioned into regions of 8 × 8 pixels. Each region of 8 × 8 pixels can now be examined for homogeneity of predefined property such as gray values, contrast, and texture. If the histogram of the predefined property for the region is unimodal, the region is said to be homogeneous. Two neighborhood regions can be merged if they are homogeneous and satisfy a predefined similarity criterion. The similarity criterion imposes constraints on the value of the property with respect to its mean and variance values. For example, two homogeneous regions can be merged if the difference between their mean gray values is within 10% of the entire dynamic range and the difference between their variances is within 10% of the variance in the image. These thresholds may be selected heuristically or through probabilistic models (10, 13). It is interesting to note that the above criterion can be easily implemented as a conditional rule in a knowledge-based system. Region-merging or region-splitting (described in the next section) methods have been implemented using a rule-based system for image segmentation (23).

Model-based systems typically encode knowledge of anatomy and image acquisition parameters. Anatomical knowledge can be modeled symbolically, describing the properties and relationships of individual structures; geometrically, either as masks or templates of anatomy; or by using an atlas (16, 17, 23, 24).

Figure 10.7 shows an MR brain image and the segmented regions for ventricles. The knowledge of the anatomical locations of ventricles was used to establish the initial seed points for region-growing. A feature-adaptive region-growing method was used for segmentation.

10.3.2 Region-Splitting

Region-splitting methods examine the heterogeneity of a predefined property of the entire region in terms of its distribution and the mean, variance, minimum, and maximum values. If the region is evaluated as heterogeneous, that is, it fails the similarity or homogeneity criterion, the original region is split into two or more regions. The region-splitting process continues until all regions satisfy the homogeneity criterion individually.

In the region-splitting process, the original region R is split into $R_1, R_2, \ldots, R_n$ subregions such that the following conditions are met (2):

1. Each region, R_i; $i = 1, 2, \ldots, n$ is connected.
2. $\bigcup_{i=1}^{n} R_i = R$
3. $R_i \cap R_j = O$ for all i, j; $i \neq j$
4. $H(R_i) = $ TRUE for $i = 1, 2, \ldots, n$.
5. $H(R_i \cup R_j) = $ FALSE for $i \neq j$

where $H(R_i)$ is a logical predicate for the homogeneity criterion on the region R_i.

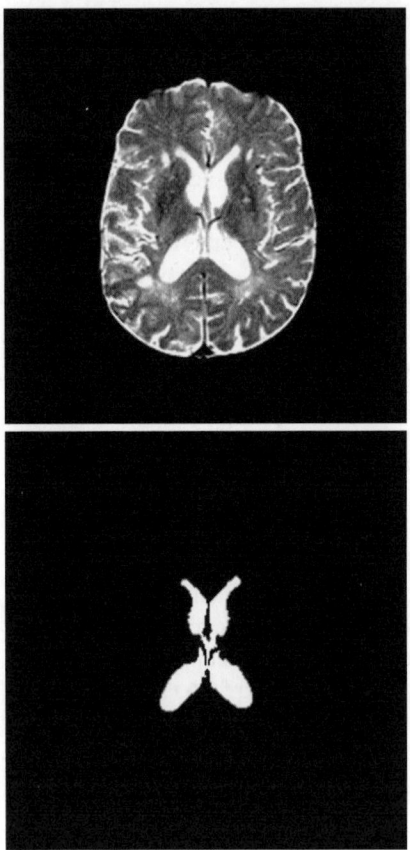

Figure 10.7 A T_2-weighted MR brain image (top) and the segmented ventricles (bottom) using the region-growing method.

Region-splitting methods can also be implemented by rule-based systems and quad trees. In the quad tree-based region-splitting method, the image is partitioned into four regions that are represented by nodes in a quad tree. Each region is checked for the homogeneity and evaluated for the logical predicate $H(R_i)$. If the region is homogeneous, no further action is taken for the respective node. If the region is not homogeneous, it is further split into four regions. Figure 10.8 shows a quad-tree structure. The image was initially split into four regions, R_1, R_2, R_3, and R_4. Regions R_1 and R_3 were found to be homogeneous and therefore no further split was needed. Regions R_2 and R_4 failed the homogeneous predicate test and were therefore further split into four regions respectively.

10.4. ADVANCED SEGMENTATION METHODS

The problem of segmenting medical images into anatomically and pathologically meaningful regions has been addressed using various approaches, including model-based estimation methods and rule-based systems (11, 15–25). Nevertheless,

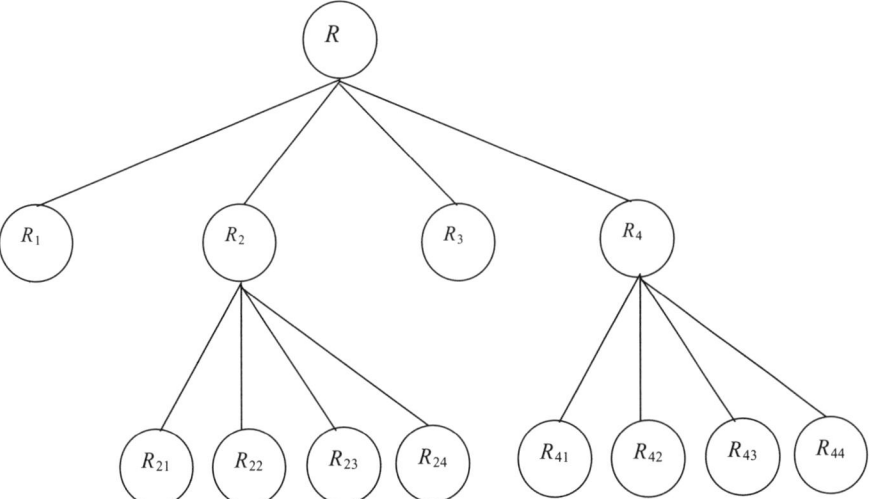

Figure 10.8 An image with quad region-splitting process (top) and the corresponding quad-tree structure (bottom).

automatic (or semi-automatic with minimal operator interaction) segmentation methods for specific applications are still current topics of research. This is due to the great variability in anatomical structures and the challenge of finding a reliable, accurate, and diagnostically useful segmentation.

A rule-based low-level segmentation system for automatic identification of brain structures from MR images has been described by Raya (16). Neural network-based classification approaches have also been applied for medical image segmentation (10, 26, 27).

10.4.1 Estimation-Model Based Adaptive Segmentation

A multilevel adaptive segmentation (MAS) method is used to segment and classify multiparameter MR brain images into a large number of classes of physiological

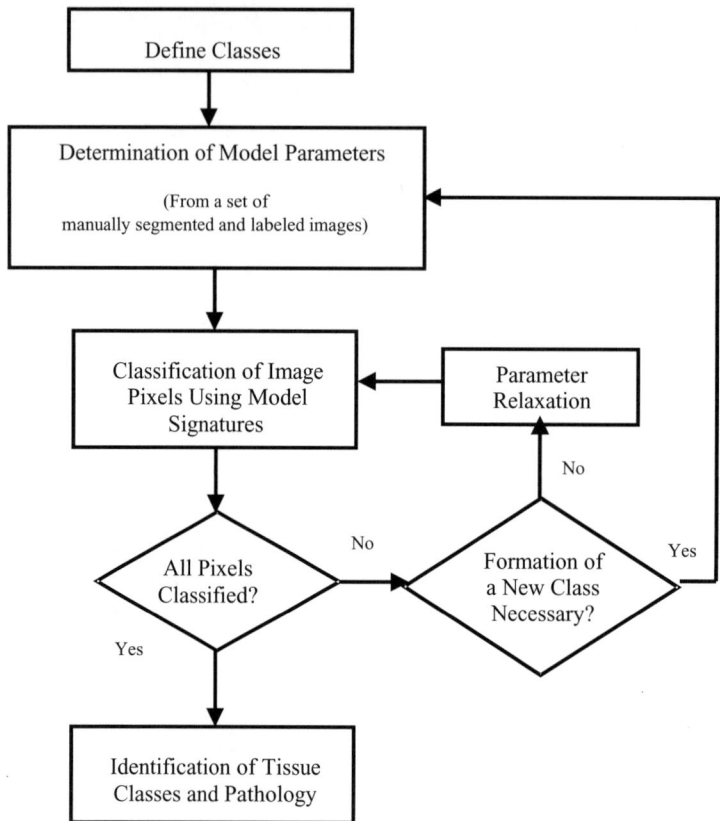

Figure 10.9 The overall approach of the MAS method.

and pathological interest (22). The MAS method is based on an estimation of signatures for each segmentation class for pixel-by-pixel classification. It can also create new classes, if necessary, when there is a significant discrepancy between the measured parameters of the image and the model signatures. The MAS method consists of a five-step procedure for generating brain model signatures, as illustrated in Figure 10.9 (22).

Let us represent a multiparameter image to be segmented with a pair of random variables

$$\{C_{m,n}, X_{m,n}\} \tag{10.31}$$

where $C_{m,n}$ is the class of the pixel (m, n) representing the spatial variability of the brain classes, and can take the values in the discrete set $\{1, 2, \ldots, K\}$ representing a specific class, and $X_{m,n}$ is a d-dimensional random variable representing the data vector of pixel (m, n) with dimension d that is based on the number of imaging parameters, such as T_1, T_2, proton density, and $G_d + T_1$.

The required parameters to develop an estimation model can be obtained using a priori knowledge or manual segmentation on a set of training images. Let us

10.4. ADVANCED SEGMENTATION METHODS

assume an ensemble of brain images manually classified; the parameters were estimated in the following way. The ith class mean vectors, $\hat{\mu}_i$, is

$$\hat{\mu}_i = \frac{1}{n}\sum_j x_j \qquad (10.32)$$

where n is the number of pixels in the ith class, and x_j is the jth of n multidimensional vectors that comprise the class. The dimension of x_j corresponds to the number of image modalities used in the analysis. The covariance matrix of class i, $\hat{\Sigma}_i$, is

$$\hat{\Sigma}_i = \frac{1}{n-1}\sum_j (x_j - \hat{\mu}_i)(x_j - \hat{\mu}_i)^t \qquad (10.33)$$

The summations in Equations 10.29 and 10.30 are expressed over all the pixels belonging to the ith class.

Given that $C_{m,n} = i$, the distribution of $X_{m,n}$ is estimated to satisfy the multivariate normal distribution described by the density function

$$\hat{p}_i(x) = \frac{1}{(2\pi)^{d/2}|\hat{\Sigma}_i|^{1/2}}\exp\left[\frac{-(x-\hat{\mu}_i)}{2\hat{\Sigma}_i(x-\hat{\mu}_i)}\right] \qquad (10.34)$$

where x is a d-element column vector, $\hat{\mu}_i$ is a d-element estimated mean vector for the class i calculated from Equation 10.29, $\hat{\Sigma}_i$ is the estimated $d \times d$ covariance matrix for class i calculated from Equation 10.30, and d is the dimension of multi-parameter data.

Four transition matrices $P_r(m, n) = [p_{ijr}(m, n)]$ can be estimated, where r is a direction index (with four spatial connectedness directions) and $p_{ijr}(m, n)$ are the transition probabilities defined by

$$p_{ij1}(m, n) = P\{C_{m,n} = j \mid C_{m,n-1} = i\}$$
$$p_{ij2}(m, n) = P\{C_{m,n} = j \mid C_{m+1,n} = i\}$$
$$p_{ij3}(m, n) = P\{C_{m,n} = j \mid C_{m,n+1} = i\}$$
$$p_{ij4}(m, n) = P\{C_{m,n} = j \mid C_{m-1,n} = i\}. \qquad (10.35)$$

Transition probabilities, in general, can be given by

$$p_{ij1}(m, n) = \frac{\sum_b \{\text{pix} \mid C_{m,n} = j, C_{m,n-1} = i\}}{\sum_b \{\text{pix} \mid C_{m,n-1} = i\}} \qquad (10.36)$$

where $\sum_b\{\text{pix} \mid P\}$ denotes the number of pixels with the property P in the ensemble of brains used to generate the model.

Due to the relatively small number of brain images in the training set, averaging over a small neighborhood of pixels around the pixel of interest (m, n) is performed. Thus, the estimate can be expressed as

$$p_{ij1}(m, n) = \frac{\sum_b \sum_n \{\text{pix} \mid C_{m,n} = j, C_{m,n-1} = i\}}{\sum_b \sum_n \{\text{pix} \mid C_{m,n-1} = i\}} \qquad (10.37)$$

where $\sum_n$ indicates the averaging over the neighborhood.

The equilibrium transition probabilities are estimated using a similar procedure and are

$$\pi_i(mn) = \frac{\sum_b \sum_n \{pix|C_{m,n} = i\}}{\sum_b \sum_n \{pix\}}. \tag{10.38}$$

To perform maximum likelihood discriminant analysis, the class random variable $C_{m,n}$ is assumed to constitute a K-state Markov random field. Rows and columns of $C_{m,n}$ constitute segments of K-state Markov chains. Chains are specified by the $K \times K$ transition matrix $P = [p_{ij}]$ where

$$p_{ij} = P\{C_{m,n} = j | C_{m,n-1} = i\} \tag{10.39}$$

with the equilibrium probabilities $(\pi_1, \pi_2, \ldots, \pi_K)$.

Thus, the probability that a pixel belongs to a specific class i is

$$P\{C_{m,n} = i | x_{kl}, (k,l) \in N(m,n)\} \tag{10.40}$$

where $N(m, n)$ is some neighborhood of the pixel (m, n).

The conditional probabilities can now be expressed as

$$P\{C_{m,n} = i | x_{kl}, (k,l) \in N(m,n)\} = \frac{P\{C_{m,n} = i, X_{m,n} | X_{m\pm1,n}, X_{m,n\pm1}\}}{P\{X_{m,n} | X_{m\pm1,n}, X_{m,n\pm1}\}}$$

and

$$P\{C_{m,n} = i | x_{kl}, (k,l) \in N(m,n)\} =$$
$$\frac{P\{X_{m,n} | C_{m,n} = i, X_{m\pm1,n}, X_{m,n\pm1}\} P\{C_{m,n} = i | X_{m\pm1,n}, X_{m,n\pm1}\}}{P\{X_{m,n} | X_{m\pm1,n}, X_{m,n\pm1}\}} \tag{10.41}$$

where

$$P\{\circ | X_{m\pm1,n}, X_{m,n\pm1}\} \equiv P\{\circ | X_{m-1,n}\} P\{\circ | X_{m,n-1}\} P\{\circ | X_{m+1,n}\} P\{\circ | X_{m,n+1}\} \tag{10.42}$$

Using class conditional independence of x_{mn} and applying Bayes' rule, Equation 10.38 can be rewritten as

$$P\{C_{m,n} = i | x_{kl}, (k,l) \in N(m,n)\} =$$
$$\frac{P\{X_{m,n} | C_{m,n} = i\} P\{X_{m\pm1,n}, X_{m,n\pm1} | C_{m,n} = i\} P\{C_{m,n} = i\}}{P\{X_{m,n} | X_{m\pm1,n}, X_{m,n\pm1}\} P\{X_{m\pm1,n}, X_{m,n\pm1}\}} \tag{10.43}$$

with

$$P\{X_{m-1,n} | C_{m,n} = i\} = \sum_{j=1}^{N} P\{X_{m-1,n} | C_{m-1,n} = j\} P\{C_{m-1,n} = j | C_{m,n} = i\} \equiv H_{m-1,n}(i). \tag{10.44}$$

With substitutions, the probability that the current pixel, mn, belongs to class i given the characteristics of the pixels in the neighborhood of mn is expressed as

$$P\{C_{m,n} = i | x_{kl}, (k,l) \in N(m,n)\} =$$
$$\frac{P\{C_{m,n} = i | X_{m,n}\} P\{X_{m,n}\} H_{m-1,n}(i) H_{m,n-1}(i) H_{m+1,n}(i) H_{m,n+1}(i)}{P\{X_{m,n} | X_{m\pm1,n}, X_{m,n\pm1}\} P\{X_{m\pm1,n}, X_{m,n\pm1}\}}. \tag{10.45}$$

The brain model consists of class probabilities, transition probabilities, mean vectors, and covariance matrices of class clusters in d dimensions (T_1, T_2, proton density, $G_d + T_1$, and perfusion) space. After the model is developed, an image to be segmented is automatically classified on a pixel-by-pixel basis using the model signatures. The multiparameter measurement vector of each pixel in the image to be classified is compared with the model signature vector of each brain class. A pixel is classified in a particular class if its distance from the model signature is less than some predefined threshold. Thus, pixel classification is done using the distances in the corresponding multidimensional metric space from the model class signatures. The thresholds here are selected in such a way as to classify pixels with relatively pure content of the corresponding class. This step provides a successful classification of a limited number of pixels that are well inside the spatial extents of brain tissue regions.

The next level of processing deals with data on the neighborhood level. For the remaining unclassified pixels, a spatial neighborhood is identified. The spatial distribution of the neighboring pixels that have been classified in the first step is now taken into consideration with the class and transitional probabilities. This processing step allows relaxation of the model signature parameters (mean and covariance) to help classification of those pixels that are in the neighborhood of already classified pixels. The relaxation results in additional pixels being classified in this step.

After the relaxation step, there may still be some unclassified pixels that belong to the edges of tissue regions. Pixels that exist on tissue boundaries will have a neighborhood composed of pixels in different classes. Because of limited resolution, the pixel itself may be a mixture of two or more tissue classes. Therefore, for boundary pixels, it is necessary to perform unmixing. Unmixing is the process of determining the set of classes, and the contribution of each, that compose a boundary or a mixed pixel. The unmixing process uses the labels of the already classified neighborhood pixels to determine the candidate set of classes that compose the unclassified pixel. Using the background class model signatures, mixing model analysis is performed for the unclassified pixels. The unmixing analysis can be based on a linear mixing model (22).

Using the background classes, the linear least squares method is used to determine the fraction of the candidate background classes in an unclassified pixel. This analysis is particularly useful in classifying pixels belonging to the boundary of two or more connected tissue regions. The linear mixing model can be expressed as:

$$\mathbf{R} = \mathbf{e}C \quad (10.46)$$

where $\mathbf{R}$ is multiparameter vector of the measured values of a pixel, $\mathbf{e}$ is the matrix consisting of all signature vectors of candidate background classes, and C is the set of unknown coefficients representing the fraction of the pixel corresponding to each candidate background class. The least squared error solution can be given by

$$C = (\mathbf{e}^T \mathbf{e})^{-1} \mathbf{e}^T \mathbf{R}. \quad (10.47)$$

If all coefficients of C are not positive, the candidate background list is renewed by eliminating the background class with minimum coefficient value. Only coefficients meeting a certain threshold requirement, such as 0.25 (which means that the minimum acceptable fraction for a background class is 25% of the pixel), are kept in the final analysis.

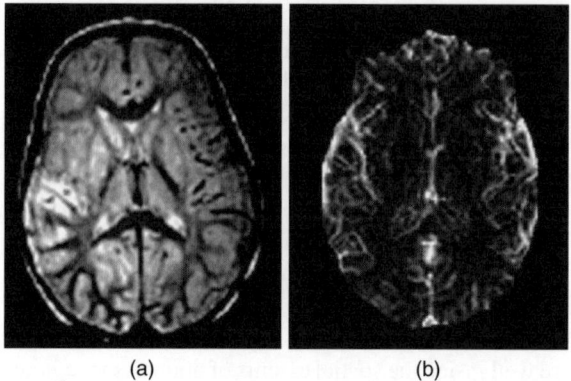

Figure 10.10 (a) Proton density MR and (b) perfusion image of a patient 48 h after stroke.

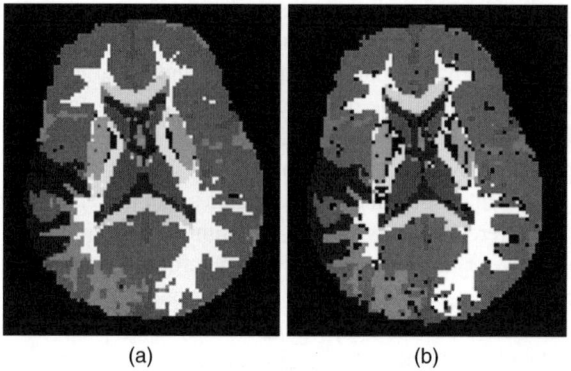

Figure 10.11 Results of MAS method with 4×4 pixel probability cell size and 4 pixel wide averaging. (a) Pixel classification as obtained on the basis of maximum probability and (b) as obtained with $P > 0.9$.

After the mixing analysis is completed, all remaining unlabeled pixels are examined for pathology detection and identification if a database of pathology signatures exists. If such a database does not exist or if an unlabeled pixel defies pathology classification, a new class is created. Figure 10.10 shows the proton density and perfusion MR brain images of a patient 48 hours after a stroke. This image was segmented using a model of 15 tissue classes. The model was developed for 15 classes of normal tissues with no information for stroke-affected lesion and edema tissues. The MAS method developed three new classes and segmented the image into 18 classes. The segmented image, using different classification probability criteria, are shown in Figure 10.11.

10.4.2 Image Segmentation Using Neural Networks

Neural networks provide another pixel classification paradigm that can be used for image segmentation (10, 26, 27). Neural networks do not require underlying class probability distribution for accurate classification. Rather, the decision boundaries for pixel classification are adapted through an iterative training process. Neural network-based segmentation approaches may provide good results for medical images with considerable variance in structures of interest. For example, angiographic images show a significant variation in arterial structures and are therefore difficult to segment. The variation in image quality among various angiograms and introduction of noise in the course of image acquisition emphasizes the importance of an adaptive, nonparametric segmentation method. Neural network paradigms such as backpropagation, radial basis function (RBF), and self-organizing feature maps have been used to segment medical images (10, 26, 27).

Neural networks learn from examples in the training set in which the pixel classification task has already been performed using manual methods. A nonlinear mapping function between the input features and the desired output for labeled examples is learned by neural networks without using any parameterization (34–38). After the learning process, a pixel in a new image can be classified for segmentation by the neural network.

It is important to select a useful set of features to be provided to the neural network as input data for classification. The selection of training examples is also very important, as they should represent a reasonably complete statistical distribution of the input data. The structure of the network and the distribution of training examples play a major role in determining its performance for accuracy, generalization, and robustness. In its simplest form, the input to a neural network can be the gray values of pixels in a predefined neighborhood in the image. Thus, the network can classify the center pixel of the neighborhood based on the information of the entire set of pixels in the corresponding neighborhood. As the neighborhood window is translated in the image, the pixels in the central locations of the translated neighborhoods are classified.

10.4.2.1 Backpropagation Neural Network for Classification

The backpropagation network is the most commonly used neural network in signal processing and classification applications. It uses a set of interconnected neural elements that process the information in a layered manner. A computational neural element, also called perceptron, provides the output as a thresholded weighed sum of all inputs. The basic function of the neural element, as shown in Figure 10.12, is analogous to the synaptic activities of a biological neuron. In a layered network structure, the neural element may receive its input from an input vector or from other neural elements. A weighted sum of these inputs constitutes the argument of a nonlinear activation function such as a sigmoidal function. The resulting thresholded value of the activation function is the output of the neural element. The output is distributed along weighted connections to other neural elements.

To learn a specific pattern of input vectors for classification, an iterative learning algorithm, such as the least mean square (LMS) algorithm, often called the Widrow–Hoff delta rule (35), is used with a set of preclassified training examples that are labeled with the input vectors and their respective class outputs. For example, if there are two output classes for classification of input vectors, the weighted sum of all input vectors may be thresholded to a binary value, 0 or 1. The output 0 represents class 1, while the output 1 represents class 2. The learning algorithm repeatedly presents input vectors of the training set to the network and forces the

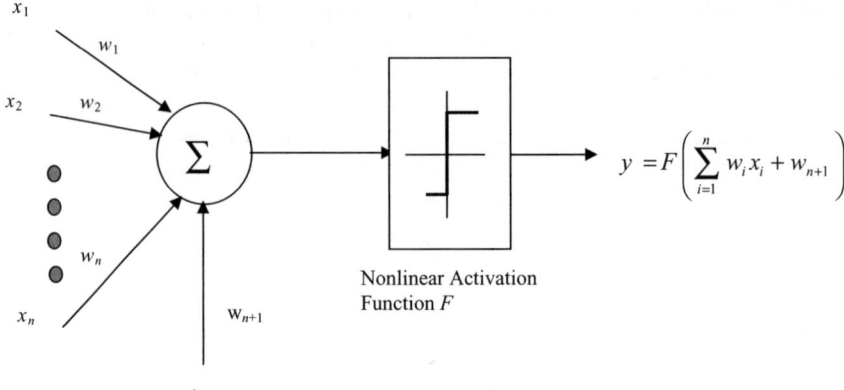

Figure 10.12 A basic computational neural element or perceptron for classification.

network output to produce the respective classification output. Once the network converges on all training examples to produce the respective desired classification outputs, the network is used to sort new input vectors into the learned classes.

The computational output of a neural element can be expressed as

$$y = F\left(\sum_{i=1}^{n} w_i x_i + w_{n+1}\right) \quad (10.48)$$

where F is a nonlinear activation function that is used to threshold the weighted sum of inputs x_i, and w_i is the respective weight. A bias is added to the element as w_{n+1}, as shown in Figure 10.12.

Let us assume a multilayer feed-forward neural network with L layers of N neural elements (perceptrons) in each layer such that

$$\mathbf{y}^{(k)} = F\left(\mathbf{W}^k \mathbf{y}^{(k-1)}\right) \quad \text{for } k = 1, 2, \ldots L \quad (10.49)$$

where $\mathbf{y}^{(k)}$ is the output of the kth layer neural elements with $k = 0$ representing the input layer, and $W^{(k)}$ is the weight matrix for the kth layer such that

$$\mathbf{y}^{(0)} = \begin{bmatrix} x_1 \\ x_2 \\ \cdot \\ x_N \\ 1 \end{bmatrix}; \quad \mathbf{y}^{(k)} = \begin{bmatrix} y_1^{(k)} \\ y_2^{(k)} \\ \cdot \\ y_N^{(k)} \\ y_{(N+1)}^{(k)} \end{bmatrix}$$

and

$$\mathbf{W}^{(k)} = \begin{bmatrix} w_{11}^{(k)} & w_{12}^{(k)} & \cdot & w_{1N}^{(k)} & w_{1(N+1)}^{(k)} \\ w_{21}^{(k)} & w_{22}^{(k)} & \cdot & w_{2N}^{(k)} & w_{2(N+1)}^{k} \\ \cdot & \cdot & \cdot & \cdot & \cdot \\ w_{N1}^{(k)} & w_{N2}^{(k)} & \cdot & w_{NN}^{(k)} & w_{N(N+1)}^{(k)} \\ w_{(N+1)1}^{(k)} & w_{(N+1)2}^{(k)} & \cdot & w_{(N+1)N}^{(k)} & w_{(N+1)(N+1)}^{(k)} \end{bmatrix} \quad (10.50)$$

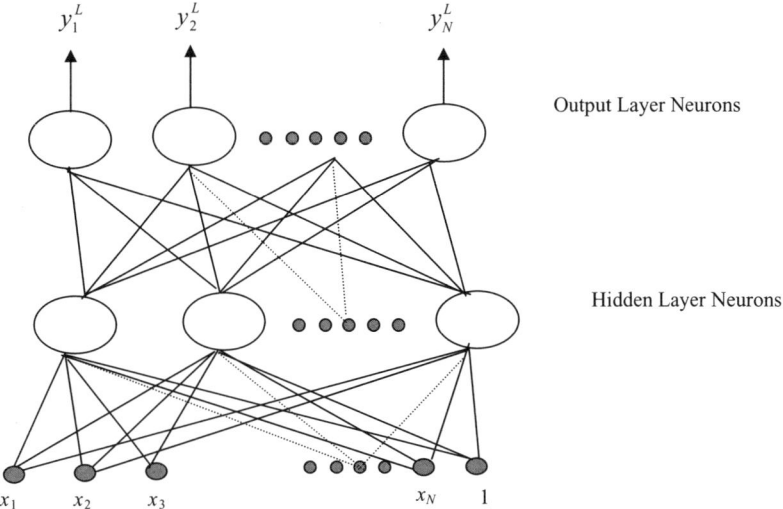

Figure 10.13 A feed-forward backpropagation neural network with one hidden layer.

The neural network is trained by presenting classified examples of input and output patterns. Each example consists of the input and output vectors $\{\mathbf{y}^{(0)}, \mathbf{y}^L\}$ or $\{\mathbf{x}, \mathbf{y}^L\}$ that are encoded for the desired classes. The objective of the training is to determine a weight matrix that would provide the desired output, respectively, for each input vector in the training set. The LMS error algorithm (35, 36) can be implemented to train a feed-forward neural network (Fig. 10.13) using the following steps:

1. Assign random weights in the range of $[-1, +1]$ to all weights w_{ij}^k.
2. For each classified pattern pair $\{\mathbf{y}^{(0)}, \mathbf{y}^L\}$ in the training set, do the following steps:
    a. Compute the output values of each neural element using the current weight matrix.
    b. Find the error $\mathbf{e}^{(k)}$ between the computed output vector and the desired output vector for the classified pattern pair.
    c. Adjust the weight matrix using the change $\Delta \mathbf{W}^{(k)}$ computed as
    $$\Delta W^{(k)} = \alpha e^{(k)}[y^{(k-1)}] \text{ for all layers } k = 1, .., L$$
    where α is the learning rate that can set be set between 0 and 1.
3. Repeat step 2 for all classified pattern pairs in the training set until the error vector for each training example is sufficiently low or zero.

The nonlinear activation function is an important consideration in computing the error vector for each classified pattern pair in the training set. A sigmoidal activation function can be used as

$$F(y) = \frac{1}{1+e^{-y}}. \quad (10.51)$$

The above described gradient descent algorithm for training a feed-forward neural network, also called backpropagation neural network (BPNN), is sensitive to the selection of initial weights and noise in the training set that can cause the algorithm to get stuck in local minima in the solution pace. This causes a poor generalization performance of the network when it is used to classify new patterns. Another problem with the BPNN is to find the optimal network architecture with the consideration of the optimal number of hidden layers and neural elements in each of them. A cascade-correlation neural network architecture has been proposed by Fahlman (36) that finds the best architecture by correlating the error patterns with the inclusion or deletion of neural elements in the hidden layers based on the learning vectors in the training set.

10.4.2.2 The RBF Network

The RBF network is based on the principle of regularization theory for function approximation. Unlike the backpropagation network, it does not suffer from problems such as sticking in the local minimum and sensitivity to the network architecture. In addition, RBF networks provide more reliable and reproducible results (37–39).

Since the RBF network is a special class of regularization networks, it provides better generalization and estimation properties for function approximation applications than traditional feed-forward neural architectures (37–39). The basic RBF network contains an input layer for input signal distribution, a hidden layer to provide the RBF processing, and an output layer (Fig. 10.14). The RBF representation can be obtained by clustering the input training data to obtain the centroid vector, c_i for all clusters. An RBF (generally a Gaussian function) is applied to the Euclidean distance between the input vector, x_j, and its own centroid. The output of each RBF unit is then weighted and summed through a linear combiner to provide the final output of the network. The final output of the network $f(x)$ can be given as:

$$f(\mathbf{x}) = \sum_{i=1}^{K} w_i \Phi(\mathbf{x}, i)$$

$$\text{with } \Phi(\mathbf{x}, i) = \frac{\exp\left(-\frac{\|\mathbf{x} - \mathbf{c}_i\|}{2\sigma_i}\right)}{\sum_{j=1}^{K} \exp\left(-\frac{\|\mathbf{x} - \mathbf{c}_j\|}{2\sigma_j}\right)} \quad (10.52)$$

where c_i represents the K centers, σ_i represents the satandard deviation of ith cluster, and w_i represents the K weighted connections from the hidden layer units to the output unit.

Within the basic topology, the system can be represented in state-space by $\mathbf{y} = (\mathbf{F}\,\mathbf{w})$ where $\mathbf{F}$ is the matrix of activation functions

$$F = \begin{pmatrix} \Phi(\mathbf{x}_1, 1) & \cdots & \Phi(\mathbf{x}_1, K) \\ \cdots & \cdots & \cdots \\ \Phi(\mathbf{x}_N, 1) & \cdots & \Phi(\mathbf{x}_N, K) \end{pmatrix} \quad (10.53)$$

10.4. ADVANCED SEGMENTATION METHODS

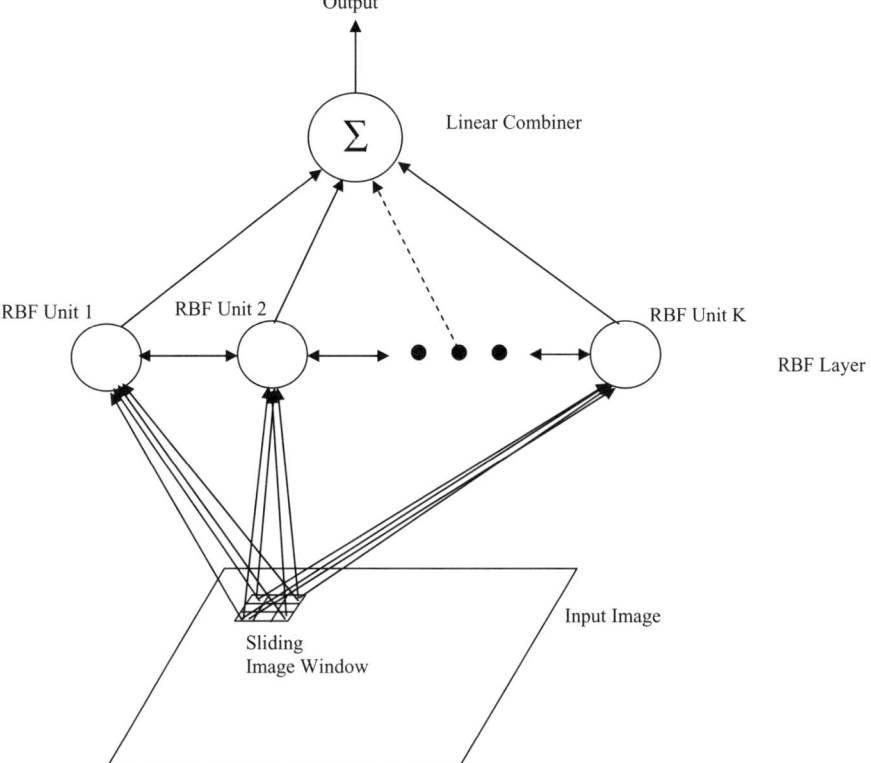

Figure 10.14 An RBF network classifier for image segmentation.

The weight can be calculated from the Moore–Penrose inverse (33)

$$\mathbf{w} = (\mathbf{F}^T \cdot \mathbf{F} + \alpha \cdot I)^{-1} \cdot \mathbf{F}^T \cdot \mathbf{y} \qquad (10.54)$$

where α is a small value, such as 0.1.

It has been shown (39) that the matrix inversion would be singular if repetitive data is applied to the inputs of the neural system during training. The major issues for implementation of the RBF network are the location of the centroids and the structure of the RBF. The locations of the RBF depend on the data being presented to the network. The optimal number of clusters can be obtained from the statistical evaluation of the population density and variance parameters of initial clusters through an adaptive k-means or fuzzy clustering method (31–33).

10.4.2.3 Segmentation of Arterial Structure in Digital Subtraction Angiograms
The arterial structure in a digital subtraction angiogram is characterized by fading ridges and a nonuniform distribution of gray values that makes the segmentation task difficult. Specific features with information about gray values, edges, and local contrast of the pixels are needed for effective segmentation using

a neural network-based classifier (26, 27). The edge features, including ridges, can be obtained using a second-order derivative function such as Laplacian or LOG as described in Chapter 9. The contrast value of a pixel can be simply computed from the largest difference in gray value between a pixel and its 8-connected neighbors. Alternately, feature-adaptive neighborhood processing can be used to obtain a contrast value of the central pixel as used in adaptive feature enhancement method discussed in Chapter 9. In addition, a multiresolution approach can be applied to improve accuracy and efficiency (26).

The feature vector consists of the gray values of the center pixel and its neighbors, combined with the contrast value at the center pixel. The ridge information can be obtained from the first- and second-order derivative operations. A pixel is labeled as a ridge if the first derivative taken along the direction of the second derivative has a zero crossing sufficiently close to the center pixel. The contrast information is computed using the feature adaptive neighborhood processing for the specified neighborhood window. All features are normalized to unit variance to be used in the RBF network classifier.

A training set of example images is prepared with a large number of pixels that are manually classified as belonging to the background or to the arterial structure. Using the respective features of all pixels, feature vectors are prepared and scaled to have a unit variance for fuzzy c-means clustering. The centers of the clusters become the locations of RBFs that are used in RBF network-based classification.

Using the fuzzy c-means clustering method for the training feature vectors, the RBF network classifier can be developed and trained for classifying pixels into two classes: background and arterial structure. Figure 10.15 shows the results of the RBF network-based arterial segmentation of an angiogram of a pig phantom image.

In the segmentation methods described above, gray values and histogram statistics of pixels in an image have been used as primary features. The histogram statistics may include the mean and variance of the gray values of pixels in the entire image or a specified neighborhood region (40, 41). In region-based segmentation algorithms, additional features may be used to include edge, contrast, and texture information computed from the specified neighborhood of pixels in the image (42). The edge features, including ridges, can be obtained using a second-order derivative function such as Laplacian or LOG as described in Chapter 9. The contrast features are also described in Chapter 9. These features can be effectively used in rule-based systems (16, 23) as well as neural network classifiers for image segmentation (10, 26, 27).

Features representing individual pixels or regions (groups of pixels) in an image play a critical role in image segmentation, analysis, and classification. A general structure of hierarchical knowledge representation for image classification and understanding starts with the properties or features associated with pixels and goes through regions to describe objects present in the image. Features associated with region and object representation for image analysis and understanding are described in the next chapter.

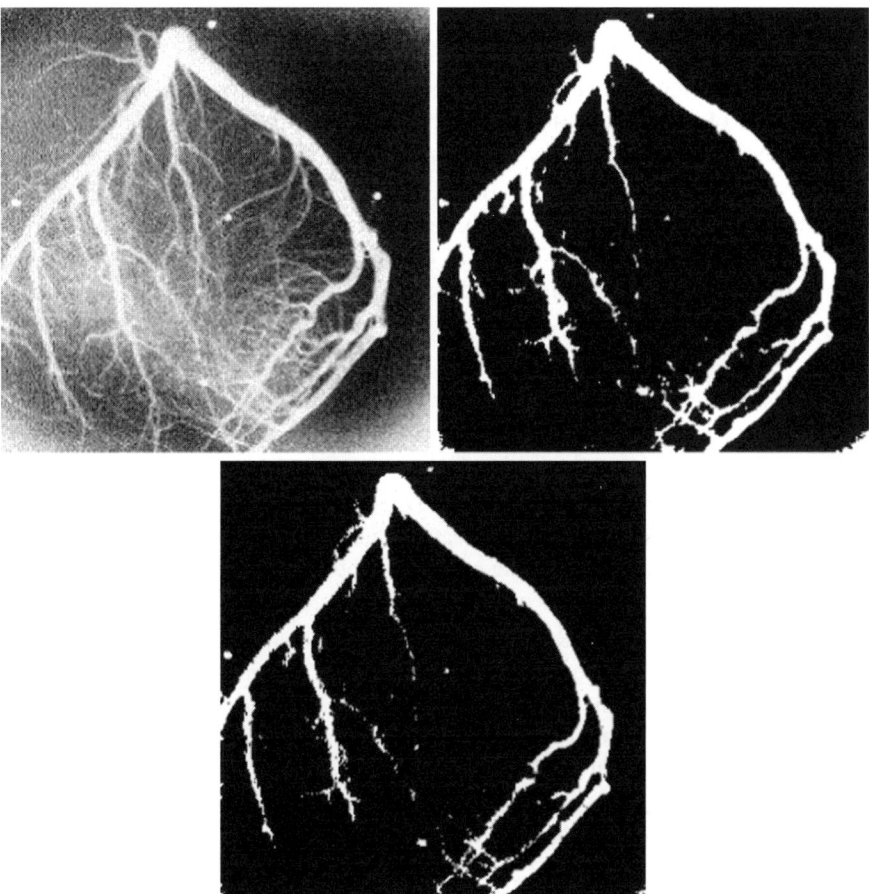

Figure 10.15 RBF segmentation of angiogram data of pig-cast phantom image (top left) using a set of 10 clusters (top right) and 12 clusters (bottom), respectively.

10.5. EXERCISES

10.1. What is the purpose of image segmentation? Why is it a significant step in image analysis?

10.2. What are the major approaches for image segmentation? Describe an image segmentation method of your preference. Explain the reasons for selecting your method.

10.3. How does edge information play a role in region-based segmentation?

10.4. What are the advantages and disadvantages of the Laplacian of Gaussian (LOG) edge detector compared with the Laplacian operator?

10.5. In the MATLAB environment, apply the LOG operator for edge detection on an X-ray mammography image. Threshold the output image at different levels to extract prominent edges. Comment on the effect of thresholding. How can you select the best threshold for this image?

10.6. Use the same image used in Exercise 10.5 and apply optimal gray value thresholding method for segmentation. Compare the resultant segmented image with the edge-based segmentation obtained in Exercise 10.5.

10.7. Select an MR brain image from the database and apply k-means clustering on the image with $k = 5$. Obtain segmented regions through pixel classification using the clustered classes. Compare the segmented regions with those obtained from the optimal gray value thresholding method.

10.8. Repeat Exercise 10.7 with $k = 9$ and compare your results with those obtained using $k = 5$.

10.9. Using the center of the clusters as obtained in Exercise 10.7, use a region-growing method to obtain segmented regions. Compare the segmented regions with those obtained in Exercise 10.7.

10.10. Write a simple algorithm for image segmentation using a maximum-likelihood-based pixel classification method. Comment on the relative advantages and disadvantages of this approach over the region-growing method for image segmentation.

10.11. Select a classified MR brain image from the database and use it to train a backpropagation neural network (BPNN) for image segmentation through pixel classification. Apply the trained BPNN to classify a new MR brain image for segmentation. Compare the segmented regions with those obtained from gray value thresholding method.

10.12. Explain a fuzzy c-means clustering method. How is it different from the k-means clustering method?

10.13. Select a classified MR brain image from the database and use it to train a radial basis function neural network (RBFNN) for image segmentation through pixel classification. Apply the trained RBFNN to classify a new MR brain image for segmentation. Compare the segmented regions with those obtained from fuzzy c-means clustering ($c = 5$) method.

10.6. REFERENCES

1. R. Jain, R. Kasturi and B.G. Schunck, *Machine Vision*, McGRaw Hill, Inc., New York, 1995.
2. R.C. Gonzalez and R.E. Woods, *Digital Image Processing*, 2nd Edition, Prentice Hall, Englewood Cliffs, NJ, 2002.
3. D. Marr and E.C. Hildreth, "Theory of edge detection," *Proc. R. Soc. Lond. B*, Vol. 207, pp. 187–217, 1980.
4. R.M. Haralick and L.G. Shapiro, "Image segmentation techniques," *Comp. Vis. Graph. Imaging Process.*, Vol. 7, pp. 100–132, 1985.
5. Y. Ohta, *Knowledge Based Interpretation of Output Natural Color Scenes*, Pittman Advanced Pub., New York, 1985.
6. S.A. Stansfield, "ANGY: A rule-based expert system for automatic segmentation of coronary vessels from digital subtracted angiograms," *IEEE Trans. Patten Anal. Mach. Intell.*, Vol. 8, pp. 188–199, 1986.

7. R. Ohlander, K. Price and D.R. Reddy, "Picture segmentation using a recursive region splitting method," *Comp. Vis. Graph. Imaging Process.*, Vol. 8, pp. 313–333, 1978.
8. S. Zucker, "Region growing: Childhood and adolescence," *Comp. Vis. Graph. Imaging Process.*, Vol. 5, pp. 382–399, 1976.
9. A.P. Dhawan and A. Sicsu, "Segmentation of images of skin lesions using color and texture information of surface pigmentation," *Comp. Med. Imaging Graph.*, Vol. 16, pp. 163–177, 1992.
10. A.P. Dhawan and L. Arata, "Segmentation of medical images through competitive learning," *Comp. Methods Prog. Biomed.*, Vol. 40, pp. 203–215, 1993.
11. S.R. Raya, "Low-level segmentation of 3-D magnetic resonance brain images," *IEEE Trans. Med. Imaging*, Vol. 9, pp. 327–337, 1990.
12. Z. Liang, "Tissue classification and segmentation of MR images," *IEEE Eng. Med. Biol. Mag.*, Vol. 12, pp. 81–85, 1993.
13. B.M. Dawant and A.P. Zijdenbos, "Image segmentation," in M. Sonka and J. M. Fitzpatrick (Eds), *Handbook of Medical Imaging, Volume 2: Medical Image Processing and Analysis*, SPIE Press, Bellingham, WA, 2000, pp. 71–128.
14. D.H. Ballard, "Generalizing the Hough transform to detect arbitrary shapes," *Pattern Recognit.*, Vol. 13, pp. 111–122, 1981.
15. M. Bomans, K.H. Hohne, U. Tiede, and M. Riemer, "3-D segmentation of MR images of the head for 3-D display," *IEEE Trans. Med. Imaging*, Vol. 9, pp. 177–183, 1990.
16. S.R. Raya, "Low-level segmentation of 3-D magnetic resonance brain images: A rule based system," *IEEE Trans. Med. Imaging*, Vol. 9, No. 1, pp. 327–337, 1990.
17. H.E. Cline, W.E. Lorensen, R. Kikinis, and F. Jolesz, "Three-dimensional segmentation of MR images of the head using probability and connectivity," *J. Comput. Assist. Tomogr.*, Vol. 14, pp. 1037–1045, 1990.
18. L. Clarke, R. Velthuizen, S. Phuphanich, J. Schellenberg, J. Arrington, and M. Silbiger, "MRI: Stability of three supervised segmentation techniques," *Magn. Reson. Imaging*, Vol. 11, pp. 95–106, 1993.
19. L.O. Hall, A.M. Bensaid, L.P. Clarke, R.P. Velthuizen, M.S. Silbiger, and J.C. Bezdek, "A comparison of neural network and fuzzy clustering techniques in segmenting magnetic resonance images of the brain," *IEEE Trans. Neural Netw.*, Vol. 3, pp. 672–682, 1992.
20. M. Vannier, T. Pilgram, C. Speidel, L. Neumann, D. Rickman, and L. Schertz, "Validation of magnetic resonance imaging (MRI) multispectral tissue classification," *Comput. Med. Imaging Graph.*, Vol. 15, pp. 217–223, 1991.
21. H.S. Choi, D.R. Haynor, and Y. Kim, "Partial volume tissue classification of multichannel magnetic resonance images—A mixed model," *IEEE Trans. Med. Imaging*, Vol. 10, pp. 395–407, 1991.
22. A. Zavaljevski, A.P. Dhawan, S. Holland, W. Ball, M. Giskill-Shipley, J. Johnson, and S. Dunn, "Multispectral MR brain image classification," *Comput. Med. Imaging Graph. Image Process.*, Vol. 24, pp. 87–98, 2000.
23. A.M. Nazif and M.D. Levine, "Low-level image segmentation: An expert system," *IEEE Trans. Pattern Anal. Mach. Intell.*, Vol. 6, pp. 555–577, 1984.
24. L.K. Arata, A.P. Dhawan, A.V. Levy, J. Broderick, and M. Gaskil, Three-dimensional anatomical model based segmentation of MR brain images through prinicpal axes registration," *IEEE Trans. Biomed. Eng.*, Vol. 42, pp. 1069–1078, 1995.
25. L. Xu, M. Jackowski, A. Goshtasby, C. Yu, D. Roseman, A.P. Dhawan, and S. Bines, "Segmentation of skin cancer images," *Image Vis. Comput.*, Vol. 17, pp. 65–74, 1999.
26. A. Sarwal and A.P. Dhawan, "Segmentation of coronary arteriograms through radial basis function neural network," *J. Comput. Inf. Technol.*, Vol. 6, pp. 135–148, 1998.
27. M. Ozkan, B.M. Dawant, and R.J. Maciunas, "Neural-network-based segmentation of multi-modal medical images: A comparative and prospective study," *IEEE Trans. Med. Imaging*, Vol. 12, pp. 534–544, Sept. 1993.
28. N.J. Nilson, *Principles of Artificial Intelligence*, Springer Verlag, New York, 1982.
29. P.H. Winston, *Artificial Intelligence*, 3rd Edition, Addison Wesley, Reading, MA, 1992.
30. R.O. Duda and P.E. Hart, *Pattern Classification and Scene Analysis*, John Wiley & Sons, New York, 1973.

31. T. Kanungo, D.M. Mount, N.S. Netanvahu, C.D. Piatko, R. Silverman, and A.Y. Xu, "An efficient k-means algorithm: Analysis and implementation," *IEEE Trans. Pattern Anal. Mach. Intell.*, Vol. 24, pp. 881–892, 2002.
32. X.L. Xie and G. Beni, "A validity measure for fuzzy clustering," *IEEE Trans. Pattern Anal. Mach. Intell.*, Vol. 13(8), pp. 841–847, August 1991.
33. A. Bezdek, *Pattern Recognition with Fuzzy Objective Function Algorithms*, Plenum, New York, 1981.
34. D.L. Pham and J.L. Prince, "Adaptive fuzzy segmentation of magnetic resonance images," *IEEE Trans. Med. Imaging*, Vol. 18, pp. 737–752, 1999.
35. J.M. Zurada, *Introduction to Artificial Neural Systems*, West Publishing Co., Boston, 1992.
36. S.E. Fahlman and C. Lebeire, *The Cascade-Correlation Learning Architecture*, Tech. Report, School of Computer Science, Carnegie Mellon University, 1990.
37. S. Chen, C.F.N. Cowan, and P.M. Grant, "Orthogonal least squares learning for radial basis function networks," *IEEE Trans. Neural Netw.*, Vol. 2, No. 2, pp. 302–309, 1991.
38. T. Poggio and F. Girosi, "Networks for approximation and learning," *Proc. IEEE*, Vol. 78, No. 9, pp.1481–1497, 1990.
39. I.R.H. Jacobson, "Radial basis functions: A survey and new results," In D. C. Handscomb (Ed), *The Mathematics of Surfaces III*, Clarendon Press, Gloucestershire, 1989, pp. 115–133.
40. S. Loncaric, A.P. Dhawan, T. Brott, and J. Broderick, "3-D image analysis of intracerebral brain hemorrhage," *Comput. Methods Prog. Biomed.*, Vol. 46, pp. 207–216, 1995.
41. J. Broderick, S. Narayan, A.P. Dhawan, M. Gaskil, and J. Khouri, "Ventricular measurement of multifocal brain lesions: Implications for treatment trials of vascular dementia and multiple sclerosis," *Neuroimaging*, Vol. 6, pp. 36–43, 1996.
42. P. Schmid, "Segmentation of digitized dermatoscopic images by two-dimensional color clustering," *IEEE Trans. Med. Imaging*, Vol. 18, pp. 164–171, 1999.

CHAPTER 11

IMAGE REPRESENTATION, ANALYSIS, AND CLASSIFICATION

An image is considered a representation of objects with specific properties that are utilized in the imaging process. The characterization (or appearance) of objects in the image depends on their specific properties and interaction with the imaging process. For example, an image of an outdoor scene captured by a photographic camera provides a characterization of objects using the reflected light from their surfaces. Thus, the appearance of objects in the image will depend on the reflective properties of surfaces, illumination, viewing angle, and the optics of the photographic camera. As described in Chapters 4–7, different medical imaging modalities provide different characterizations of the physiological objects based on their properties and the type and parameters of the imaging modality. For example, a T_1-weighted magnetic resonance (MR) image of the brain would show a different contrast of soft tissue, ventricles, and cerebrospinal fluid than its T_2-weighted MR image.

In order to perform a computerized analysis of an image, it is important to establish a hierarchical framework of processing steps representing the image (data) and knowledge (model) domains. The hierarchical image representation with bottom-up and top-down analysis approaches is schematically presented in Figure 11.1. A scenario consists of a multiple image data set involving multidimensional, multimodality, or multisubject images and can be represented as a set of scenes consisting of specific objects in the corresponding images. The objects can be represented into surface regions (S-regions) consisting of one or more regions formed by contours and edges defining specific shapes of object structures.

The bottom-up analysis starts with the analysis at the pixel-level representation and moves up toward the understanding of the scene or the scenario (in the case of multiple images). The top-down analysis starts with the hypothesis of the presence of an object and then moves toward the pixel-level representation to verify or reject the hypothesis using the knowledge-based models. It is difficult to apply a complete bottom-up or top-down approach for efficient image analysis and understanding. Usually, an appropriate combination of both approaches provides the best results. Pixel-level analysis, also known as low-level analysis, can incorporate a bottom-up approach for the edge and region segmentation. The characteristic features of

---

Medical Image Analysis, Second Edition, by Atam P. Dhawan
Copyright © 2011 by the Institute of Electrical and Electronics Engineers, Inc.

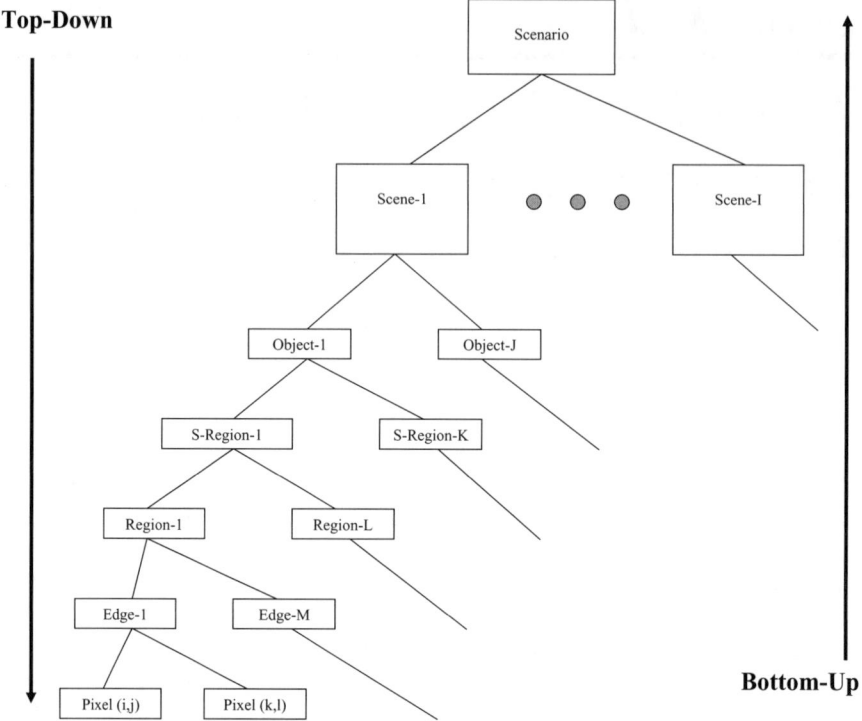
Figure 11.1 A hierarchical representation of image features.

segmented regions can be extracted for preliminary region and object analysis. Features can then be analyzed for object identification and classification using knowledge-based models with a top-down approach.

Figure 11.2 shows a paradigm of image analysis with associated structure of knowledge-based models that can be used at different stages of processing. The knowledge of physical constraints and tissue properties can be very useful in imaging and image reconstruction. For example, knowledge of the interaction of a radioactive pharmaceutical drug with body tissue is an important consideration in nuclear medicine imaging modalities. To improve contrast in proton density-based MR imaging, a paramagnetic contrast agent such as gadolinium (Gd) is used. The imaging sequences in MR imaging are specifically modified using knowledge of the physical properties of tissues and organs to be imaged. Anatomical locations of various organs in the body often impose a challenge in imaging the desired tissue or part of the organ. Using knowledge of physical regions of interest, data collection image reconstruction methods can be modified. The performance of image reconstruction algorithms can be improved using some physical models and properties of the imaging process. The pixel-level image analysis for edge and region segmentation can also be improved using probabilistic and knowledge-based models of expected regions and objects. For example, Hough transform can be used to extract specific regions of target shapes. A model-based tissue segmentation algorithm is described

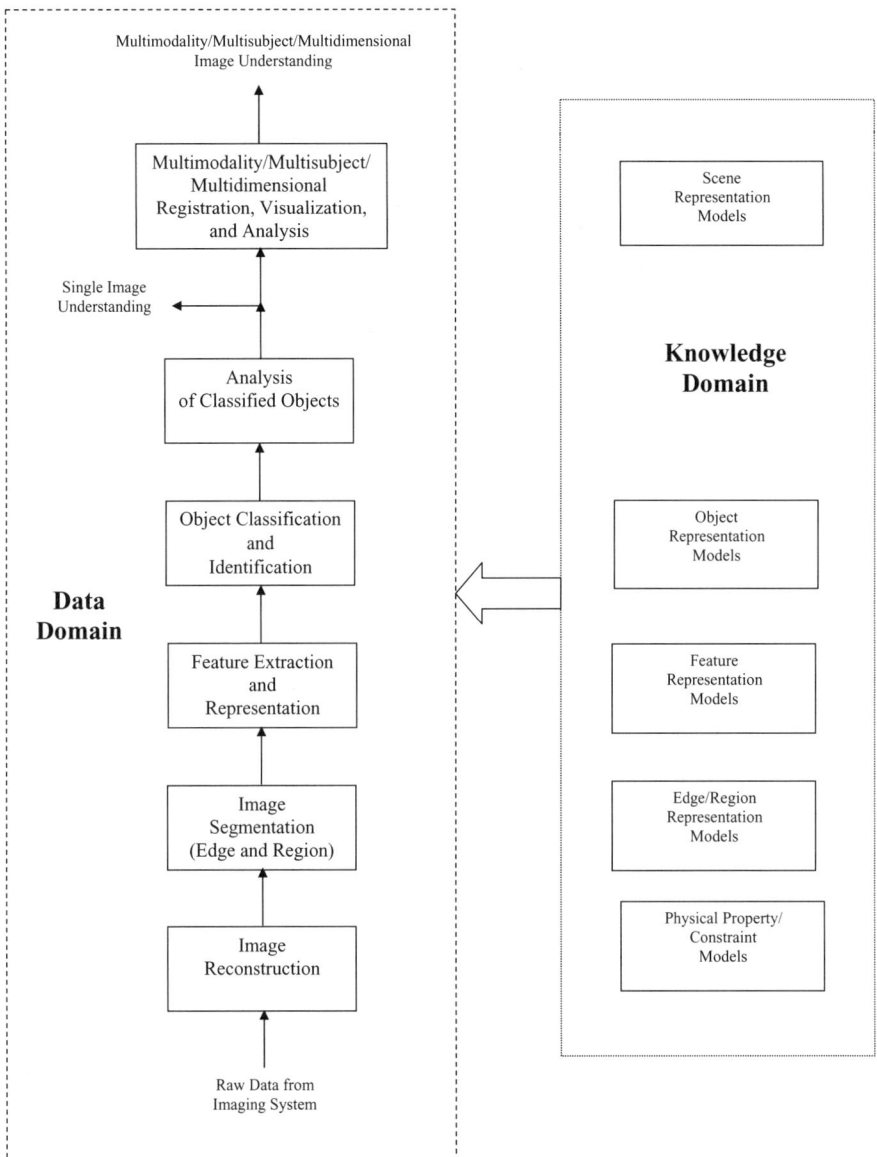

Figure 11.2 A hierarchical structure of medical image analysis.

in Chapter 10. Furthermore, the characteristic features of segmented regions can be efficiently analyzed and classified using probabilistic and knowledge-based models of expected objects. An object representation model usually provides the knowledge about the shape or other characteristic features of a single object for the classification analysis. In addition, the scene interpretation models can provide knowledge about the geometrical and relational features of other objects present in the image. For example, a three-dimensional (3-D) anatomical chest cavity model can provide shape and relational information of the major cardiac chambers (left ventricle, right ventricle, left atrium, and right atrium) along with the cardiac cage, lungs, and liver. Such models are quite useful in improving the classification and understanding of occluded objects in the image.

This chapter describes feature extraction methods for region representation followed by classification methods for object identification and understanding.

11.1. FEATURE EXTRACTION AND REPRESENTATION

As described above, after segmentation, specific features representing the characteristics and properties of the segmented regions in the image need to be computed for object classification and understanding. Features are also important for measurements of parameters leading to direct image understanding. For example, a quantitative analysis of MR perfusion time-series images provides information about the parameters of cerebral perfusion. A complete feature representation of the segmented regions is critical for object classification and analysis. There are four major categories of features for region representation:

1. **Statistical Pixel-Level (SPL) Features:** These features provide quantitative information about the pixels within a segmented region. The SPL features may include mean, variance, and histogram of the gray values of pixels in the region. In addition, SPL features may include the area of the region and information about the contrast of pixels within the region and edge gradient of boundary pixels.
2. **Shape Feature:** These features provide information about the characteristic shape of the region boundary. The shape-based features may include circularity, compactness, moments, chain-codes, and Hough transform. Recently, morphological processing methods have also been used for shape description.
3. **Texture Features:** These features provide information about the local texture within the region or the corresponding part of the image. The texture features may be computed using the second-order histogram statistics or co-occurrence matrices. In addition, wavelet processing methods for spatio-frequency analysis have been used to represent local texture information.
4. **Relational Features:** These features provide information about the relational and hierarchical structure of the regions associated with a single object or a group of objects.

11.1.1 Statistical Pixel-Level Features

Once the regions are segmented in the image, gray values of pixels within the region can be used for computing the following SPL features (1, 2):

1. The histogram of the gray values of pixels in the image as

$$p(r_i) = \frac{n(r_i)}{n} \quad (11.1)$$

where $p(r_i)$ and $n(r_i)$ are, respectively, the probability and number of occurrences of a gray value r_i in the region and n is the total number of pixels in the region.

2. Mean m of the gray values of the pixels in the image can be computed as

$$m = \frac{1}{n}\sum_{i=0}^{L-1} r_i p(r_i) \tag{11.2}$$

where L is the total number gray values in the image with $0, 1, \ldots, L-1$.

3. Variance and central moments in the region can be computed as

$$\mu_n = \sum_{i=0}^{L-1} p(r_i)(r_i - m)^n \tag{11.3}$$

where the second central moment μ_2 is the variance of the region. The third and fourth central moments can be computed, respectively, for $n = 3$ and $n = 4$. The third central moment is a measure of noncentrality, while the fourth central moment is a measure of flatness of the histogram.

4. Energy: Total energy E of the gray values of pixels in the region is given by

$$E = \sum_{i=0}^{L-1} [p(r_i)]^2. \tag{11.4}$$

5. Entropy: The entropy Ent as a measure of information represented by the distribution of gray values in the region is given by

$$Ent = -\sum_{i=0}^{L-1} p(r_i) \log_2(r_i). \tag{11.5}$$

6. Local contrast corresponding to each pixel can be computed by the difference between the gray value of the center pixel and the mean of the gray values of the neighborhood pixels. An adaptive method for computing contrast values is described in Chapter 7. The normalized local contrast $C(x, y)$ for the center pixel can also be computed as

$$C(x,y) = \frac{|P_c(x,y) - P_s(x,y)|}{\max\{P_c(x,y), P_s(x,y)\}} \tag{11.6}$$

where $P_c(x, y)$ and $P_s(x, y)$ are the average gray-level values of the pixels corresponding to the center and the surround regions respectively centered on the pixel (Chapter 9).

7. Additional features such as maximum and minimum gray values can also be used for representing regions.

8. The features based on the statistical distribution of local contrast values in the region also provide useful information about the characteristics of the regions representing objects. For example, features representing the mean, variance, energy, and entropy of contrast values in the segmented regions contribute significantly in classification analysis of X-ray mammograms (3).

9. Features based on the gradient information for the boundary pixels of the region are also an important consideration in defining the nature of edges. For example, the fading edges with low gradient form a characteristic feature of malignant melanoma and must be included in the classification analysis of images of skin lesions (4, 5).

11.1.2 Shape Features

There are several features that can be used to represent the geometric shape of a segmented region. The shape of a region is basically defined by the spatial distribution of boundary pixels. A simple approach for computing shape features for a two-dimensional (2-D) region is representing circularity, compactness, and elongatedness through the minimum bounded rectangle that covers the region. For example, Figure 11.3 shows a segmented region and its minimum bounded rectangle ABCD.

Several features using the boundary pixels of the segmented region can be computed as

1. Longest axis GE
2. Shortest axis HF
3. Perimeter and area of the minimum bounded rectangle ABCD
4. Elongation ratio: GE/HF
5. Perimeter p and area A of the segmented region
6. Hough transform of the region using the gradient information of the boundary pixels of the region (as described in Chapter 7)
7. Circularity ($C = 1$ for a circle) of the region computed as

$$C = \frac{4\pi A}{p^2}. \tag{11.7}$$

8. Compactness C_p of the region computed as

$$C_p = \frac{p^2}{A}. \tag{11.8}$$

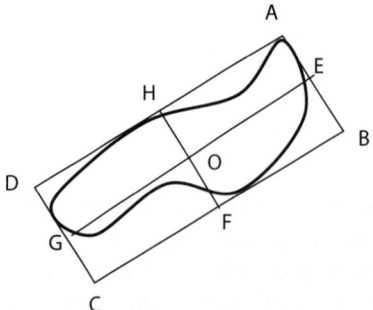

Figure 11.3 A segmented region with a minimum bounded region.

9. Chain code for boundary contour as obtained using a set of orientation primitives on the boundary segments derived from a piecewise linear approximation
10. Fourier descriptor of boundary contours as obtained using the Fourier transform of the sequence of boundary segments derived from a piecewise linear approximation
11. Central moments-based shape features for the segmented region
12. Morphological shape descriptors as obtained though morphological processing on the segmented region

Shape features using the chain code, Fourier descriptor, central moments, and morphological processing are described below.

11.1.2.1 Boundary Encoding: Chain Code Let us define a neighborhood matrix with orientation primitives with respect to the center pixel as shown in Figure 11.4. The codes of specific orientation are set for 8-connected neighborhood directions based on the location of the end of the boundary segment with respect to its origin at the center x_c. Thus, the orientation directions are coded with a numerical value ranging from 0 to 7. To apply these orientation codes to describe a boundary, the boundary contour needs to be approximated as a list of segments that have preselected length and directions. For example, the boundary of the region shown in Figure 11.5 is approximated in segments using the directions of 8-connected neighborhood and orientation codes shown in Figure 11.4. To obtain boundary segments representing a piecewise approximation of the original boundary contour, a discretization method, such as "divide and conquer," is applied. The divide and conquer method for curve approximation selects two points on a boundary contour as vertices. These vertices can be selected arbitrarily or on the basis of gradient information. Usually points with a significant change in the gradient direction are selected as potential vertices. A straight line joining the two selected vertices can be used to approximate the respective curve segment if it satisfies a maximum-deviation criterion for no further division of the curve segment. The maximum-deviation criterion is based on the perpendicular distance between any point on the original curve segment between the selected vertices and the corresponding approximated straight-line segment. If the perpendicular distance or deviation of any point on the curve

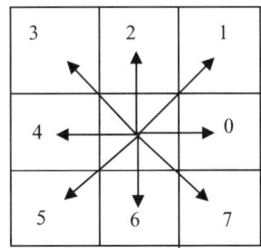

Figure 11.4 The 8-connected neighborhood codes (left) and the orientation directions (right) with respect to the center pixel x_c.

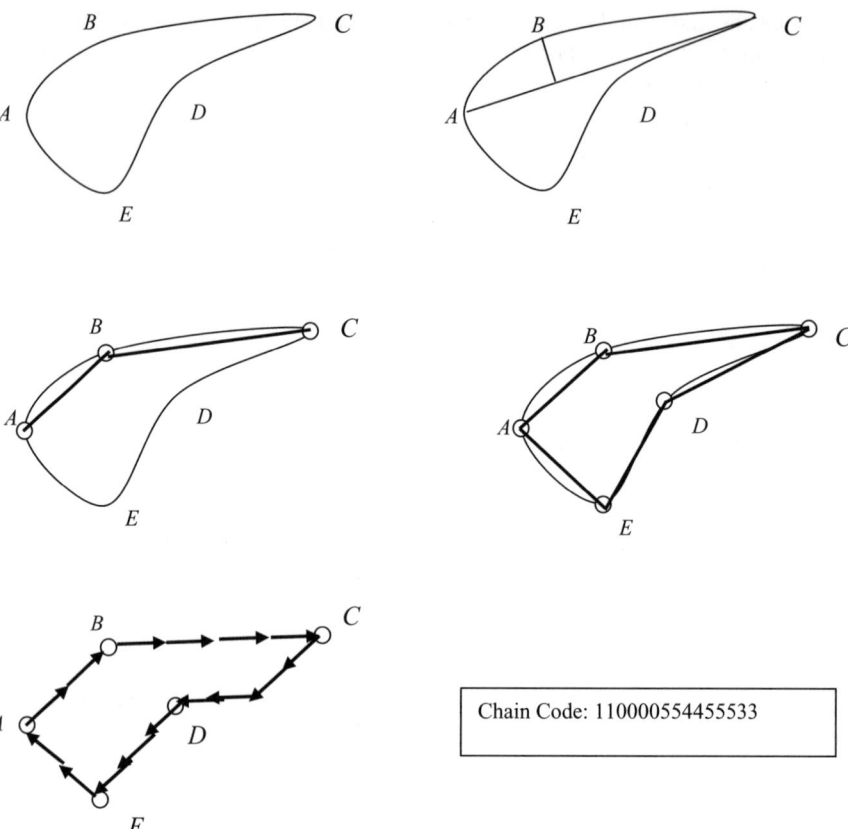

Figure 11.5 A schematic example of developing chain code for a region with boundary contour *ABCDE*. From top left to bottom right: the original boundary contour, two points *A* and *C* with maximum vertical distance parameter *BF*, two segments *AB* and *BC* approximating the contour *ABC*, five segments approximating the entire contour *ABCDE*, contour approximation represented in terms of orientation primitives, and the respective chain code of the boundary contour.

segment from the approximated straight-line segment exceeds a preselected deviation threshold, the curve segment is further divided at the point of maximum deviation. This process of dividing the segments with additional vertices continues until all approximated straight-line segments satisfy the maximum-deviation criterion. For example, two points *A* and *C* on the boundary contour *ABCDE* shown in Figure 11.5 have significant change in the direction of their respective gradients and are therefore taken as initial vertices for curve approximation. It can be seen in the example shown in Figure 11.5 that the approximated straight-line segment *AC* does not satisfy the maximum-deviation criterion, that is, the perpendicular distance BF is more than an acceptable threshold. The boundary arc segment *AC* is then further divided into two segments *AB* and *AC* with their respective approximated straight-line segments. As shown in Figure 11.5, this process is continued until a final approximation of five straight-line segments, *AB*, *BC*, *CD*, *DE*, and *EA* is obtained.

This representation is further approximated using the orientation primitives of the 8-connected neighborhood as defined in Figure 11.4. The chain code descriptor of the boundary can now be obtained using the orientation primitive based approximated representation. The boundary segment shown in Figure 11.5 can thus have a chain code *110000554455533*. It should be noted that though this code is starting at the vertex A, it is circular in nature. Two parameters can change the chain code: number of orientation primitives and the maximum-deviation threshold used in approximating the curve. However, other methods for approximating curves can also be used before orientation primitives are applied to obtain chain codes (1, 5, 6).

11.1.2.2 Boundary Encoding: Fourier Descriptor

Fourier series may be used to approximate a closed boundary of a region. Let us assume that the boundary of an object is expressed as a sequence of N points (or pixels) with the coordinates $\mathbf{u}[n] = \{x(n), y(n)\}$ such that

$$u(n) = x(n) + iy(n); \quad n = 0, 1, 2, \ldots, N-1. \tag{11.9}$$

The discrete Fourier transform (DFT) of the sequence $\mathbf{u}[n]$ is the Fourier descriptor $\mathbf{F}_d[n]$ of the boundary and is defined as

$$\mathbf{F}_d[m] = \frac{1}{N} \sum_{n=0}^{N-1} u(n) e^{-2\pi i m/N} \quad \text{for } 0 \leq m \leq N-1. \tag{11.10}$$

Rigid geometric transformation of a boundary such as translation, rotation, and scaling can be represented by simple operations on its Fourier transform. Thus, the Fourier descriptors can be used as shape descriptors for region matching dealing with translation, rotation, and scaling. Fourier descriptor-based boundary representation models have been used in medical imaging for segmentation and object identification (7).

11.1.2.3 Moments for Shape Description

The shape of a boundary or contour can be represented quantitatively by the central moments for matching. The central moments represent specific geometrical properties of the shape and are invariant to translation, rotation, and scaling. The central moments μ_{pq} of a segmented region or binary image $f(x, y)$ are given by (8, 9)

$$\mu_{pq} = \sum_{i=1}^{L} \sum_{j=1}^{L} (x_i - \overline{x})^p (y_j - \overline{y})^q f(x, y)$$

where

$$\overline{x} = \sum_{i=1}^{L} \sum_{j=1}^{L} x_i f(x_i, y_j)$$

$$\overline{y} = \sum_{i=1}^{L} \sum_{j=1}^{L} y_j f(x_i, y_j). \tag{11.11}$$

For example, the central moment μ_{21} represents the vertical divergence of the shape of the region indicating the relative extent of the bottom of the region compared with the top. The normalized central moments are then defined as where

$$\eta_{pq} = \frac{\mu_{pq}}{(\mu_{00})^\gamma}$$

$$\gamma = \frac{p+q}{2} + 1. \tag{11.12}$$

The seven invariant moments $\phi_1 - \phi_7$ for shape matching are defined as (9)

$$\phi_1 = \eta_{20} + \eta_{02}$$
$$\phi_2 = (\eta_{20} - \eta_{02})^2 + 4\eta_{11}^2$$
$$\phi_3 = (\eta_{30} - 3\eta_{12})^2 + (3\eta_{21} - \eta_{03})^2$$
$$\phi_4 = (\eta_{30} + \eta_{12})^2 + (\eta_{21} + \eta_{03})^2$$
$$\phi_5 = (\eta_{30} - 3\eta_{12})(\eta_{30} + \eta_{12})[(\eta_{30} + \eta_{12})^2 - 3(\eta_{21} + \eta_{03})^2]$$
$$\quad + (3\eta_{21} - \eta_{03})(\eta_{21} + \eta_{03})[3(\eta_{30} + \eta_{12})^2 - (\eta_{21} + \eta_{03})^2]$$
$$\phi_6 = (\eta_{20} - \eta_{02})[(\eta_{30} + \eta_{12})^2 - (\eta_{21} + \eta_{03})^2] + 4\eta_{11}(\eta_{30} + \eta_{12})(\eta_{21} + \eta_{03})$$
$$\phi_7 = (3\eta_{21} - \eta_{03})(\eta_{30} + \eta_{12})[(\eta_{30} + \eta_{12})^2 - 3(\eta_{21} + \eta_{03})^2]$$
$$\quad + (3\eta_{12} - \eta_{30})(\eta_{21} + \eta_{03})[3(\eta_{30} + \eta_{12})^2 - (\eta_{21} + \eta_{03})^2]. \tag{11.13}$$

The invariant moments are used extensively in the literature for shape matching and pattern recognition (2, 6–10).

11.1.2.4 Morphological Processing for Shape Description

Mathematical morphology is based on set theory. It provides basic tools to process images for filtering, thinning, and pruning operations. These tools are useful in the description of region shape, involving boundary and skeleton representations.

There are two fundamental operations in morphological processing: dilation and erosion. Most of the morphological processing algorithms are based on specific combinations of the dilation and erosion operations. Let us define two sets, A and B, belonging to an n-dimensional space Z^n. For gray-level images, the parameter n is equal to 3 considering 2-D space for x- and y-scoordinates and the third dimension for the gray values of pixels in the image. For a binary or segmented image with regions, the parameter n takes the value of 2 since the sets A and B can represent the boolean values of "1" (within the set) and "0" (outside the set). For simplicity, only binary or region-based ssegmented images are considered here with a 2-D representation of sets A and B. However, they can be extended to 3-D space for gray-level morphological image processing.

The set A can be assumed to be the binary image while the set B is considered to be the structuring element of the same dimensions. For example, Figure 11.6 shows a large region representing the set A and a smaller region representing the set B for the structuring element. The dilation of set A by the set B, $D(A, B)$ is denoted by $A \oplus B$ and defined by the Minkowski set addition as

$$D(A,B) = A \oplus B = \bigcup_{b \in B} A + b. \tag{11.14}$$

11.1. FEATURE EXTRACTION AND REPRESENTATION

Set A

Set B

Figure 11.6 A large region with square shape representing the set A and a small region with rectangular shape representing the structuring element set B.

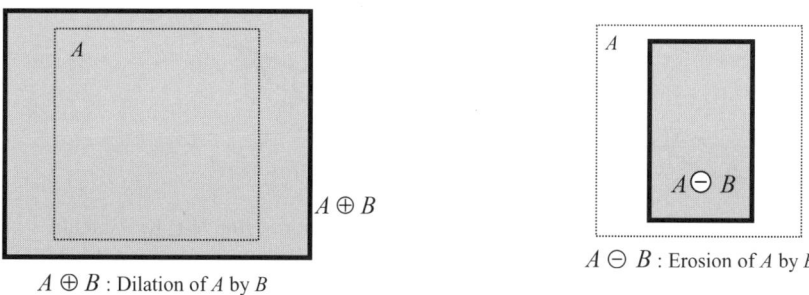

$A \oplus B$: Dilation of A by B

$A \ominus B$: Erosion of A by B

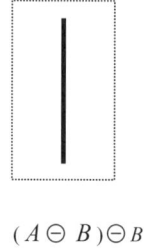

$(A \ominus B) \ominus B$

Figure 11.7 The dilation of set A by the structuring element set B (top left), the erosion of set A by the structuring element set B (top right), and the result of two successive erosions of set A by the structuring element set B (bottom).

It can be shown that

$$A \oplus B = \{x | (\breve{B})_x \cap A \neq 0\} \qquad (11.15)$$

where $\breve{B} = \{-b | b \in B\}$ is the reflection set of B with respect to its origin.

Equation 11.15 states that the dilation of a set (shape) A by a structuring element B comprises all points x such that the reflected structuring element $\breve{B}$ translated to x intersects A. Figure 11.7 shows the dilation of a shape (of a region) A by the structuring element B.

As all operations in set theory have their respective dual operations, the dual operation of dilation is erosion. The erosion of set (shape) A by the set B (structuring

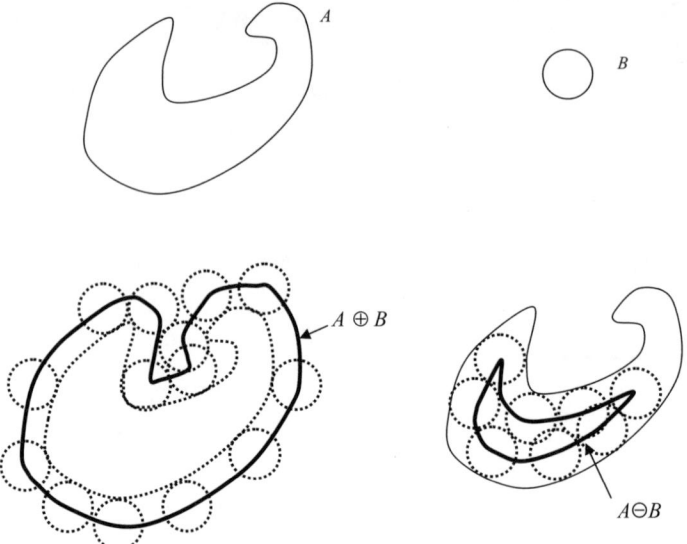

Figure 11.8 Dilation and erosion of an arbitrary shape region A (top left) by a circular structuring element B (top right): dilation of A by B (bottom left) and erosion of A by B (bottom right).

element), $E(A, B)$, is denoted by $A \ominus B$ and is defined by the Minkowski set subtraction as

$$E(A, B) = A \ominus B = \bigcap_{b \in B} A - b. \qquad (11.16)$$

It can be shown that

$$A \ominus B = \{x \mid (B)_x \subseteq A\}. \qquad (11.17)$$

Equation 11.17 states that the erosion of a set (shape) A by the structuring element B comprises all points x such that the structuring element B located at x is entirely inside A.

The dilation and erosion of an arbitrary shape region A by a circular structuring element set B is shown in Figure 11.8. It can be seen that the dilation operation provides the property of increasingness (dilated regions are larger) while the erosion provides the property of decreasingness (eroded regions are smaller).

As mentioned above, the dilation and erosion are dual operations to each other, that is,

$$A \oplus B = \left(A^c \ominus \breve{B}\right)^c$$

and

$$A \ominus B = \left(A^c \oplus \breve{B}\right)^c \qquad (11.18)$$

where A^c represents the complement of set A.

Both of these operations also provide translation variance and distributive properties as

$$(A+x) \oplus B = A \oplus (B+x) = (A \oplus B) + x \quad \text{Translation invariance of dilation}$$
$$(A_1 \cup A_2) \oplus B = (A_1 \oplus B) \cup (A_2 \oplus B) \quad \text{Distributivity of union of dilation}$$

$$(A+x) \ominus B = A \ominus (B-x) = (A \ominus B) + x \quad \text{Translation invariance of dilation}$$
$$(A_1 \cap A_2) \ominus B = (A_1 \ominus B) \cap (A_2 \ominus B) \quad \text{Distributivity of intersection of erosion}$$
(11.19)

Dilation and erosion operations successively change the shape of the region or binary image. The successive application of erosion as shown in Figure 11.7 can be used to describe the shape of the region. However, combinations of dilation and erosion such as opening and closing operations can also be used effectively for shape description (11–14).

The morphological opening of set A by the structuring element set B, $A \circ B$, is defined as the composition of erosion followed by dilation as

$$A \circ B = (A \ominus B) \oplus B. \tag{11.20}$$

The morphological closing of set A by the structuring element set B, $A \circ B$, is defined as the composition of erosion followed by dilation as

$$A \bullet B = (A \oplus B) \ominus B. \tag{11.21}$$

The advantage of using morphological opening and closing operations in shape description is that successive applications of these operations do not change the shape of the image or region. It can be shown that the union of openings is an opening, whereas the intersection of closings is a closing (11). Figure 11.9

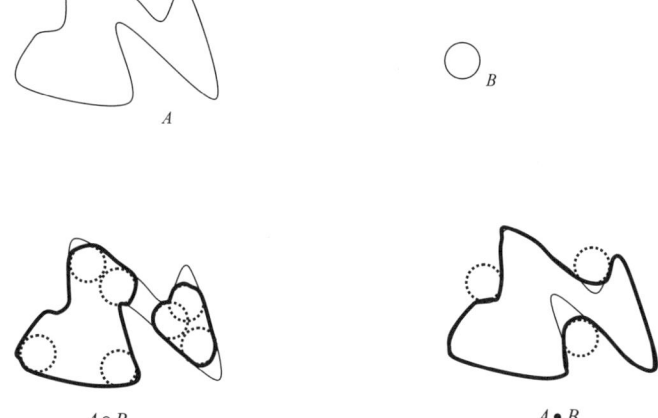

Figure 11.9 The morphological opening and closing of set A (top left) by the structuring element set B (top right): opening of A by B (bottom left) and closing of A by B (bottom right).

shows the opening and closing of an arbitrary shape by a circular structuring element.

Morphological decomposition methods have been used for shape representation and description (11–14) and applied in 3-D computed tomography (CT) image analysis of intracerebral brain hemorrhage (15). Let F be an input binary image or a segmented region and S be a structuring element for a shape decomposition process. Using a multiscale representation with a scale parameter r, a shape description of an image F can be given by (14, 15)

$$Z(r,0), \ldots, Z(r,N-1)$$
$$\text{with } Z(r,n) = \mathbf{M}(r,F,S^n) \tag{11.22}$$

where $\mathbf{M}$ is a morphological operation such as erosion, dilation, opening, or closing; r is the scale parameter; and $n = 0, 1, \ldots, N-1$ is a parameter that controls the size and shape of the structuring element S.

Morphological shape descriptors using a specific set of structuring elements on multiple scales can provide a translation, size, and rotation invariant shape representation (14, 16).

A popular method for shape description is using morphological operations for skeleton representation of regions of interest. A skeleton $K(A)$ of a set A using the structuring element set B can be computed using the erosion and opening operations as

$$K(A) = \bigcup_{n=0}^{N} K_n(A)$$

with

$$K_n(A) = (A \ominus nB) - (A \ominus nB) \circ B \tag{11.23}$$

where $(A \ominus nB)$ represents n successive erosions of the set A by the structuring element set B, and N denotes the last iterative step before the set A erodes to an empty set.

Figure 11.7 shows the skeleton of the set A that is obtained by two successive erosions by the structuring element set B. It should be noted that in this example, a customized shape of the structuring element is used which happens to provide the skeleton representation in just two erosions. In practice, a predefined set of structuring elements can be tried on a set of training shapes to determine the best structuring element (16) that can provide a good skeleton representation using the method described in Equation 11.23.

Morphological operations can also be used in image processing such as image smoothing, segmentation, boundary detection, and region filling. For example, morphological erosion can significantly reduce the background noise in the image. An opening operation can remove the speckle noise and provide smooth contours to the spatially distributed structures in the image. A closing operation preserves the peaks and reduces the sharp variations in the signal such as dark artifacts. Thus, a morphological opening followed by closing can reduce the bright and dark artifacts and noise in the image. The morphological gradient image can be obtained by subtracting

11.1. FEATURE EXTRACTION AND REPRESENTATION

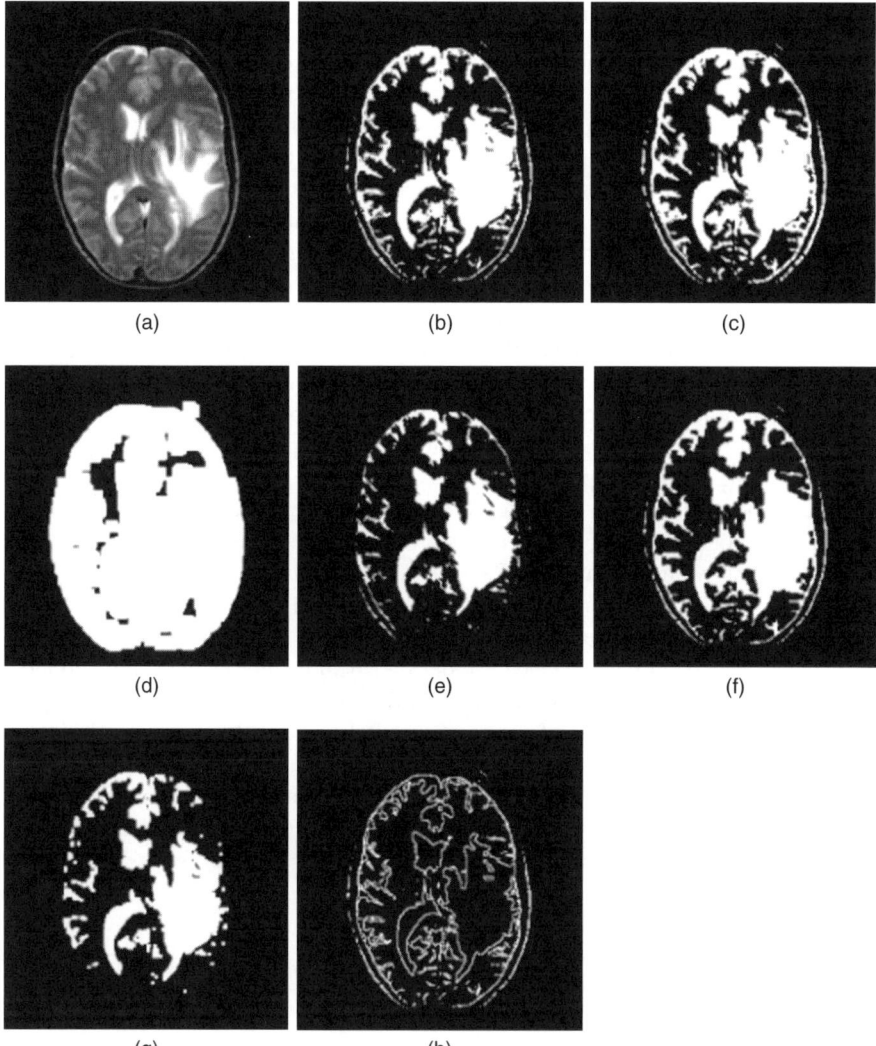

Figure 11.10 Example of morphological operations on MR brain image using a structuring element of $\begin{bmatrix} 1 & 0 \\ 0 & 1 \end{bmatrix}$ (a) the original MR brain image; (b) the thresholded MR brain image for morphological operations; (c) dilation of the thresholded MR brain image; (d) resultant image after five successive dilations of the thresholded brain image; (e) erosion of the thresholded MR brain image; (f) closing of the thresholded MR brain image; (g) opening of the thresholded MR brain image; and (h) morphological boundary detection on the thresholded MR brain image.

the eroded image from the dilated image. Edges can also be detected by subtracting the eroded image from the original image.

Figure 11.10 shows an MR brain image and the results of morphological operations applied to thresholded MR brain image.

11.1.3 Texture Features

Texture is an important spatial property that can be used in region segmentation as well as description. There are three major approaches to represent texture: statistical, structural, and spectral. Since texture is a property of the spatial arrangements of the gray values of pixels, the first-order histogram of gray values provides no information about the texture. Statistical methods representing the higher-order distribution of gray values in the image are used for texture representation. The second approach uses structural methods such as arrangements of prespecified primitives in texture representation. For example, a repetitive arrangement of square and triangular shapes can produce a specific texture. The third approach is based on spectral analysis methods such as Fourier and wavelet transforms. Using spectral analysis, texture is represented by a group of specific spatio-frequency components.

The gray-level co-occurrence matrix (GLCM) exploits the higher-order distribution of gray values of pixels that are defined with a specific distance or neighborhood criterion. In the simplest form, the GLCM $P(i, j)$ is the distribution of the number of occurrences of a pair of gray values i and j separated by a distance vector $d=[dx, dy]$. For example, Figure 11.11 shows a matrix representation of an image with three gray values with its GLCM $P(i, j)$ for $d=[1, 1]$.

The GLCM can be normalized by dividing each value in the matrix by the total number of occurrences, providing the probability of occurrence of a pair of gray values separated by a distance vector. Statistical texture features are computed from the normalized GLCM as the second-order histogram $H(y_q, y_r, d)$ representing the probability of occurrence of a pair of gray values yq and yr separated by a distance vector d. Texture features can also be described by a difference histogram, $H_d(y_s, d)$, where $y_s = |y_q - y_r|$. $H_d(y_s, d)$ indicates the probability that a difference in gray levels exists between two distinct pixels. Commonly used texture features based on the second-order histogram statistics are as follows.

1. Entropy of $H(y_q, y_r, d)$, S_H:

$$S_H = - \sum_{y_q=y_1}^{y_t} \sum_{y_r=y_1}^{y_t} H(y_q, y_r, d) \log_{10}[H(y_q, y_r, d)]. \qquad (11.24)$$

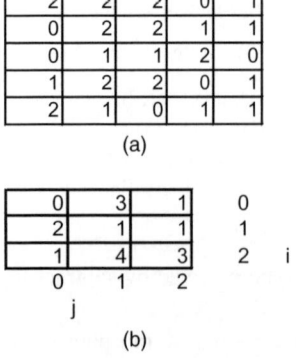

Figure 11.11 (a) A matrix representation of a 5 × 5 pixel image with three gray values; (b) the GLCM $P(i, j)$ for $d = [1, 1]$.

Entropy is a measure of texture nonuniformity. Lower entropy values indicate greater structural variation among the image regions.

2. Angular second moment of $H(y_q, y_r, d)$, ASM_H:

$$ASM_H = \sum_{y_q=y_1}^{y_t} \sum_{y_q=y_1}^{y_t} [H(y_q, y_r, d)]^2. \tag{11.25}$$

The ASM_H indicates the degree of homogeneity among textures, and is also representative of the energy in the image. A lower value of ASM_H is indicative of finer textures.

3. Contrast of $H(y_q, y_r, d)$:

$$Contrast = \sum_{y_q=y_1}^{y_t} \sum_{y_q=y_1}^{y_t} \partial(y_q, y_r) H(y_q, y_r, d) \tag{11.26}$$

where $\partial(y_q, y_r)$ is a measure of intensity similarity and is defined by $\partial(y_q, y_r) = (y_q - y_r)^2$. Thus, the contrast characterizes variation in pixel intensity.

4. Inverse difference moment of $H(y_q, y_r, d)$, IDM_H:

$$IDM_H = \sum_{y_q=y_1}^{y_t} \sum_{y_q=y_1}^{y_t} \frac{H(y_q, y_r, d)}{1 + \partial(y_q, y_r)}, \tag{11.27}$$

where $\partial(y_q, y_r)$ is defined as before. The $IDMH$ provides a measure of the local homogeneity among textures.

5. Correlation of $H(yq, yr, d)$:

$$Cor_H = \frac{1}{\sigma_{y_q} \sigma_{y_r}} \sum_{y_q=y_1}^{y_t} \sum_{y_q=y_1}^{y_t} (y_q - \mu_{y_q})(y_r - \mu_{y_r}) H(y_q, y_r, d), \tag{11.28}$$

where μ_{y_q}, μ_{y_r}, σ_{y_q}, and σ_{y_r} are the respective means and standard deviations of yq and yr. The correlation can also be expanded and written in terms of the marginal distributions of the second-order histogram, which are defined as

$$H_m(y_q, d) = \sum_{y_r=y_1}^{y_t} H(y_q, y_r, d),$$

$$H_m(y_r, d) = \sum_{y_q=y_1}^{y_t} H(y_q, y_r, d). \tag{11.29}$$

The correlation attribute is greater for similar elements of the second-order histogram.

6. Mean of $H(y_q, y_r, d)$: μ_{H_m}:

$$\mu_{H_m} = \sum_{y_q=y_1}^{y_t} y_q H_m(y_q, d). \tag{11.30}$$

The mean characterizes the nature of the gray-level distribution. Its value is typically small if the distribution is localized around $y_q = y_1$.

7. Deviation of $H_m(y_q, d)$: σ_{H_m}:

$$\sigma_{H_m} = \sqrt{\sum_{y_q=y_1}^{y_t}\left[y_q - \sum_{y_r=y_1}^{y_t} y_r H_m(y_r,d)\right]^2 H_m(y_q,d)}. \quad (11.31)$$

The deviation indicates the amount of spread around the mean of the marginal distribution. The deviation is small if the histogram is densely clustered about the mean.

8. Entropy of $H_d(y_q, d)$: $S_{H_d(y_s,d)}$:

$$S_{H_d(y_s,d)} = -\sum_{y_s=y_1}^{y_t} H_d(y_s,d) \log_{10}[H_d(y_s,d)]. \quad (11.32)$$

9. Angular second moment of $H_d(y_s, d)$: $ASM_{H_d(y_s,d)}$:

$$ASM_{H_d(y_s,d)} = \sum_{y_s=y_1}^{y_t} [H_d(y_s,d)]^2. \quad (11.33)$$

10. Mean of $H_d(y_s, d)$: $\mu_{H_d(y_s,d)}$:

$$\mu_{H_d(y_s,d)} = \sum_{y_s=y_1}^{y_t} y_s [H_d(y_s,d)]. \quad (11.34)$$

The features computed using the difference histogram, $Hd(ys, d)$, have the same significance as those attributes determined by the second-order statistics.

Figure 11.12a,b shows two images from digitized X-ray mammograms, with, respectively, regions of benign lesion and malignant cancer of the breast. Their respective second-order histograms computed from the gray-level co-occurrence matrices are shown in Figure 11.12c,d. It can be seen that the second-order gray-level histogram statistics have better correlation with the classification of breast cancer images than the first-order histogram (16).

11.1.4 Relational Features

Relational features provide information about adjacencies, repetitive patterns, and geometrical relationships among regions of an object. Such features can also be extended to describe the geometrical relationships between objects in an image or a scene. The relational features can be described in the form of graphs or rules using a specific syntax or language. The geometric properties of images using linear quad-trees (where one parent node is divided into four children nodes) are described by Samet and Tamminen (17). Figure 11.13 shows a block (pixel)-based image representation of the letter "A" with its quad-tree representation. The quad-tree-based region descriptor can directly provide quantitative features such as perimeter, area, and Euler number by tracking the list of nodes belonging to the region of interest (17). The adjacent relationships of the elements of the quad-tree are translation invariant and can be treated as rotational invariant under specific conditions. The quad-tree-based region descriptors can also be used for object recognition and classification using the tree matching algorithms (18).

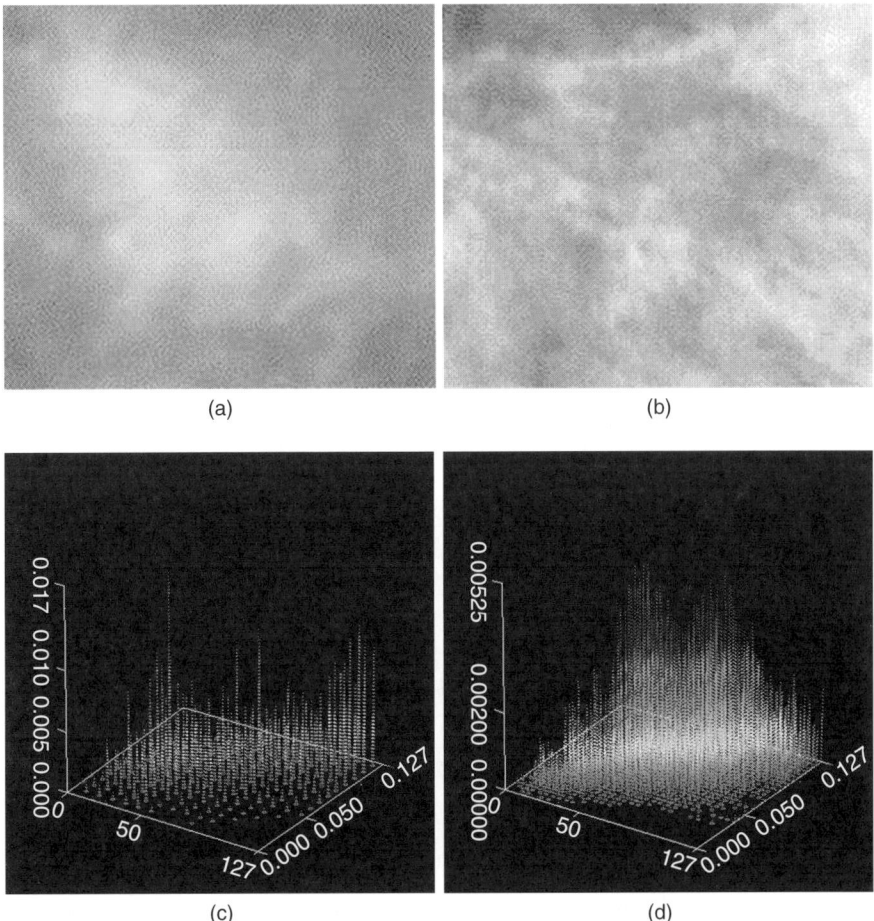

Figure 11.12 (a) A part of a digitized X-ray mammogram showing a region of benign lesion; (b) a part of a digitized X-ray mammogram showing a region of malignant cancer of the breast; (c) a second-order histograms of (a) computed from the gray-level co-occurrence matrices with a distance vector of [1, 1]; and (d) a second-order histogram of (b) computed from the gray-level co-occurrence matrices with a distance vector of [1, 1].

Tree and graph structures have been used effectively for knowledge representation and developing models for object recognition and classification. Figure 11.14 shows a tree structure representation of brain ventricles for applications in brain image segmentation and analysis (19, 20).

11.2. FEATURE SELECTION FOR CLASSIFICATION

A feature classification system can be viewed as a mapping from input features representing the given image to an output variable representing one of the categories or

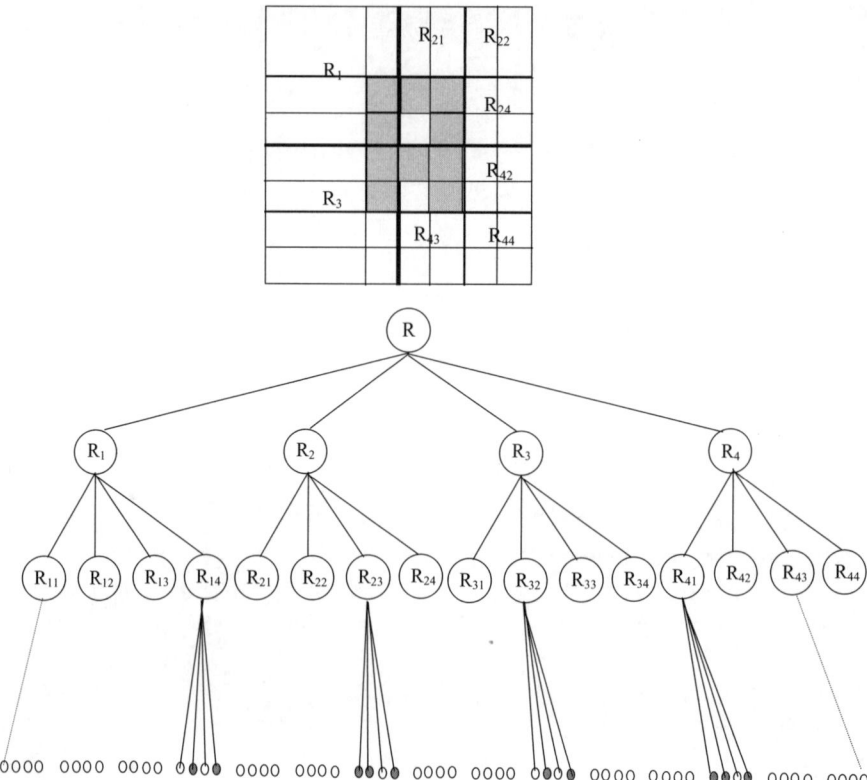

Figure 11.13 A block representation of an image with major quad partitions (top) and its quad-tree representation.

classes. For image analysis and classification task to interpret a medical image for diagnostic evaluation, a raw medical image may be first preprocessed with image enhancements and noise removal operations (described in Chapter 9). The preprocessed image is then analyzed for segmentation and extraction of features of interest. Usually, a large number of features with potential correlation to object classification can be computed. It is usually advantageous to select meaningful features that are well correlated to the task of object classification. Feature selection is the process of identifying the most effective subset of the correlated features for final feature representation and classification. Selection of correlated features leads to dimensionality reduction in the classification task, which improves the computational efficiency and classification performance, as only well-correlated features are used in the classifier.

The final set of features for classification can be determined through data correlation, clustering, and analysis algorithms to explore similarity patterns in the training data. Features that provide well separated clusters or clusters with minimum overlaps can be used for classification. The redundant and uncorrelated features are abandoned to reduce dimensionality for better classification. Data clustering methods such as agglomerative hierarchical clustering, k-means, fuzzy c-means, and adaptive fuzzy c-means clustering algorithms have been described in Chapter 10. Commonly

11.2. FEATURE SELECTION FOR CLASSIFICATION

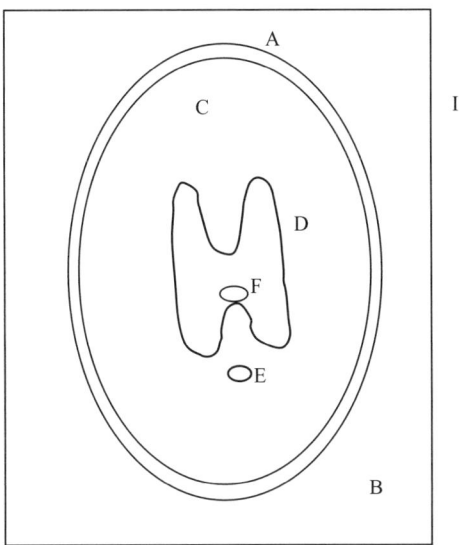

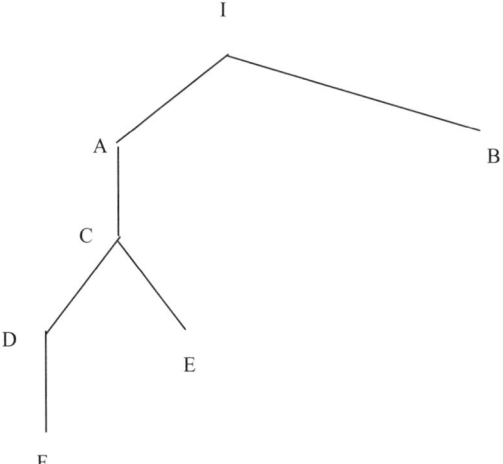

Figure 11.14 A 2-D brain ventricles and skull model (top) and region-based tree representation.

used approaches for feature selection and dimensionality reduction include linear discriminant analysis, principal component analysis (PCA), and genetic algorithm (GA)-based optimization methods. These methods are described below.

11.2.1 Linear Discriminant Analysis

Linear discriminant analysis methods are used to find a linear combination of features that can provide best possible separation among classes of data in the feature

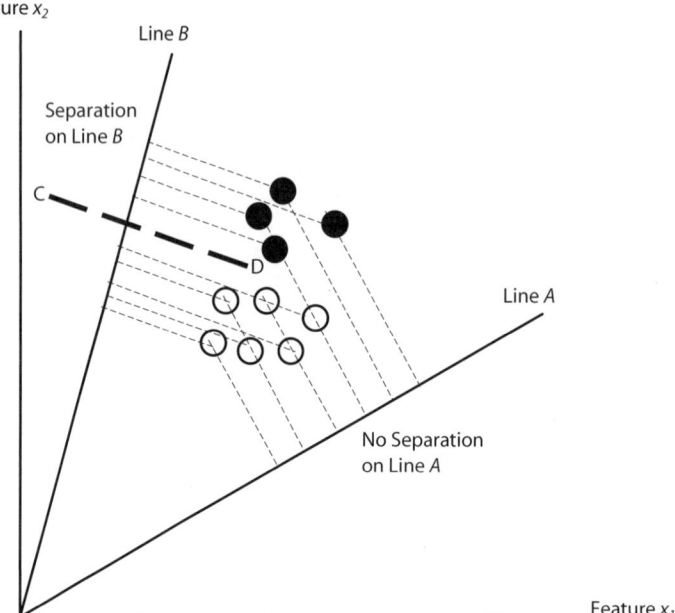

Figure 11.15 Projection of features or data points for two-class classification on two lines A and B in two-dimensional space. Open circles represent data points for class-1, while the black circles represent class-2 data points. Projections on line A are not separable, while projections on line B are well separated. The separating o decision boundary is shown by the dotted line CD.

space. A linear combination of features thus obtained reduces dimensionality for classification and provides better classification performance with a linear classifier. For example, let us assume that a d-dimensional set of features can be projected on an arbitrary line as shown in Figure 11.15. The projection of features onto the line can now be analyzed for separation among classes. Figure 11.15 shows 2-D feature space for two-class (e.g., benign and malignant) classification. It can be seen that the projections on line A are not separable while they become well separated if the line A is rotated to position B.

Let us assume that there is n number of d-dimensional features vectors, $\mathbf{x}$, in a d-dimensional space $(x_1, x_2, \ldots x_d)$, in the training set that is projected onto a line in the direction $\mathbf{w}$ as an n-dimensional vector $\mathbf{y} = (y_1, y_2, \ldots, y_n)$ as

$$y = \mathbf{w}^T \mathbf{x}. \qquad (11.35)$$

It can be noted that each y_i is the projection of each $\mathbf{x}_i$ onto the line in the direction $\mathbf{w}$, if $\|\mathbf{w}\| = 1$.

Considering first the case of two classes (C_i; $i = 1, 2$), a line in the direction $\mathbf{w}$ has to be found such that the projected points from each class on the line must form two clusters that are well separated with respect to their mean and variances. Let μ_i be the mean of two d-dimensional samples (features or data points in two classes with n_i; $i = 1, 2$ number of samples in each class) as

11.2. FEATURE SELECTION FOR CLASSIFICATION

$$\mu_i = \frac{1}{n_i} \sum_{x \in C_i} x \tag{11.36}$$

The projected points on the line may be represented with respective mean values $\tilde{\mu}_i$ as

$$\tilde{\mu}_i = \frac{1}{n_i} \sum_{y \in C_i} y = \frac{1}{n_i} \sum_{x \in C_i} \mathbf{w}^T \mathbf{x} = \mathbf{w}^T \mathbf{\mu}_i. \tag{11.37}$$

Thus, the separation between the two classes with respect to their mean values can be expressed as

$$|\tilde{\mu}_1 - \tilde{\mu}_2| = |\mathbf{w}^T(\mathbf{\mu}_1 - \mathbf{\mu}_2)|. \tag{11.38}$$

Let us define scatter $\tilde{s}_i^2$ of projected points within a class as

$$\tilde{s}_i^2 = \sum_{y \in C_i} (y - \tilde{\mu}_i^2) \tag{11.39}$$

The Fisher linear discriminant is then defined as the linear function $y = \mathbf{w}^T \mathbf{x}$ for which a criterion function $J(\mathbf{w})$ based on the separation of mean values and within-class scatter $(\tilde{s}_1^2 + \tilde{s}_2^2)$ is maximized. The criterion function $J(\mathbf{w})$ can be defined as (21)

$$J(\mathbf{w}) = \frac{|\tilde{\mu}_1 - \tilde{\mu}_2|^2}{\tilde{s}_1^2 + \tilde{s}_2^2}. \tag{11.40}$$

Considering within-class scatter, a within-class matrix S_w can be defined as

$$S_w = \sum_{x \in C_1} (\mathbf{x} - \mathbf{\mu}_1)(\mathbf{x} - \mathbf{\mu}_1)^T + \sum_{x \in C_2} (\mathbf{x} - \mathbf{\mu}_2)(\mathbf{x} - \mathbf{\mu}_2)^T. \tag{11.41}$$

A between-class scatter matrix S_B based on the separation of mean values can be defined as

$$S_B = (\mathbf{\mu}_1 - \mathbf{\mu}_2)(\mathbf{\mu}_1 - \mathbf{\mu}_2)^T. \tag{11.42}$$

A generalized expression for two-class Fisher linear discriminant can be expressed in terms of S_W and S_B as

$$J(\mathbf{w}) = \frac{\mathbf{w}^T S_B \mathbf{w}}{\mathbf{w}^T S_W \mathbf{w}}. \tag{11.43}$$

It can be shown that a vector $\mathbf{w}$ that maximizes the criterion function $J(\mathbf{w})$ can be solved using the eigenvalues λ as (assuming S_w to be nonsingular):

$$S_W^{-1} S_B \mathbf{w} = \lambda \mathbf{w}. \tag{11.44}$$

The above representation leads to a general solution as

$$\mathbf{w} = S_W^{-1}(\mathbf{\mu}_1 - \mathbf{\mu}_2). \tag{11.45}$$

It should be noted that the above solution leads to many-to-one mapping that may not always minimize the classification error. However, it can be shown that if the conditional probability density functions for both classes are considered to be multivariate normal with equal covariance matrix Σ, the optimal linear discriminant function with a decision boundary for classification can be expressed as

$$\mathbf{w}^T\mathbf{x} + w_0 = 0 \tag{11.46}$$

where $\mathbf{w} = \Sigma^{-1}(\mu_1 - \mu_2)$ and w_0 is a contant involving prior probabilities.

The above described two-class fisher linear discriminant analysis can be extended and generalized for multiclass discriminant analysis to provide projection of a d-dimensional space to $(C - 1)$ dimensional space where C is the total number of classes with

$$y_i = \mathbf{w}_i^T\mathbf{x} \quad i = 1, 2, \ldots, (C-1). \tag{11.47}$$

The between-class and within-class scatter matrices can now be defined as

$$S_B = \sum_{i=1}^{C} n_i (\mu_i - \mu)(\mu_i - \mu)^T$$

$$S_W = \sum_{i=1}^{C} \sum_{\mathbf{x} \in C_i} (\mathbf{x} - \mu_i)(\mathbf{x} - \mu_i)^T. \tag{11.48}$$

For multiple classes, the mapping from d-dimensional space to $(C - 1)$-dimensional space involves a transformation matrix $\mathbf{W}$ such that the criterion function $J(\mathbf{W})$ is expressed as

$$J(\mathbf{W}) = \frac{|\mathbf{W}^T S_B \mathbf{W}|}{|\mathbf{W}^T S_W \mathbf{W}|}. \tag{11.49}$$

11.2.2 PCA

Principal component analysis is an efficient method to reduce the dimensionality of a data set that consists of a large number of interrelated variables (22). The goal here is to map vectors $\mathbf{x}$ in a d-dimensional space $(x_1, x_2, \ldots x_d)$ onto vectors $\mathbf{z}$ in an M-dimensional space $(z_1, z_2, \ldots z_M)$ where $M < d$. Without loss of generality, we express vector $\mathbf{x}$ as a linear combination of a set of d orthonormal vectors $\mathbf{u}_i$

$$\mathbf{x} = \sum_{i=1}^{d} x_i \mathbf{u}_i \tag{11.50}$$

where the vectors $\mathbf{u}_i$ satisfy the orthonormality relation

$$\mathbf{u}_i^T \mathbf{u}_j = \delta_{ij} \tag{11.51}$$

Therefore, the coefficient in Equation 11.50 can be expressed as

$$x_i = \mathbf{u}_i^T \mathbf{x}. \tag{11.52}$$

Let us suppose that only a subset of $M < d$ of the basis vectors $\mathbf{u}_i$ are to be retained, so that only M coefficients of x_i are used. Let us assume a set of new basis vectors, $\mathbf{v}_i$, which meet the orthonormality requirement. As above, only M coefficients from x_i are used and the remaining coefficients are replaced by b_i. The vector x can now be approximated as

11.2. FEATURE SELECTION FOR CLASSIFICATION

$$\tilde{\mathbf{x}} = \sum_{i=1}^{M} x_i \mathbf{v}_i + \sum_{i=M+1}^{d} b_i \mathbf{v}_i \qquad (11.53)$$

The next step is to minimize the sum of squares of errors over the entire data set as

$$E_M = \frac{1}{2} \sum_{i=M+1}^{d} \mathbf{v}_i^T A \mathbf{v}_i \qquad (11.54)$$

where A is the covariance matrix for vector $\mathbf{x}$.

Now the error E_M should be minimized with respect to the choice of basis vectors $\mathbf{v}_i$. A minimum value is obtained when the basis vectors satisfy the condition:

$$A\mathbf{v}_i = \beta_i \mathbf{v}_i \qquad (11.55)$$

where $\mathbf{v}_i$ with $i = M + 1 \ldots d$ represents the eigenvectors of the covariance matrix.

It can be shown that

$$E_M = \frac{1}{2} \sum_{i=M+1}^{d} \beta_i. \qquad (11.56)$$

Therefore, the minimum error is achieved by rejecting the $(d-M)$ smallest eigenvalues and their corresponding eigenvectors. As the first M largest eigenvalues are retained, each of the associated eigenvectors $\mathbf{v}_i$ is called a principal component.

For computer implementation, singular value decomposition (SVD) algorithm can be employed to calculate the eigenvalues and its corresponding eigenvectors (21, 22). In addition, several algorithms are available for implementation of the PCA method (22). However, the PCA method may not provide optimal selection of features for the data with sparse distribution and noise. GA-based optimization methods have been used to find more practical solutions to feature selection that can provide the best classification results.

11.2.3 GA-Based Optimization

A GA is a robust optimization and search method based on the natural selection principles. GA provide improved performance by exploiting past information and promoting competition for survival. A fundamental feature of GA is that they can adapt to specific problem parameters. These parameters are typically encoded as binary strings that are associated with a measure of goodness or fitness value. As in natural evolution, GA favors the survival of the fittest through selection and recombination. Through the process of reproduction, individual strings are copied according to their degree of fitness. In crossover operations, strings are probabilistically mated by swapping all variables located after a randomly chosen position. Mutation is a secondary genetic operator that randomly changes the value of a string position to introduce variation to the population and recover lost genetic information (23).

Genetic algorithms maintain a population of structures that are potential solutions to an objective function. Let us assume that features are encoded into binary strings that can be represented as $A = a_1, a_2, \ldots, a_L$ where L is the specified string length or the number of representative bits. A simple GA operates on these strings according to the following iterative procedure:

1. Initialize a population of binary strings.
2. Evaluate the strings in the population.
3. Select candidate solutions for the next population and apply mutation and crossover operators to the parent strings.
4. Allocate space for new strings by removing members from the population.
5. Evaluate the new strings and add them to the population.
6. Repeat steps 3–5 until the stopping criterion is satisfied.

The structure of the GA is based on the encoding mechanism used to represent the variables in the optimization problem. The candidate solutions may encode any number of variable types, including continuous, discrete, and boolean variables. Although different string coding methods may be used (23), a simple binary encoding mechanism provides quite useful results. The allele of a gene in the chromosome indicates whether or not a feature is significant in the problem. The objective function evaluates each chromosome in a population to provide a measure of the fitness of a given string. Since the value of the objective function can vary widely between problems, a fitness function is used to normalize the objective function within the range of 0 to 1. The selection scheme uses this normalized value, or fitness, to evaluate a string.

One of the most basic reproduction techniques is proportionate selection, which is carried out by the roulette wheel selection scheme. In roulette wheel selection, each chromosome is given a segment of a roulette wheel whose size is proportionate to the chromosome's fitness. A chromosome is reproduced if a randomly generated number falls in the chromosome's corresponding roulette wheel slot. Since more fit chromosomes are allocated larger wheel portions, they are more likely to generate offspring after a spin of the wheel. The process is repeated until the population for the next generation is completely filled. However, due to sampling errors, the population must be very large in order for the actual number of offspring produced for an individual chromosome to approach the expected value for that chromosome.

In proportionate selection, a string is reproduced according to how its fitness compares with the population average, in other words, as $f_i/\bar{f}$, where f_i is the fitness of the string and $\bar{f}$ is the average fitness of the population. This proportionate expression is also known as the selective pressure on an individual. The mechanics of proportionate selection can be expressed as: A_i receives more than one offspring on average if $f_i > \bar{f}$; otherwise, A_i receives less than one offspring on average. Since the result of applying the proportionate fitness expression will always be a fraction, this value represents the expected number of offspring allocated to each string, not the actual number.

Once the parent population is selected through reproduction, the offspring population is created after application of genetic operators. The purpose of recombination, also referred to as crossover, is to discover new regions of the search space, rather than relying on the same population of strings. In recombination, strings are randomly paired and selected for crossover. If the crossover probability condition is satisfied, then a crossover point along the length of the string pair is randomly chosen. The offspring are generated by exchanging the portion of the parent strings beyond the crossover position. For a string of length l, the $l-1$ possible crossover positions may be chosen with equal probability.

Mutation is a secondary genetic operator that preserves the random nature of the search process and regenerates fit strings that may have been destroyed or lost during crossover or reproduction. The mutation rate controls the probability that a bit value will be changed. If the mutation probability condition is exceeded, then the selected bit is inverted.

An example of a complete cycle for the simple GA is illustrated in Table 11.1. The initial population contains four strings composed of 10 bits. The objective function determines the number of 1s in a chromosome, and the fitness function normalizes the value to lie in the range of 0 to 1.

The proportional selection method allocates 0, 1, 1, and 2 offspring to the initial offspring in their respective order. After selection, the offspring are randomly paired for crossover so that strings 1 and 3 and strings 2 and 4 are mated. However, since the crossover rate is 0.5, only strings 1 and 3 are selected for crossover, and the other strings are left intact. The pair of chromosomes then exchanges their genetic material after the fifth bit position, which is the randomly selected crossover point. The final step in the cycle is mutation. Since the mutation rate is selected to be 0.05, only two bits out of the 40 present in the population are mutated. The second

TABLE 11.1 A Sample Generational Cycle of the Simple Genetic Algorithm

	Chromosome	Fitness value	Average fitness
Population P_1 (initial population)	0001000010	0.2	
	0110011001	0.5	0.50
	1010100110	0.5	
	1110111011	0.8	
Population P_2 (after selection)	0110011001	0.5	
	1010100110	0.5	0.65
	1110111011	0.8	
	1110111011	0.8	
Population P_3 (after crossover)	01100|11011	0.6	
	1010100110	0.5	0.65
	11101|11001	0.7	
	1110111011	0.8	
Population P_4 (after mutation)	0110011011	0.6	
	1110100110	0.6	0.70
	1110111001	0.7	
	1111111011	0.9	

bit of string 2 and the fourth bit of string 4 are randomly selected for mutation. As can be seen from the Table 11.1, the average fitness of Population P_4 is significantly better than the initial fitness after only one generational cycle.

The average fitness value in the initial stages of a GA is typically low. Thus, during the first few generations the proportionate selection scheme may assign a large number of copies to a few strings with relatively superior fitness, known as super individuals. These strings will eventually dominate the population and cause the GA to converge prematurely. The proportionate selection procedure also suffers from decreasing selective pressure during the last generations when the average fitness value is high. Scaling techniques and ranking selection can help alleviate the problems of inconsistent selective pressure and domination by superior individuals.

Ranking selection techniques assign offspring to individuals by qualitatively comparing levels of fitness. The population is sorted according to their fitness values and allotted offspring based on their rank. In ranking selection, subsequent populations are not influenced by the balance of the current fitness distributions so that selective pressure is uniform. Each cycle of the simple GA produces a completely new population of offspring from the previous generation, known as generational replacement. Thus, the simple GA is naturally slower in manipulating useful areas of the search space for a large population. Steady-state replacement is an alternative method that typically replaces one or more of the worst members of the population each generation. Steady-state replacement can be combined with an elitist strategy, which retains the best strings in the population (23).

Genetic algorithms are global optimization techniques that are highly suited to searching in nonlinear, multidimensional problem spaces, and used for medical image analysis for computer-aided diagnosis such as analysis of mammographic microcalcification images for diagnosis of breast cancer (23–25). An example of such analysis is described in the last section of this chapter.

11.3. FEATURE AND IMAGE CLASSIFICATION

Features selected for image representation are classified for object recognition and characterization. For example, features representing mammographic microcalcifications are analyzed and classified for the detection of breast cancer. In the analysis of medical images, features and measurements can also be used for region segmentation to extract meaningful structures, which are then interpreted using knowledge-based models and classification methods.

11.3.1 Statistical Classification Methods

Statistical classification methods are broadly defined into two categories: unsupervised and supervised. The unsupervised methods cluster the data based on their separation in the feature space. Data clustering methods such as k-means and fuzzy clustering methods are commonly used for unsupervised classification. Probabilistic methods such as nearest neighbor classifier and Bayesian classifier can be used for supervised classification.

11.3.1.1 Nearest Neighbor Classifier

A popular statistical method for classification is the nearest neighbor classifier, which assigns a data point to the nearest class model in the feature space. It is apparent that the nearest neighbor classifier is a supervised method as it uses labeled clusters of training samples in the feature space as models of classes. Let us assume that there are C number of classes represented by c_j; $j = 1, 2, \ldots, C$. An unknown feature vector $\mathbf{f}$ is to be assigned to the class that is closest to the class model developed from clustering the labeled feature vectors during the training. A distance measure $D_j(\mathbf{f})$ is defined by the Euclidean distance in the feature space as

$$D_j(\mathbf{f}) = \|\mathbf{f} - \mathbf{u}_j\| \qquad (11.57)$$

where $\mathbf{u}_j = \dfrac{1}{N_j} \sum_{f_j \in c_j} \mathbf{f}_j$, $j = 1, 2, \ldots C$ is the mean of the feature vectors for the class c_j and N_j is the total number of feature vectors in the class c_j.

The unknown feature vector is assigned to the class c_i if

$$D_j(\mathbf{f}) = \min_{i=1}^{C}[D_i(\mathbf{f})]. \qquad (11.58)$$

11.3.1.2 Bayesian Classifier

A probabilistic approach can be applied to the task of classification to incorporate a priori knowledge to improve performance. Bayesian and maximum likelihood methods have been widely used in object recognition and classification for different applications. A maximum likelihood method for pixel classification for brain image segmentation is presented in Chapter 10.

Let us assume that the probability of a feature vector $\mathbf{f}$ belonging to the class c_i is denoted by $p(c_i/\mathbf{f})$. Let an average risk of wrong classification for assigning the feature vector to the class c_j be expressed by $r_j(\mathbf{f})$ as

$$r_j(\mathbf{f}) = \sum_{k=1}^{C} Z_{kj} p(c_k / \mathbf{f}) \qquad (11.59)$$

where Z_{kj} is the penalty of classifying a feature vector to the class c_j when it belongs to the class c_k.

It can be shown that

$$r_j(\mathbf{f}) = \sum_{k=1}^{C} Z_{kj} p(\mathbf{f} / c_k) p(c_k) \qquad (11.60)$$

where $p(c_k)$ is the probability of occurrence of class c_k.

A Bayes classifier assigns an unknown feature vector to the class c_i if

$$r_j(\mathbf{f}) < r_i(\mathbf{f})$$

or

$$\sum_{k=1}^{C} Z_{kj} p(\mathbf{f} / c_k) p(c_k) < \sum_{q=1}^{C} Z_{qi} p(\mathbf{f} / c_q) p(c_q) \quad \text{for } i = 1, 2, \ldots, C. \qquad (11.61)$$

11.3.2 Rule-Based Systems

The decision making process of classification can be implemented using a rule-based system. A rule-based system analyzes the feature vector using multiple sets of rules that are designed to check specific conditions in the database of feature vectors to initiate an action. The rules are comprised of two parts: condition premises and actions. They are based on expert knowledge to infer the action if the conditions are satisfied. The action part of the rule may change the database or label a feature vector depending upon the state of the analysis. Usually, a rule-based system has three sets of rules: supervisory or strategy rules, focus of attention rules, and knowledge rules. The supervisory or strategy rules guide the analysis process and provide the control actions such as starting and stopping the analysis. The strategy rules also decide the rules to be scheduled and tested during the analysis process. The focus-of-attention rules provide specific features into analysis by accessing and extracting the required information or features from the database. These rules bring the information from the input database into the activity center where the execution of knowledge rules is scheduled. The knowledge rules analyze the information with respect to the required conditions and implement an action causing changes in the output database. These changes lead to the classification and labeling of the feature vectors for object recognition. Figure 11.16 presents a schematic diagram of a general-purpose rule-based system for image analysis.

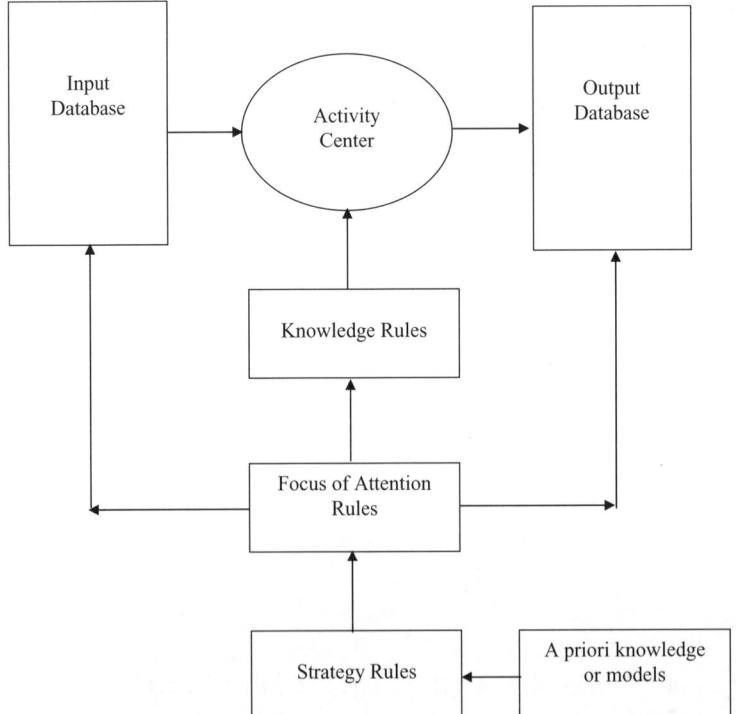

Figure 11.16 A schematic diagram of a rule-based system for image analysis.

Rule-based systems have been used for image segmentation (26) for biomedical applications (4, 27, 28). The examples of strategy, focus of attention, and knowledge rules for segmentation of CT images of the human chest are as follows (27). The symbols used in the analysis are shown in the capital case.

Strategy Rule SR1:
   If
      NONE REGION is ACTIVE
      NONE REGION is ANALYZED
   Then
      ACTIVATE FOCUS in SPINAL_CORD AREA

Strategy Rule SR2:
   If
      ANALYZED REGION is in SPINAL_CORD AREA
      ALL REGIONS in SPINAL_CORD AREA are NOT ANALYZED
   Then
      ACTIVATE FOCUS in SPINAL_CORD AREA

Strategy Rule SR3:
   If
      ALL REGIONS in SPINAL_CORD AREA are ANALYZED
      ALL REGION in LEFT_LUNG AREA are NOT ANALYZED
   Then
      ACTIVATE FOCUS in LEFT_LUNG AREA

Focus of Attention Rule FR1:
   If
      REGION-X is in FOCUS AREA
      REGION-X is LARGEST
      REGION-X is NOT ANALYZED
   Then
      ACTIVATE REGION-X

Focus of Attention Rule FR2:
   If
      REGION-X is in ACTIVE
      MODEL is NOT ACTIVE
   Then
      ACTIVATE KNOWLEDGE_MERGE rules

Knowledge Rule: Merge_Region_KR1
   If
      REGION-1 is SMALL
      REGION-1 has HIGH ADJACENCY with REGION-2
      DIFFERENCE between AVERAGE VALUE of REGION-1 and REGION-2 is LOW or VERY LOW
      REGION-2 is LARGE or VERY LARGE
   Then
      MERGE REGION-1 in REGION-2
      PUT_STATUS ANALYZED in REGION-1 and REGION-2

It should be noted that the sequence of execution of rules directly affects the sequential changes in the database. Thus, a different sequence of execution of rules may produce very different results. To avoid this problem, all rules in the system must be statistically independent. This condition is usually unrealistic because it is difficult to translate the expert-domain knowledge into statistically independent rules. Condition probability-based Bayes models and fuzzy inference may help the inference by execution of rules for better performance and robustness. Nevertheless, the formation of knowledge rules along with the probabilistic models is usually a very involved task.

11.3.3 Neural Network Classifiers

Several artificial neural network paradigms have been used for feature classification for object recognition and image interpretation. The paradigms include backpropagation, radial basis function, associative memories, and self-organizing feature maps. The backpropagation neural network (BPNN) and the radial basis function neural network (RBFNN) are described in Chapter 10 for pixel classification for image segmentation (28). Recently, fuzzy system-based approaches have been applied in artificial neural networks for better classification and generalization performance (29–32). A neuro-fuzzy pattern classifier is described here which has also been used for medical image analysis (33).

11.3.3.1 Neuro-Fuzzy Pattern Classification
Any layer in a feedforward network such as BPNN performs partitioning of the multidimensional feature space into a specific number of subspaces. These subspaces are always convex and their number can be estimated (29). A computational neural element is shown in Figure 11.17 with an input vector X, nonlinearity function $f(\varphi)$, and the final output vector Y. The input synapses represented by X are linearly combined through connection weights w_i to provide the postsynaptic signal φ as:

$$\varphi = \sum_{i=1}^{d} x_i w_i + w_0 \qquad (11.62)$$

where d is the total number of input synapses or features.

For $\varphi = 0$ (or any other constant), Equation 11.62 represents a $(d-1)$-dimensional hyperplane H in the d-dimensional input space separating two regions defined by the connection weights w_i (28, 29):

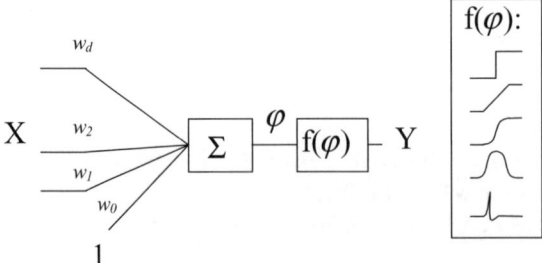

Figure 11.17 A computational neuron model with linear synapses.

$$(H: \varphi = 0) \Rightarrow \left(H: \sum_{i=1}^{d} x_i w_i + w_0 = 0 \right). \quad (11.63)$$

Each network layer comprises many hyperplanes that intersect to create a finite number of the aforementioned convex subspaces. Therefore, there is a direct relationship between the connection weight values and the obtained d-dimensional convex subspaces. The process of network training can be assumed as an attempt at finding an optimal dichotomy of the input space into these convex regions. Moreover, it can also be said that finding the optimal dichotomy of input space into convex subspaces is equivalent to network training. The classes are separated in the feature space by computing the homogeneous nonoverlapping closed convex subsets. The classification is obtained by placing separating hyperplanes between neighboring subsets representing classes. This completes the design of a network hyperplane layer. Since the hyperplane separation of the subsets results in the creation of the homogenous convex regions, the consecutive network layer is to determine in which region an unknown input pattern belongs.

In the approach presented by Grohman and Dhawan (33), a fuzzy membership function M_f is devised for each convex subset ($f = 1, 2, \ldots, K$). The classification decision is made by the output layer based on the "winner-take-all" principle. The resulting category C is the convex set category with the highest value of membership function for the input pattern. Thus, the neuro-fuzzy pattern classifier (NFPC) design method includes three stages: convex set creation, hyperplane placement (hyperplane layer creation), and construction of the fuzzy membership function for each convex set (generation of the fuzzy membership function layer). The architecture of the NFPC is shown in Figure 11.18.

There are two requirements for computing the convex sets: they have to be homogeneous and nonoverlapping. To satisfy the first condition, one needs to devise a method of finding one-category points within another category's hull. Thus, two

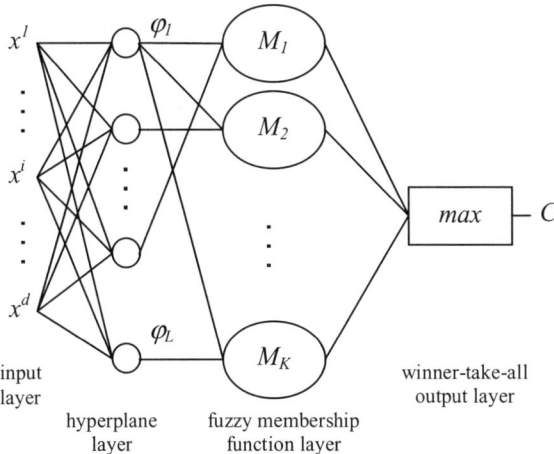

Figure 11.18 The architecture of the neuro-fuzzy pattern classifier.

problems can be defined: (1) how to find whether the point P lies inside of a convex hull (CH) of points; and (2) how to find out if two CH of points are overlapping. The second problem is more difficult to examine because hulls can be overlapping over a common (empty) space that contains no points from either category. When training samples are not completely noise-free, a compromise between computational efficiency and accuracy may be desirable. The following algorithm A1 addresses the first problem using the separation theorem, which states that for two closed non-overlapping convex sets S_1 and S_2 there always exists a hyperplane that separates the two sets.

Algorithm A1: Checking if the point P lies inside of a CH:

1. Consider P as origin.
2. Normalize points of CH (the vectors $V = (v_1, v_2, \ldots, v_n)$ from the origin).
3. Find min. and max. vector coordinates in each dimension.
4. Find set E of all vectors V that have at least one extreme coordinate.
5. Compute mean and use it as projection vector ϕ:

$$\phi = (\overline{v_i} \mid \forall\ v_i \in E).$$

6. Set a maximum number of allowed iterations (usually = $2n$).
7. Find a set $U = (u_1, u_2, \ldots, u_m)$ (where $m \leq n$) of all points in CH that have negative projection on ϕ.
8. If U is empty (P is outside of CH), exit, or else proceed to step 9.
9. Compute coefficient ψ as

$$\psi = \phi^T \overline{U}$$
$$\overline{U} = \frac{1}{m} \sum_{i=1}^{m} u_i.$$

10. Calculate correction vector $\delta\phi$ by computing all of its k-dimensional components $\delta\phi^k$:

$$\begin{pmatrix} \overline{U}^k \neq 0 \Rightarrow \delta\phi^k = \dfrac{\psi}{\overline{U}^k d} \\ \overline{U}^k = 0 \Rightarrow \delta\phi^k = \dfrac{\psi}{d} \end{pmatrix}, \quad k = 1, 2, \ldots, d$$

where d is the dimension of the feature space.

11. Update ϕ: $\phi = \phi - \eta \cdot \delta\phi$, where $\eta > 1$ is a training parameter.
12. If iteration limit exceeded exit (assume P inside of CH), otherwise go to 7.

The value of the training parameter η should be close to 1, so even the points lying outside but close to the hull can be found. Heuristically it has been found that the values of α should fall in the range $1.0001 < \eta < 1.01$. They are, however, dependent on the precision of the training data and should be adjusted accordingly. The main objective of the algorithm is to find the hyperplane (defined by its orthogonal vector ϕ) separating P and CH. If such a hyperplane is found within a certain amount of iterations, the point is definitely outside of CH. If the hyperplane has not been found, it is assumed that P is inside. Now, having found the solution to problem 1, the convex subsets can be created using the algorithm A2 as follows.

Algorithm A2: Convex subset creation:

1. Select one category from the training set and consider all data points in the category. This is a positive set of samples. The training points from all the remaining categories constitute a negative set. Both sets are in d-dimensional linear space L. Mark all positive points as "not yet taken" and order them in a specific way. For example, choose an arbitrary starting point in the input space and order all positive points according to their Euclidean distance from that point. Use an index array Λ to store the order.

2. Construct the convex subsets:

    Initialize current subset S by assigning to it the first point in Λ. Loop over ordered positive category points (in Λ) until there are no more points remaining. Consider only points that have not yet been "taken":

    a. Add the current point P to the subset S.

    b. Loop over points from negative category. Consider only negative points that are closer than P to the middle of the current subset. Using A1, look for at least one negative point inside of conv S. If there is one, disregard the latest addition to S. Otherwise mark the current point P as "taken."

    c. Update Λ. Reorder the "not yet taken" positive category points according to their distance from the mean of points in the current subset.

3. If all points in the category have been assigned to a subset, proceed to step 4, otherwise go back to step 2 and create the next convex subset. The starting point is the first "not yet taken" point in the list.

4. Check if all categories have been divided into convex subsets. If not, go back to step 1 and create subsets of the next category.

In step 2b, it is not always necessary to use algorithm A1 to check the presence of every single negative point within the current convex subset. Once a separating hyperplane is found for one negative point it should be used to eliminate all other negative points that lie on the opposite side of the hyperplane than the convex subset, from the checklist. Thus both presented algorithms should be used together in order to save computations.

Once the nonoverlapping convex subsets are found, hyperplanes are paced to separate two neighboring subsets. The NPFC hyperplane layer comprises a set of all hyperplanes needed to fully separate all convex subsets from different categories. The hyperplanes define the convex regions constructed from the training samples. The fuzzy membership function M_f to reflect the true shape of the convex subset f ($f = 1, 2, \ldots, K$) can be computed as:

$$M_f(\mathbf{x}) = \sqrt[L_f]{\prod_{i=1}^{L_f} \theta_i}, \quad \theta_i = \frac{1}{\left(1 + e^{\lambda_{if}\varphi_i \mathbf{x}}\right)} \tag{11.64}$$

where L_f is the number of separating hyperplanes for the subset f; φ_i is the ith separating hyperplane function for the subset, in the vector form; $\mathbf{x}$ is the input vector in the augmented form; and λ_{if} is the steepness (scaling) coefficient for the ith hyperplane in the subset f.

The value of λ_{if} depends on the depth of convex subset f, as projected onto the separating hyperplane H_i (defined by ϕ_i):

$$\lambda_{if} = \frac{-\log\left(\frac{1-\chi}{\chi}\right)}{\mu_{if}}, \quad \mu_{if} = \frac{1}{n}\sum_{j=1}^{n}\varphi_i \mathbf{x}_j \quad (11.65)$$

where n is the number of training points in the convex subset f; ϕ_i is the ith hyperplane equation in the vector form; μ_{if} is the depth of the convex subset f, as projected onto the ith hyperplane; $\mathbf{x}_j$ is augmented coordinate vector of the jth point in the subset; and χ is the center value of the membership function.

The structure of the fuzzy membership function described above is shown in Figure 11.19. Scaling and multiplication stages are represented by Equations 11.65 and 11.64, respectively.

The output O of the classifier is the category C of the convex set fuzzy membership function M_i that attains the highest value for the specified input pattern x, that is:

$$\left(O = C \,\middle|\, \begin{array}{c} \forall \\ 1 \leq f \leq K \; M_f(x) < M_i(x), \; M_i \in C \\ f \neq i \end{array}\right) \quad (11.66)$$

where K is the number of convex sets obtained during training (number of fuzzy function neurons in the fuzzy membership function layer), M_i is the highest fuzzy membership function value for the input x, and C is the category of convex subset used to construct membership function M_i.

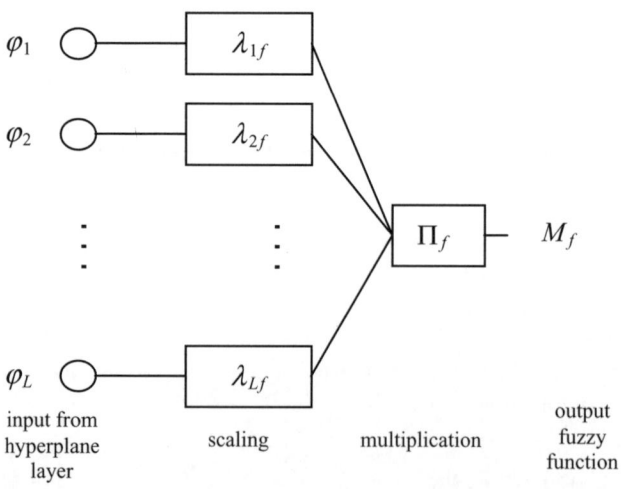

Figure 11.19 The structure of the fuzzy membership function.

In other words, the output is based on the winner-take-all principle, with the convex set category corresponding to M_i determining the output. A decision surface for each category can be determined by the fuzzy union of all of the fuzzy membership functions for the convex subsets belonging to the category. Thus the decision surface for a particular category can be defined as:

$$\left(M_{category}(x) = \max(M_i(x)) \;\middle|\; \begin{matrix}\forall\\ i, M_i \in category\end{matrix} \right) \quad (11.67)$$

where $M_{category}(x)$ is the decision surface for the category and M_i is the fuzzy membership function for the convex cluster i.

Figure 11.20 shows an example of classification with two categories: dark and white dots. The hyperplanes are placed to separate two convex subsets of the black category from the convex subset of the white category. Figure 11.21a,b shows the fuzzy membership functions $M_1(x)$ and $M_2(x)$ for black category subsets. Figure 11.22 illustrates the membership function $M_3(x)$ for the white category. The resulting decision surface $M_{black}(x)$ for the black category is shown in Figure 11.23.

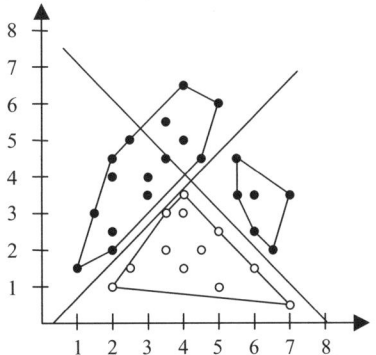

Figure 11.20   Convex set-based separation of two categories.

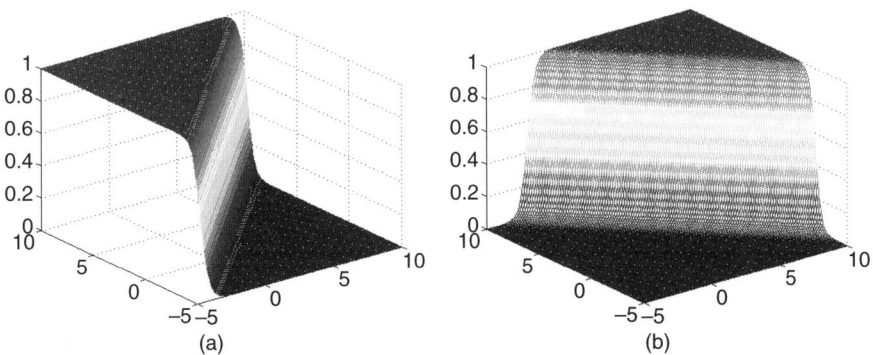

Figure 11.21   (a) Fuzzy membership function $M_1(x)$ for the subset #1 of the black category. (b) Fuzzy membership function $M_2(x)$ for the subset #2 of the black category.

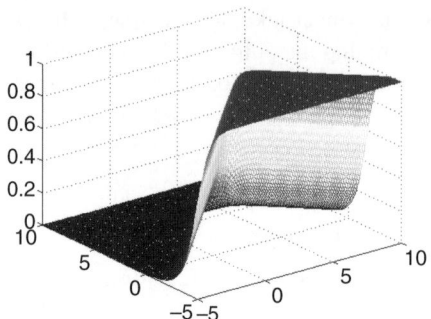

Figure 11.22 Fuzzy membership function $M_3(x)$ (decision surface) for the white category membership.

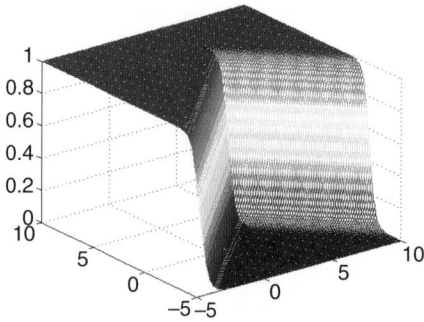

Figure 11.23 Resulting decision surface $M_{black}(x)$ for the black category membership function.

11.3.4 Support Vector Machine for Classification

As described above, the winner-take-all strategy can be effectively used for multi-classification. A set of prototypes such as fuzzy membership functions in the above described approach can be defined. A scoring function $\phi : \chi \times M \rightarrow \Re$ is also defined measuring the similarity of an input feature vector, an element in χ with M_i prototypes defined in space M. Thus, a most similar prototype is selected to assign the respective class C, from a set $\{\gamma\}$, to the feature vector for classification. A multi-prototype approach for multiclass classification using the winner-take-all method can thus be expressed as (34–37)

$$H(\mathbf{x}) = C\left(\arg\max_{i \in \Omega} \phi(\mathbf{x}, M_i)\right) \quad (11.68)$$

where **x** is an input feature vector, Ω is the set of prototypes indexes, M_i ($i = 1, 2, \ldots k$) are prototypes, and $C : \Omega \rightarrow \{\gamma\}$ is the function to assign the class associated with a given prototype.

Use of large margin kernels for search of a linear discriminant model in high-dimensional feature space for pattern classification has been investigated by several investigators (34–37). For example, a radial basis function (RBF) can be used as a kernel function as

$$k(\mathbf{x},\mathbf{y}) = \exp\left(-\lambda \|\mathbf{x}-\mathbf{y}\|^2\right), \quad \lambda \geq 0. \tag{11.69}$$

A generalized kernel function can be expressed as

$$k(\mathbf{x},\mathbf{y}) = (\langle\mathbf{x},\mathbf{y}\rangle + u)^d, \quad u \geq 0, d \in \mathrm{N} \tag{11.70}$$

where d is the dimensionality of classification space.

The relevance vector machine (RVM) (35) uses a model prototype for regression and classification exploiting a probabilistic Bayesian principle. There are several other models investigated for pattern classification using theoretic approaches from kernel-based classifier to linear programming perturbation-based methods (34–37).

A single prototype per class (as described above) can be used for multiclass classification using a Bayesian probabilistic model. For a correct classification using a multiclass classifier, the prototype of the correct class should have a larger score than the maximum scores related to all other incorrect classes. The multiclass margin for input vector $\mathbf{x}_i$ is then defined as (34)

$$p(\mathbf{x}_i, c_i \mid \mathbf{M}) = \langle M_{y_i}, \mathbf{x}_i \rangle - \max_{r \neq y_i} \langle M_r, \mathbf{x}_i \rangle \tag{11.71}$$

where y_i chosen such that $C(y_i) = c_i$, is the index of the prototype associated to the correct label for the training example $\mathbf{x}_i$. In the single prototype case, the associated class indices may be coincident, that is $y_i = c_i$.

It follows that for a correct classification of $\mathbf{x}_i$ with a margin greater than or equal to 1, the following condition has to be satisfied as described in Reference (34):

$$\langle M_{y_i}, \mathbf{x}_i \rangle \geq \theta_i + 1 \quad \text{where} \quad \theta_i = \max_{r \neq y_i} \langle M_r, \mathbf{x}_i \rangle. \tag{11.72}$$

Recently, the above single-prototype-based approach has been extended to multiprototype-based support vector machine (SVM) for multiclass classification by Aiolli and Sperduti (34).

11.4. IMAGE ANALYSIS AND CLASSIFICATION EXAMPLE: "DIFFICULT-TO-DIAGNOSE" MAMMOGRAPHIC MICROCALCIFICATIONS

Breast microcalcifications are often fuzzy and poorly defined structures. In such cases, it is difficult to distinguish between benign and malignant microcalcifications associated with breast cancer. There have been a number of approaches used in the computer-aided analysis of mammographic microcalcifications (2, 25, 38–41). Artificial neural networks and fuzzy logic-based feature analysis have also been used for detection (2, 25, 41).

In the analysis of difficult-to-diagnose mammographic microcalcifications, Dhawan et al. used the second-order histogram statistics and wavelet processing to represent texture feature for classification into benign and malignant cancer categories. Two sets of 10 wavelet features were computed for the discrete Daubechies filter prototypes, D_6 and D_{20}, where the subscripts indicate the size of the filter. In total, 40 features were extracted and used in a GA-based feature reduction and correlation analysis. The initial set of 40 features included 10 binary segmented microcalcification cluster features (Feature #1–10), 10 global texture-based image structure features (Feature #11–20), and 20 wavelet analysis-based local texture features (Feature #21–40). These features are listed below (2).

1. Number of microcalcifications
2. Average number of pixels per microcalcification (area)
3. Standard deviation of number of gray levels per pixel
4. Average gray level per microcalcification
5. Standard deviation of gray levels
6. Average distance between microcalcifications
7. Standard deviation of distances between microcalcifications
8. Average distance between calcification and center of mass
9. Standard deviation of distances between calcification and center of mass
10. Potential energy of the system using the product of the average gray level and the area.
11. Entropy of $H(y_q, y_r, d)$
12. Angular second moment of $H(y_q, y_r, d)$
13. Contrast of $H(y_q, y_r, d)$
14. Inverse difference moment of $H(y_q, y_r, d)$
15. Correlation of $H(y_q, y_r, d)$
16. Mean of $H(y_q, y_r, d)$
17. Deviation of $H_m(y_q, d)$
18. Entropy of $H_d(y_s, d)$
19. Angular second moment of $H_d(y_s, d)$
20. Mean of $H_d(y_s, d)$
21. Energy for the D_6 wavelet packet at level 0
22. Energy for the D_6 low-low wavelet packet at level 1
23. Energy for the D_6 low-high wavelet packet at level 1
24. Energy for the D_6 high-low wavelet packet at level 1
25. Energy for the D_6 high-high wavelet packet at level 1
26. Entropy for the D_6 wavelet packet at level 0
27. Entropy for the D_6 low-low wavelet packet at level 1
28. Entropy for the D_6 low-high wavelet packet at level 1
29. Entropy for the D_6 high-low wavelet packet at level 1
30. Entropy for the D_6 high-high wavelet packet at level 1
31. Energy for the D_{20} wavelet packet at level 0
32. Energy for the D_{20} low-low wavelet packet at level 1
33. Energy for the D_{20} low-high wavelet packet at level 1

34. Energy for the D_{20} high-low wavelet packet at level 1
35. Energy for the D_{20} high-high wavelet packet at level 1
36. Entropy for the D_{20} wavelet packet at level 0
37. Entropy for the D_{20} low-low wavelet packet at level 1
38. Entropy for the D_{20} low-high wavelet packet at level 1
39. Entropy for the D_{20} high-low wavelet packet at level 1
40. Entropy for the D_{20} high-high wavelet packet at level 1

Genetic algorithms were used to select the best subset of features from the binary cluster, global, and local textural representations.

Using the GA, the initial set of 40 features was reduced to the two best correlated set of 20 features: VP1 (using the proportional selection in GA), and VR1 (using the ranking selection in GA). These feature sets are shown in Table 11.2, with the Feature number from the above list.

Selected features were used as inputs to the radial basis function for subsequent classification of the microcalcifications. Although the best chromosomes, and thus the feature inputs, were chosen on the basis of fitness, the ultimate measure of performance is the area under the receiver operating characteristic (ROC) curve. The optimal network architecture was determined heuristically for the combined feature set for different numbers of samples in the training and test sets. The maximum and average area over 40 partitions of the data are indicated in Table 11.3 for the

TABLE 11.2 Lists of Two Best Sets of Features Selected Through Genetic Algorithm Using Proportional Selection (VP1) and Ranking Selection (VR1)

Experiment	Feature list
VP1	1,3,5,8,11,13,16,20,21,22,23,25,26, 27,28,30,31,35,37,39
VR1	1,3,4,5,7,13,15,16,22,23,24,25.27,29,31,32,36,37,39,40

TABLE 11.3 ROC Performance of the Radial Basis Function Network Trained on Various Combined Input Sets and Number of Training Samples Using Proportional and Ranking Selection and K-Means Clustering to Place the Basis Units

Experiment	Network architecture	Maximum area	Average area	Standard deviation
VP-1	A	0.743	0.712	0.046
	B	0.824	0.773	0.048
	C	0.801	0.732	0.049
	D	0.829	0.795	0.047
	E	0.857	0.81	0.045
VR-1	A	0.77	0.738	0.047
	B	0.751	0.725	0.049
	C	0.794	0.737	0.047
	D	0.827	0.798	0.047
	E	0.874	0.83	0.044

combined feature set using both the proportional and ranking selection schemes for the input parameters selected by the GA. Only the performance of the combined feature set is presented in this chapter. It can be seen in Table 11.3 that the discrimination ability of each experiment typically increases with increasing numbers of training samples. Computer-aided analysis of mammographic microcalcifications seems to have the potential to help reduce the false positive rate without reducing the true positive rate for difficult-to-diagnose cases (2, 23–25).

11.5. EXERCISES

11.1. Describe a basic paradigm of image analysis and classification. Why is it important to compute feature to represent regions?

11.2. What do you understand by hierarchical representation of features? Explain with the help of an example.

11.3. How do knowledge models improve image analysis and classification tasks?

11.4. How can Hough transform be used in shape representation and analysis?

11.5. Explain the difference between the chain code and Fourier descriptor for boundary representation.

11.6. Show that Fourier boundary descriptors are size, rotation, and translation invariant.

11.7. What is the role of higher-order moments in shape representation and analysis?

11.8. Describe the seven invariant moments for shape description.

11.9. What are the fundamental operations in morphological image processing?

11.10. What is the difference between morphological closing and opening operations?

11.11. What is the role of a structuring element in morphological image processing?

11.12. Describe a rule-based system for region merging and splitting.

11.13. Define texture in an image. What are the major features to represent image texture?

11.14. Explain why you need to select the best correlated features for image classification.

11.15. Why is a dimensionality reduction approach such as linear discriminant analysis needed before the features are classified?

11.16. Explain the method associated with principal component analysis. How is this method different than linear discriminant analysis?

11.17. What are the different paradigms of classification?

11.18. Explain in detail the nearest-neighborhood classifier. What are the limitations and shortcomings of this method?

11.19. What are the advantages and disadvantages of a neural network classifier over statistical classifiers?

11.20. Can a two-layered backpropagation neural network provide a nonlinear partitioning of multidimensional feature space for classification?

11.21. Describe a structure of a multilayered backpropagation neural network classifier with training algorithm for multiclass classification.

11.22. In the MATLAB environment, segment serial brain images for ventricles using the region growing method. Obtain ventricle boundaries in segmented images.

11.23. Develop a relational model of the hierarchical structure of ventricle shapes and assign a set of features to each ventricle. Develop this model in the MATLAB environment.

11.24. Compute a set of features for representing shapes of all ventricles for the segmented images obtained in Exercise 11.16.

11.25. Develop a nearest-neighbor classifier using the computed features for classification of ventricles segmented in Exercise 11.16.

11.26. Select a new MR brain image and perform region segmentation for ventricular structure. Select correlated features for the segmented regions and use the classifier developed in Exercise 11.19 for classification of ventricles. Comment on the success of your classifier in ventricle classification.

11.27. Select a set of five features for the classification of mammographic microcalcifications. In the MATLAB environment, compute the selected features on the labeled images of benign and malignant microcalcifications. Divide all cases into two groups: training and test. Now develop a radial basis neural network (RBFNN) for microcalcification classification using the training set. Obtain the true positive and false positive rates of the classifier on the test cases. Comment on the success of the classifier.

11.28. Repeat Exercise 11.21 using a backpropagation neural network classifier and compare the results with those obtained using the RBFNN.

11.29. What is a support vector machine (SVM)? How is it different from backpropagation and RBF neural networks?

11.30. Repeat Exercise 11.21 using a SVM and compare the results with BPNN and RBFNN.

11.6. REFERENCES

1. M.H. Loew, "Feature extraction," in M. Sonka and J.M. Fitzpatrick (Eds), *Handbook of Medical Imaging*, Volume 2: *Medical Image Processing and Analysis*, SPIE Press, Bellingham, WA, 2000.
2. A.P. Dhawan, Y. Chitre, C. Kaiser-Bonasso, and M. Moskowitz, "Analysis of mammographic microcalcifications using gray levels image structure features," *IEEE Trans. Med. Imaging*, Vol. 15, pp. 246–259, 1996.
3. L. Xu, M. Jackowski, A. Goshtasby, C. Yu, D. Roseman, A.P. Dhawan, and S. Bines, "Segmentation of skin cancer images," *Image Vis. Comput.*, Vol. 17, pp. 65–74, 1999.

4. A.P. Dhawan and A. Sicsu, "Segmentation of images of skin lesions using color and texture information of surface pigmentation," *Comput. Med. Imaging Graph.*, Vol. 16, pp. 163–177, 1992.
5. D.H. Ballard and C.M. Brown, *Computer Vision*, Prentice Hall, Englewood Cliffs, NJ, 1982.
6. R.C. Gonzalaez and R.E. Wintz, *Digital Image Processing*, Prentice Hall, Englewood Cliffs, NJ, 2002.
7. M.K. Hu, "Visual pattern recognition by moments invariants," *IRE Trans. Inf. Theo.*, Vol. 8, pp. 179–187, 1962.
8. J. Flusser and T. Suk, "Pattern recognition by affine moments invariants," *Pattern Recog.*, Vol. 26, pp. 167–174, 1993.
9. J. Serra, *Image Analysis and Mathematical Morphology*, Academic Press, San Diego, CA, 1982.
10. L.H. Staib and J.S. Duncan, "Boundary finding with parametrically deformable models," *IEEE Trans. Pattern Anal. Mach. Intell.*, Vol. 14, pp. 1061–1075, 1992.
11. S. Sternberg, L. Shapiro, and R. MacDonald, "Ordered structural shape matching with primitive extraction by mathematical morphology," *Pattern Recog.*, Vol. 20, pp. 75–90, 1987.
12. P. Maragos, "Pattern spectrum and multiscale shape representation," *IEEE Trans. Pattern Anal. Mach. Intell.*, Vol. 11, pp. 701–716, 1989.
13. S. Loncaric and A.P. Dhawan, "A morphological signature transform for shape description," *Pattern Recog.*, Vol. 26, No. 7, pp. 1029–1037, 1993.
14. S. Loncaric, A.P. Dhawan, T. Brott, and J. Broderick, "3-D image analysis of intracerebral brain hemorrhage," *Comput. Methods Prog. Biomed.*, Vol. 46, pp. 207–216, 1995.
15. S. Loncaric and A.P. Dhawan, "Optimal MST-based shape description via genetic algorithms," *Pattern Recog.*, Vol. 28, pp. 571–579, 1995.
16. H. Samet and M. Tamminen, "Computing generic properties of images represented by quadtrees," *IEEE Trans. Pattern Anal. Mach. Intell.*, Vol. 7, pp. 229–240, 1985.
17. Y. Shirari and J. Tsujii, *Artificial Intelligence: Concepts, Techniques and Applications*, John Wiley & Sons, New York, 1984.
18. A.P. Dhawan and S. Juvvadi, "A knowledge-based approach to the analysis and interpretation of CT images," *Comput. Methods Prog. Biomed.*, Vol. 33, pp. 221–239, 1990.
19. J. Broderick, S. Narayan, A.P. Dhawan, M. Gaskil, and J. Khouri, "Ventricular measurement of multifocal brain lesions: Implications for treatment trials of vascular dementia and multiple sclerosis," *Neuroimaging*, Vol. 6, pp. 36–43, 1996.
20. A.M. Nazif and M.D. Levine, "Low-level image segmentation: An expert system," *IEEE Trans. Pattern Anal. Mach. Intell.*, Vol. 6, pp. 555–577, 1984.
21. R.O. Duda, P.E. Hart, and D.G. Stork, *Pattern Classification*, 2nd Edition, John Wiley & Sons, New York, 2001.
22. I.T. Jolliffe, *Principal Component Analysis, Springer Series in Statistics*, 2nd Edition, Springer, New York, 2002.
23. C. Peck and A.P. Dhawan, "A review and critique of genetic algorithm theories," *J. Evol. Comput.*, Vol. 3, pp. 39–80, 1995.
24. Y. Chitre, A.P. Dhawan, and M. Moskowitz, "Classification of mammographic microcalcifications," in K.W. Boyer and S. Astlay (Eds), *State of the Art in Digital Mammographic Image Analysis*, World Scientific Publishing Co., New York, 1994, pp. 167–197.
25. Z. Huo, M.L. Giger, and C.J. Vyborny, "Computerized analysis of multiple mammographic views: Potential usefulness of special view mammograms in computer aided diagnosis," *IEEE Trans. Med. Imaging*, Vol. 20, pp. 1285–1292, 2001.
26. S.A. Stansfield, "ANGY: A rule based expert system for automatic segmentation of coronary vessels from digital subtracted angiograms," *IEEE Trans. Pattern Anal. Mach. Intell.*, Vol. 8, pp. 188–199, 1986.
27. L.K. Arata, A.P. Dhawan, A.V. Levy, J. Broderick, and M. Gaskil, "Three-dimensional anatomical model based segmentation of MR brain images through principal axes registration," *IEEE Trans. Biomed. Eng.*, Vol. 42, No. 11, pp. 1069–1078, 1995.
28. J.M. Zurada, *Introduction to Artificial Neural Systems*, West Publishing Co., Boston, 1992.
29. S. Mitra and S.K. Pal, "Fuzzy multi-layer perceptron, inferencing and rule generation," *IEEE Trans. Neural Netw.*, Vol. 6, No. 1, pp. 51–63, 1995.
30. L.A. Zadeh, "Fuzzy sets as a basis for a theory of possibility," *Fuzzy Sets Syst.*, Vol. 1, pp. 3–28, 1978.

31. Y.-Q. Zhang and A. Kandel, "Compensatory neurofuzzy systems with fast learning algorithms," *IEEE Trans. Neural Netw.*, Vol. 9, No. 1, pp. 83–105, 1998.
32. V. Petridis and V.G. Kaburlasos, "Fuzzy lattice neural network (FLNN): A hybrid model for learning," *IEEE Trans. Neural Netw.*, Vol. 9, No. 5, pp. 877–890, 1998.
33. W. Grohman and A.P. Dhawan, "Fuzzy convex set based pattern classification of mammographic microcalcifications," *Pattern Recog.*, Vol. 34, No. 7, pp. 119–132, 2001.
34. F. Aiolli and A. Sperduti, "Multiclass classification with multi-prototype support vector machines," *J. Mach. Learn. Res.*, Vol. 6, pp. 817–850, 2005.
35. M.E. Tipping, "Sparse Bayesian learning and the relevance vector machine," *J. Mach. Learn. Res.*, Vol. 1, pp. 211–244, 2001.
36. T. Downs, K.E. Gates, and A. Masters, "Exact simplification of support vector solutions," *J. Mach. Learn. Res.*, Vol. 2, pp. 293–297, 2001.
37. F. Aiolli and A. Sperduti, "An efficient SMO-like algortihm for multiclass SVM," in *Proceedings of IEEE Workshop on Neural Networks for Signal Processing*, IEEE Press, Piscataway, NJ, pp. 297–306, 2002.
38. W.B. Johnson Jr, "Wavelet packets applied to mammograms," in R. Acharya and D.B. Goldof (Eds), Proc. SPIE 1905, *Biomedical Image Processing and Biomedical Visualization*, SPIE Press, Bellingham, WA, 1993, pp. 504–508.
39. R.N. Strickland and H.I. Hahn, "Detection of microcalcifications using wavelets," in A.G. Gale, A.M. Astley, D.R. Dance, and A.Y. Cairns (Eds), *Digital Mammography*, Proceedings, 2nd International Workshop on Digital Mammography, Elsevier Science B.V., Amsterdam, 1994, pp. 79–88.
40. W. Qian, L.P. Clarke, M. Kallergi, H.D. Li, R.P. Velthuizen, R.A. Clarke, and M.L. Silbigier, "Tree-structured nonlinear filter and wavelet transform for microcalcification segmentation in mammography," in R. Acharya and D.B. Goldof (Eds), Proc. SPIE 1905, *Biomedical Image Processing and Biomedical Visualization*, SPIE Press, Bellingham, WA, 1993, pp. 509–521.
41. N. Mudigonda, R.M. Rangayyan, and J.E. Leo Desautals, "Detection of breast masses in mammograms by density slicing and texture flow-field analysis," *IEEE Trans. Med. Imaging*, Vol. 120, pp. 1215–1227, 2001.

CHAPTER 12

IMAGE REGISTRATION

Recent advances in medical imaging have made it possible to obtain three-dimensional (3-D) anatomical and metabolic information about the internal structure of the human body. As described in Chapters 4–7, different medical imaging modalities provide specific information about human physiology and physiological processes that is often complementary in diagnosis. To better understand physiological processes, images obtained from different modalities need to be registered. For example, anatomical images of the brain obtained from magnetic resonance imaging (MRI) modality need to be registered with metabolic images of the same brain obtained from the positron emission tomography (PET) imaging modality to analyze the metabolism within the anatomical volume of a tumor. Through the comparative quantitative and qualitative analyses of anatomical and metabolic volumes of the tumor from the registered images acquired during the treatment, the response of the treatment can be evaluated. Analysis of registered 3-D multimodality images from a control group of subjects allows the study of variance of specific features for better diagnosis, understanding of pathology, and therapeutic intervention protocols. In addition, postprocessing registration methods are useful in image-guided surgery, functional mapping, and characterization of normal versus abnormal physiological processes.

To study the variability of anatomical and functional (or metabolic) structures among the subjects, images from respective modalities can be registered to develop computerized atlases. The atlases can be broadly classified into two categories: structural computerized atlas (SCA) and functional computerized atlas (FCA). The SCA representing the anatomical variations among subjects can be developed using registered images from anatomical medical imaging modalities such as computer tomography (CT) or conventional MRI. It can be used as models for image segmentation and extraction of a structural volume of interest (VOI). It can also provide anatomical signatures for various groups of subjects for radiological studies. The FCA representing the metabolic variations among subjects for a specific pathology or function can be developed using registered images from functional medical imaging modalities such as functional MRI (fMRI), SPECT, or PET. When registered with structural images, it can be used to understand the metabolism or functional activity in a specific structural VOI. For example, the metabolism of a specific structural VOI of the brain can be studied to evaluate the cognitive functions of a subject. Figure 12.1 shows a schematic diagram of multimodality MR–PET medical

---

Medical Image Analysis, Second Edition, by Atam P. Dhawan
Copyright © 2011 by the Institute of Electrical and Electronics Engineers, Inc.

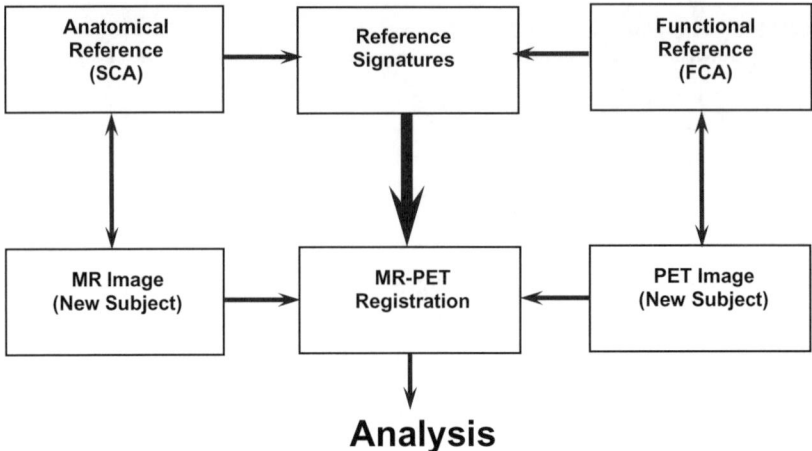

Figure 12.1 A schematic diagram of multimodality MR–PET image analysis using computerized atlases.

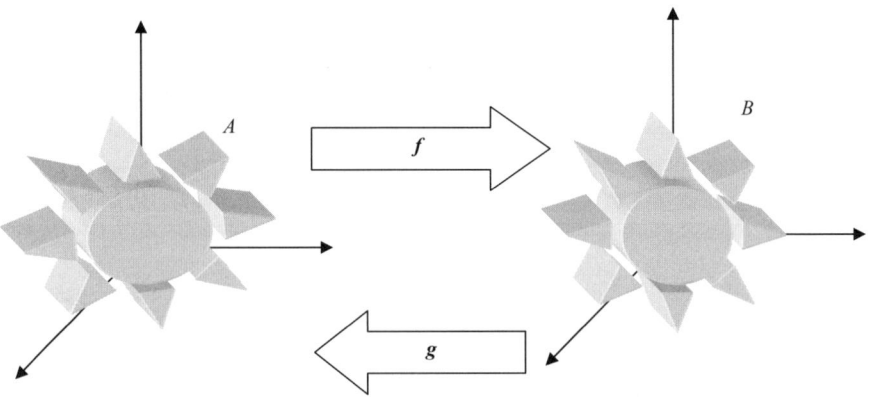

Figure 12.2 Image registration through transformation.

image analysis using the SCA and FCA. Anatomical and functional references are obtained using the SCA and FCA, respectively, for a specific physiological region such as the brain. The MR and PET brain images of a patient are then registered and analyzed in the context of the respective reference signature obtained from the atlases. As mentioned above, the atlases provide variability models for the analysis and interpretation of structural and functional images (1–6).

Image registration methods and algorithms provide transformation of a source image to the target image. The target image may be an image of the same or any other subject from any medical imaging modality. As described above, the target image could also be from an atlas. In ideal cases the transformation from source to target image should be reversible; that is, by using the inverse transformation, the source image can be recovered from the target image. Also, the transformation must preserve the topological properties of the image. Figure 12.2 shows a forward transformation f to map the source image A to the target image B and a reverse transformation g for mapping the target image B to the source image A. In ideal cases, g is the inverse of f.

Although multimodality image registration and analysis methods can be applied to any physiological region, the methods in this chapter are described in the context of registration of human brain images. The registration of human brain images is a challenging problem in multimodality brain image analysis (1–35). However, references are provided for the registration of images of other physiological regions, such as the chest (36–40).

The approaches investigated in multimodality brain image registration and analysis can be divided into three broad categories.

1. **External Markers and Stereotactic Frame-Based Landmark Registration:** The first category belongs to image registration and analysis methods, which require external markers in multiple scans or the use of stereotactic frames to establish a common coordinate system (1–3, 7–9). Stereotactic methods using special frames with markers, which are visible in different modalities, have also been used for image registration (1–9). Such external landmark-based registration methods are based on coordinate transformation (rotation, translation, and scaling) and interpolation computed from visible markers (21) by optimizing the mean squared error. Stereotatctic frames are usually uncomfortable for the patient.

2. **Rigid-Body Transformation-Based Global Registration:** The second category of multimodality image registration methods treats the brain volume as a rigid body for global registration. Levy et al. presented a principal axes transformation-based 3-D registration method, which requires no operator interaction (11–15). This method was used in PET-PET (11), MR-MR (14) and MR–PET (15) brain image registration. PET scans, because of their limited field of view, often do not cover the entire brain, while MR scans are usually obtained for the entire brain volume. In such cases, the PET volume does not match the MR volume. The principal axes transformation method therefore does not provide accurate registration of MR and PET volumes. An iterative principle axes registration method was developed by Dhawan et al. to register MR brain images with PET scans covering the partial volume of the brain (15).

3. **Image Feature-Based Registration:** A large number of algorithms have been developed for image registration based on image features involving edges, contours, surfaces, volumes, and internal landmarks (16–35). This category can be divided into two major subcategories.

   a. **Boundary and Surface Matching-Based Registration:** Image registration methods have been developed using edges, boundary, and surface information from images (16–20). Pelizzari et al. presented a surface matching-based registration method that maps a large number of points though a computer (16, 17). In this surface matching technique, 3-D models of the surface to be matched are first produced by outlining contours on serial slices of each scan. The surface or boundary matching methods may require extensive computation and often need operator interaction to guide a nonlinear optimization. With CT or MR scans, the identification of the external surface is usually not a problem. Pelizzari et al. (16) suggested the use of PET transmission scans to identify the external surface from the PET data. 3-D models of the brain surface from both scans are then corrected for possible geometrical errors. A geometric transformation is obtained by minimizing a predefined error function between the surfaces. Once the transformation is determined through surface matching, the registration information is transferred between the scans using the VOI solid model constructed from its boundary contours (16–20).

b. **Image Landmarks and Feature-Based Registration:** Recently, several image registration algorithms have been developed that utilize predefined anatomical landmarks or features that can be identified and extracted in images (23–35). Bayesian model-based probabilistic methods have been used to integrate 3-D image information for registration (23, 24) Neuroanatomical atlases have been used for elastic matching of brain images (25–30). Rohr et al. used a landmark-based elastic matching algorithm for image registration (34). Other probabilistic model-based approaches, such as maximum likelihood estimation, have been investigated in the literature (20, 35).

12.1. RIGID-BODY TRANSFORMATION

Rigid-body transformation is primarily based on translation and rotation operations. Two images of equal dimensions are registered by applying a pixel-by-pixel transformation consistently throughout the image space. In three dimensions, a rigid transformation-based mapping of a point vector x to x' is defined by

$$\mathbf{x}' = \mathbf{R}\mathbf{x} + \mathbf{t} \tag{12.1}$$

where $\mathbf{R}$ is a rotation matrix and $\mathbf{t}$ is translation vector.

The translation and rotation operations in individual dimensions of the 3-D coordinate space are shown in Figure 12.3 and can be expressed as

a. Translation along x-axis by p:

$$\begin{aligned} x' &= x + p \\ y' &= y \\ z' &= z \end{aligned} \tag{12.2}$$

b. Translation along y-axis by q:

$$\begin{aligned} x' &= x \\ y' &= y + q \\ z' &= z \end{aligned} \tag{12.3}$$

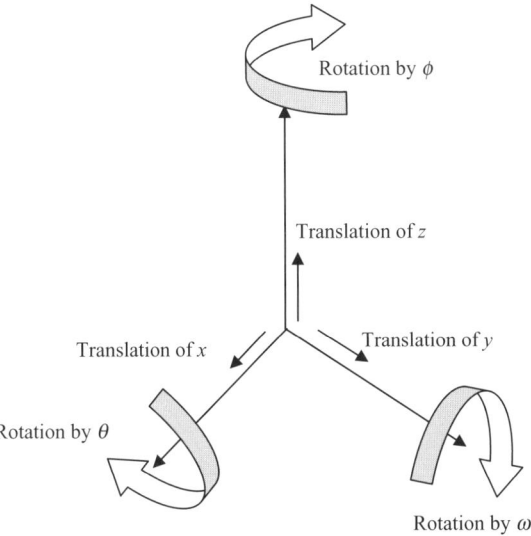

Figure 12.3 The translation and rotation operations of a 3-D rigid transformation.

c. Translation along z-axis by r:
$$x' = x$$
$$y' = y \tag{12.4}$$
$$z' = z + r$$

d. Rotation about x-axis by θ:
$$x' = x$$
$$y' = y\cos\theta + z\sin\theta \tag{12.5}$$
$$z' = -y\sin\theta + z\cos\theta$$

e. Rotation about y-axis by ω:
$$x' = x\cos\omega - z\sin\omega$$
$$y' = y \tag{12.6}$$
$$z' = x\sin\omega + z\cos\omega$$

f. Rotation about z-axis by ϕ:
$$x' = x\cos\varphi + y\sin\varphi$$
$$y' = -x\sin\varphi + y\cos\varphi \tag{12.7}$$
$$z' = z$$

It should be noted that the order of operations in the translation and rotation operations is important. Different results could be obtained if the order of translation and rotation operations is changed.

It can be shown that the rotation matrix **R** for the *x-y-z* rotational order of operation can be given as

$$\mathbf{R} = R_\theta R_\omega R_\phi = \begin{bmatrix} \cos\theta & \sin\theta & 0 \\ -\sin\theta & \cos\theta & 0 \\ 0 & 0 & 1 \end{bmatrix} \begin{bmatrix} \cos\omega & 0 & -\sin\omega \\ 0 & 1 & 0 \\ \sin\omega & 0 & \cos\omega \end{bmatrix} \begin{bmatrix} 1 & 0 & 0 \\ 0 & \cos\phi & \sin\phi \\ 0 & -\sin\phi & \cos\phi \end{bmatrix} \quad (12.8)$$

12.1.1 Affine Transformation

Affine transformation is a special case of rigid-body transformation that includes translation, rotation, and scaling operations. If the two image volumes to be registered are not at the same scale, a scaling parameter in each dimension has to be added as

$$\begin{aligned} x' &= ax \\ y' &= by \\ z' &= cz \end{aligned} \quad (12.9)$$

where a, b, and c are the scaling parameters along x-, y-, and z-directions.

The affine transformation can be expressed as:

$$\mathbf{x'} = \mathbf{A}\mathbf{x} \quad (12.10)$$

where **A** is the affine matrix that includes the translation, rotation, and scaling transformation with nine parameters.

Thus, the overall mapping can be expressed as

$$\begin{bmatrix} x' \\ y' \\ z' \\ 1 \end{bmatrix} = \begin{bmatrix} 1 & 0 & 0 & p \\ 0 & 1 & 0 & q \\ 0 & 0 & 1 & r \\ 0 & 0 & 0 & 1 \end{bmatrix} \begin{bmatrix} \cos\theta & \sin\theta & 0 & 0 \\ -\sin\theta & \cos\theta & 0 & 0 \\ 0 & 0 & 1 & 0 \\ 0 & 0 & 0 & 1 \end{bmatrix} \begin{bmatrix} \cos\omega & 0 & -\sin\omega & 0 \\ 0 & 1 & 0 & 0 \\ \sin\omega & 0 & \cos\omega & 0 \\ 0 & 0 & 0 & 1 \end{bmatrix}$$
$$\begin{bmatrix} 1 & 0 & 0 & 0 \\ 0 & \cos\phi & \sin\phi & 0 \\ 0 & -\sin\phi & \cos\phi & 0 \\ 0 & 0 & 0 & 1 \end{bmatrix} \begin{bmatrix} a & 0 & 0 & 0 \\ 0 & b & 0 & 0 \\ 0 & 0 & c & 0 \\ 0 & 0 & 0 & 1 \end{bmatrix} \begin{bmatrix} x \\ y \\ z \\ 1 \end{bmatrix} \quad (12.11)$$

12.2. PRINCIPAL AXES REGISTRATION

Principal axes registration (PAR) can be used for global matching of two binary volumes such as segmented brain volumes from CT, MR, or PET images (11–15). Let us represent a binary segmented $B(x, y, z)$ as

$$\begin{aligned} B(x, y, z) &= 1 \text{ if } (x, y, z) \text{ is in the object} \\ &= 0 \text{ if } (x, y, z) \text{ is not in the object.} \end{aligned} \quad (12.12)$$

12.2. PRINCIPAL AXES REGISTRATION

Let the centroid of the binary volume $B(x, y, z)$ be represented by (x_g, y_g, z_g) where

$$x_g = \frac{\sum_{x,y,z} xB(x,y,z)}{\sum_{x,y,z} B(x,y,z)}$$

$$y_g = \frac{\sum_{x,y,z} yB(x,y,z)}{\sum_{x,y,z} B(x,y,z)}$$

$$z_g = \frac{\sum_{x,y,z} zB(x,y,z)}{\sum_{x,y,z} B(x,y,z)}. \tag{12.13}$$

Following Goldstein (22), the principle axes of $B(x, y, z)$ are the eigenvectors of the inertia matrix I:

$$I = \begin{bmatrix} I_{xx} & -I_{xy} & -I_{xz} \\ -I_{yx} & I_{yy} & -I_{yz} \\ -I_{zx} & -I_{zy} & I_{zz} \end{bmatrix}$$

where

$$I_{xx} = \sum_{x,y,z} \left[(y-y_g)^2 + (z-z_g)^2\right] B(x,y,z)$$

$$I_{yy} = \sum_{x,y,z} \left[(x-x_g)^2 + (z-z_g)^2\right] B(x,y,z)$$

$$I_{zz} = \sum_{x,y,z} \left[(x-x_g)^2 + (y-y_g)^2\right] B(x,y,z)$$

$$I_{xy} = I_{yx} = \sum_{x,y,z} (x-x_g)(y-y_g) B(x,y,z)$$

$$I_{xz} = I_{zx} = \sum_{x,y,z} (x-x_g)(z-z_g) B(x,y,z)$$

$$I_{yz} = I_{zy} = \sum_{x,y,z} (y-y_g)(z-z_g) B(x,y,z). \tag{12.14}$$

The inertia matrix is diagonal when computed with respect to the principal axes. Thus, the centroid and the principal axes provide a method to completely describe the orientation of an arbitrary volume. The method can resolve six degrees of freedom of an object, including three rotations and three translations. Furthermore, it provides a precise way of comparing the orientations of two binary volumes through rotation, translation, and scaling.

Let us define a normalized eigenvector matrix E as

$$E = \begin{bmatrix} e_{11} & e_{12} & e_{13} \\ e_{21} & e_{22} & e_{23} \\ e_{31} & e_{32} & e_{33} \end{bmatrix}. \tag{12.15}$$

Let $\mathbf{R} = R_\alpha R_\beta R_\gamma$ represent the rotation matrix as

$$R_\alpha R_\beta R_\gamma = \begin{bmatrix} \cos\alpha & \sin\alpha & 0 \\ -\sin\alpha & \cos\alpha & 0 \\ 0 & 0 & 1 \end{bmatrix} \begin{bmatrix} \cos\beta & 0 & -\sin\beta \\ 0 & 1 & 0 \\ \sin\beta & 0 & \cos\beta \end{bmatrix} \begin{bmatrix} 1 & 0 & 0 \\ 0 & \cos\gamma & \sin\gamma \\ 0 & -\sin\gamma & \cos\gamma \end{bmatrix}. \quad (12.16)$$

where α, β, and γ are the rotation angles with respect to the x, y, and z axes, respectively.

By equating the normalized eigenvector matrix to the rotation matrix as

$$E = R_\alpha R_\beta R_\gamma. \quad (12.17)$$

It can be shown that

$$\begin{aligned} \beta &= \arcsin(e_{31}) \\ \alpha &= \arcsin(-e_{21}/\cos\beta) \\ \gamma &= \arcsin(-e_{32}/\cos\beta). \end{aligned} \quad (12.18)$$

Given two volumes, V_1 and V_2, for registration, the PAR method provides the following operations:

1. Translate the centroid of V_1 to the origin.
2. Rotate the principal axes of V_1 to coincide with the x-, y-, and z-axes.
3. Rotate the x, y, and z axes to coincide with the principal axes of V_2.
4. Translate the origin to the centroid of V_2.

Finally, the volume V_2 is scaled to match the volume V_1 using the scaling factor F_s

$$F_s = \sqrt[3]{\frac{V_1}{V_2}}. \quad (12.19)$$

Probabilistic models can be constructed by counting the occurrence of a particular binary subvolume that is extracted from the registered volumes corresponding to various images. Let $M(x, y, z)$ be a function describing the model providing the spatial probability distribution of the subvolume, then

$$M(x, y, z) = \frac{1}{n}\sum_{i=1}^{n} S_i(x, y, z). \quad (12.20)$$

where n is the total number of data sets in the model and $S_i(x, y, z)$ is the ith subvolume.

Figure 12.4 shows a model of brain ventricles that is based on the frequency of occurrence in registered brain images of 22 normal subjects using the PAR method. This composite model provides a 3-D probabilistic spatial distribution of the ventricles. The probability of spatial matching as indicated by the gray-level value ranges from 0.0455 (1/22) to 1.0 (22/22). For visualization, an opacity factor equal to the probability of matching was assigned to all gray-level values (14). The consistency of the match of the third and fourth ventricles and the variability evident in the lateral ventricles can be noted in the rotated views of the model shown in Figure 12.5.

12.3. ITERATIVE PRINCIPAL AXES REGISTRATION

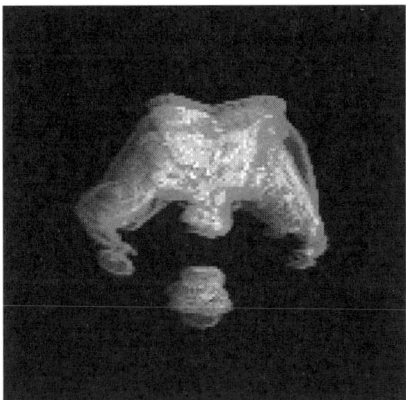

Figure 12.4 A 3-D model of brain ventricles obtained from registering 22 MR brain images using the PAR method.

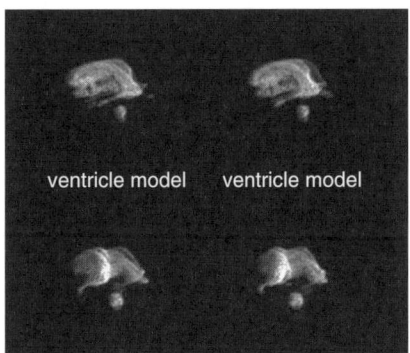

Figure 12.5 Rotated views of the 3-D brain ventricle model shown in Figure 12.3.

12.3. ITERATIVE PRINCIPAL AXES REGISTRATION

Dhawan et al. (15) developed an iterative PAR (IPAR) method for registering MR and PET brain images. The advantage of the IPAR over the conventional principal axes registration method is that the IPAR method can be used with partial volumes. This procedure assumes that the field of view (FOV) of a functional image such as PET is less than the full brain volume, while the other volume (MR image) covers the entire brain.

Let V_1 and V_2 represent two volumes to be registered. The IPAR method can be implemented using the following steps (15):

1. Find the full dynamic range of the PET data and select a threshold, T, which is about 20% of the maximum gray-level value. Threshold each PET slice to avoid streaking artifacts and overestimation of the brain regions, such that all pixels with gray-level values equal to or less than the threshold T are set to zero. Extract binary brain regions using a region-growing method on the thresholded PET slice data.

2. Threshold and extract binary brain regions from the MR data using a region-growing method.
3. Stack two-dimensional (2-D) binary segmented MR slices and interpolate as necessary to obtain cubic voxel dimensions using a shape-based interpolation algorithm (21). This is referred to as 3-D binary MR data.
4. Stack 2-D binary segmented PET slices and interpolate as necessary to obtain a cubic voxel dimension to match the voxel dimension of binary MR data using a shape-based interpolation algorithm (21). This is referred to as 3-D binary PET data.
5. Define a FOV box, FOV(0), as a parallelepiped from the slices of the interpolated binary PET data to cover the PET brain volume. Because of the smaller FOV of the PET scanner, voxels outside the binary PET brain volume will have zero values.
6. Compute the centroid and principal axes of the binary PET brain volume as described above.
7. Add n slices to the FOV(0) box (of binary PET brain volume) on the top and the bottom such that the augmented FOV(n) box will have the same number of slices as the binary MR data. The added slices are spaced equally on the top and bottom. The FOV(n) box will now be shrunk gradually back to its original size, FOV(0), through an iterative process. Initially, the whole MR brain volume is used in computing the transformation parameters using the augmented FOV(n) box. In each iteration, the FOV(n) box is reduced in size and the binary MR data is trimmed accordingly to provide the current MR brain volume. This volume is used to compute the centroid and principal axes parameters to obtain a new transformation for matching the PET FOV box to the current MR brain. The iterative process continues until the FOV box reaches its original size to provide the final transformation parameters to register MR and PET data. Figure 12.6 shows three iterations of the IPAR algorithm for registration of two volumes. The IPAR algorithm is as follows.

For $i = n$ to 0:

A. Compute the centroid and principal axes of the current binary MR brain volume. This binary MR brain volume is gradually trimmed at each step by the transformed FOV(i) box.

B. Transform the augmented FOV(i) box according to the space of the MR slices as follows.

Let c_{PET} and c_{MR} be the centroids, (x_g, y_g, z_g), of the binary PET and MR data, and let E_{PET} and E_{MR} be the normalized eigenvector matrices of the binary PET and MR data; then for any point, x_{PET}, its position, x_{MR}, in the MR space can be calculated as

$$x_{MR} = (E_{MR} E_{PET}^T (x_{PET} - c_{PET})) + c_{MR}. \tag{12.21}$$

The normalized eigenvector matrix of a binary volume will rotate the standard x-, y-, and z-axes parallel to the principal axes of the volume. If the centroid of the volume is first translated to the origin, then after rotation

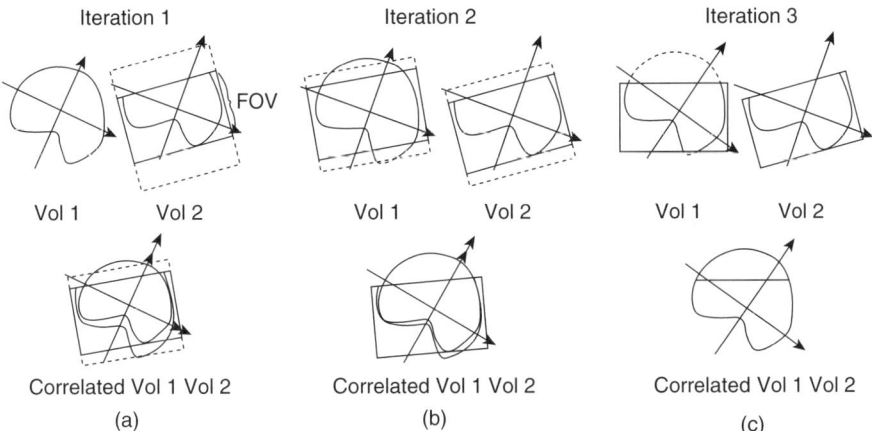

Figure 12.6 Three successive iterations of the IPAR algorithms for registration of vol 1 and vol 2: The results of the first iteration (a), the second iteration (b), and the final iteration (c). Vol 1 represents the MR data while the PET image with limited filed of view (FOV) is represented by vol 2.

by the eigenvector matrix the x-, y-, and z-axes will be coincident with the principal axes of the volume.

The PET data is registered with the MR data through the process of the required translations and rotations. The rotation angles are determined as described above. To express all points, $(x_{PET}, y_{PET}, z_{PET})$, of the PET data in the coordinate space of the MR data, the following steps must be performed:

1. Translate the centroid of the binary PET data to the origin.
2. Rotate the principal axes of the binary PET data to coincide with the x-, y-, and z-axes.
3. Rotate the x-, y-, and z-axes to coincide with the MR principal axes.
4. Translate the origin to the centroid of the binary MR data.

C. Remove all voxels of the binary MR brain that lie outside the transformed FOV(i) box. This is the new binary MR brain volume.

The final transformation parameters for registration of MR and PET data are obtained from the last iteration.

8. Interpolate the gray-level PET data to match the resolution of MR data, to prepare the PET data for registration with MR data.
9. Transform the gray-level PET data into the space of the MR slices using the last set of MR and PET centroids and principal axes. Extract the slices from the transformed gray-level PET data that match the gray-level MR image.

The IPAR algorithm allows registration of two 3-D image data sets, in which one set does not cover the entire volume but has the subvolume contained in the other data set. Figures 12.7 a–c show the MR (middle rows) and PET (bottom rows) brain

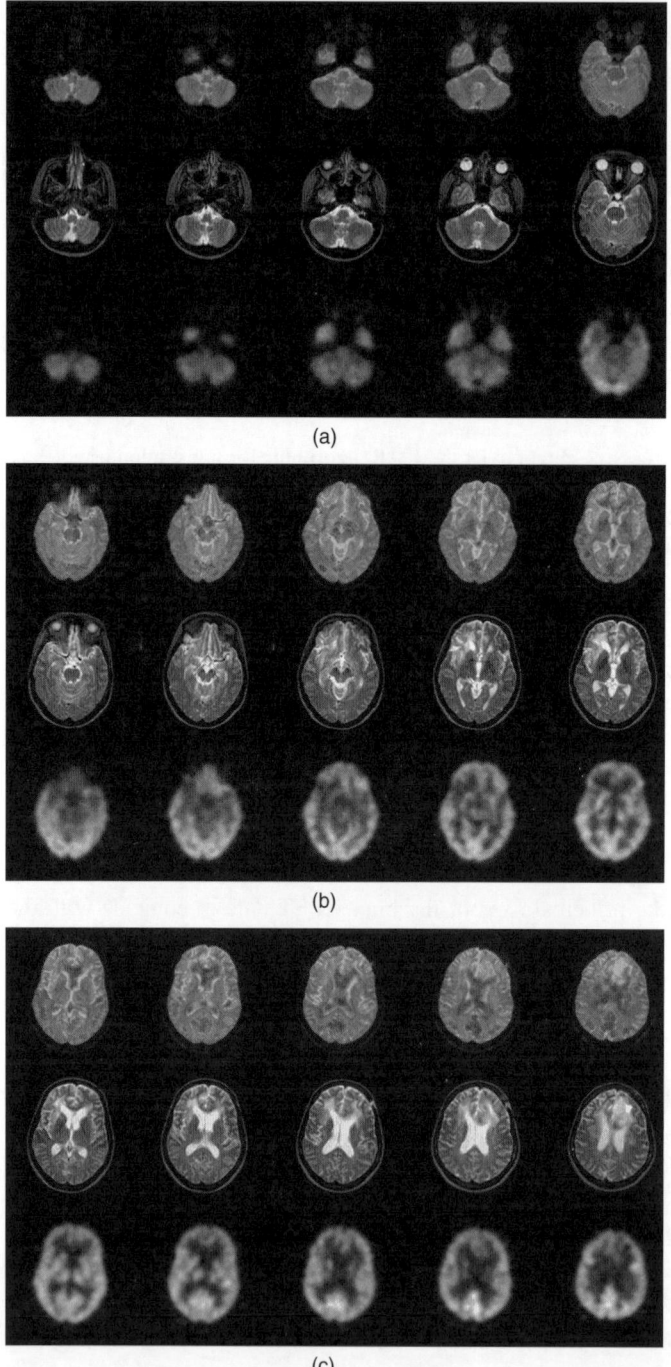

Figure 12.7 (a, b, c) Sequential slices of MR (middle rows) and PET (bottom rows) and the registered MR–PET brain images (top row) of the corresponding slices using the IPAR method.

images of a patient with a brain tumor. The 3-D MR and PET images were registered using the IPAR method. The corresponding registered overlaid MR–PET images for the respective slices are shown in the top rows. The MR data was obtained from a Philips Gyroscan S15 scanner with 256 × 256 pixel resolution corresponding to about 0.9 mm pixel size with an interslice separation of 5 mm. The PET data was obtained from a Siemens-CTI: 951 scanner as 128 × 128 pixel images with a pixel size of 1.9 mm. The interslice distance of the PET data was about 3.5 mm. The PET brain FOV was about 70% of the MR brain FOV.

12.4. IMAGE LANDMARKS AND FEATURES-BASED REGISTRATION

Rigid and nonrigid transformations have been used in image landmarks (points) and features-based medical image registration (16–20). Once the corresponding landmarks or features are identified from source and target image spaces, a customized transformation can be computed for registering the source image into the target image space. In the previous sections, global registration methods (PAR and IPAR) based on principal axes were described. These methods use the basic principle of rigid-body transformation with an additional operation of scaling. However, a number of nonrigid transformation methods that exploit the relationships of corresponding points and features such as surfaces in source and target images have been investigated for registration (16–20). Two simple algorithms for point-based registration of source and target images are described below.

12.4.1 Similarity Transformation for Point-Based Registration

Let us assume that x and y are, respectively, the corresponding points (represented as vectors) in the source and target image spaces belonging to the source X and target Y images. A nonrigid transformation $T(x)$ for registering the source image into the target image space can be defined by a combination of rotation, translation, and scaling operations to provide x' from x as (41)

$$\mathbf{x'} = s\mathbf{rx} + \mathbf{t} \tag{12.22}$$

such that the registration error E is minimized as

$$E(\mathbf{x}) = T(\mathbf{x}) - \mathbf{y} \tag{12.23}$$

where r, s, and t represent the rotation, scaling, and translation operations.

A transformation should be obtained with r, s, and t values to minimize the error function as

$$\sum_{i=1}^{N} w_i^2 \left| s\mathbf{rx}_i + \mathbf{t} - \mathbf{y}_i \right|^2 \tag{12.24}$$

where w_i are the weighting factors representing the confidence in the specific landmark (point) or feature correspondence and N is the total number of landmarks.

The following algorithm can be implemented to register the source image into the target image space:

1. Set $s = 1$.
2. Find r through the following steps:
   (a) Compute the weighted centroid of the body representing the set of landmarks (points) in each space as

   $$\bar{x} = \frac{\sum_{i=1}^{N} w_i^2 x_i}{\sum_{i=1}^{N} w_i^2}$$

   $$\bar{y} = \frac{\sum_{i=1}^{N} w_i^2 y_i}{\sum_{i=1}^{N} w_i^2} \qquad (12.25)$$

   (b) Compute the distance of each landmark from the centroid as

   $$\bar{x}_i = x_i - \bar{x}$$
   $$\bar{y}_i = y_i - \bar{y} \qquad (12.26)$$

   (c) Compute the weighted covariance matrix as

   $$Z = \sum_{i=1}^{N} w_i^2 \bar{x}_i \bar{y}_i^t \qquad (12.27)$$

   with a singular value decomposition as

   $$Z = U \Lambda V^t$$

   where $U^t U = V^t V = I$
   and

   $$\Lambda = diag(\lambda_1, \lambda_2, \lambda_3); \qquad \lambda_1 \geq \lambda_2 \geq \lambda_3 \geq 0 \qquad (12.28)$$

   (d) Compute $r = V diag(1, 1, det(VU)) U^t$ (12.29)

3. Compute the scaling factor

$$s = \frac{\sum_{i=1}^{N} w_i^2 r\bar{x}_i \cdot \bar{y}_i}{\sum_{i=1}^{N} w_i^2 r\bar{x}_i \cdot \bar{x}_i} \qquad (12.30)$$

4. Compute $t = \bar{y} - sr\bar{x}$ (12.31)

12.4.2 Weighted Features-Based Registration

Different optimization functions can be designed to improve the computation of parameters of transformation for registration of the source image into the target image space. In the above example, an error function was used for minimization to achieve the transformation parameters. In many registration methods, geometrical features or landmarks are used to register 3-D images. Defining a transformation T on x as in Equation 12.23, a disparity function can be designed as

$$d(T) = \sqrt{\sum_{i=1}^{N_s} \sum_{j=1}^{N_{X_i}} w_{ij}^2 \|T(x_{ij}) - y_{ij}\|^2} \qquad (12.32)$$

where $\{X_i\}$ for $i = 1, 2, 3, \ldots, N_s$ represents a set of corresponding data shapes in x and y spaces.

The transformation T must minimize the disparity function to register the source image into the target image space utilizing the correspondence of geometrical features.

An iterative algorithm can be implemented for registration as (42);

1. Determine the parameters for a rigid or nonrigid-body transformation T using the above algorithm in Section 12.4.1.
2. Initialize the transformation optimization loop for $k = 1$ as

$$x_{ij}^{(0)} = x_{ij}$$
$$x_{ij}^{(1)} = T^{(0)}(x_{ij}^{(0)}) \qquad (12.33)$$

3. For each shape X_i in the source space, find the closest points in the corresponding shape in the target space Y_i as

$$y_{ij}^{(k)} = C_i(x_{ij}^{(k)}, Y_i); \quad j = 1, 2, 3, \ldots, N_{X_i} \qquad (12.34)$$

where C_i is the corresponding function.

4. Compute the transformation between $\{x_{ij}^{(0)}\}$ and $\{y_{ij}^{(k)}\}$ using the weights $\{w_{ij}\}$ using the above algorithm in Section 12.4.1.
5. Use the transformation parameters for registration of the corresponding points as

$$x_{ij}^{(k+1)} = T^{(k)}(x_{ij}^{(0)}) \qquad (12.35)$$

6. Compute the disparity measure difference $d(T^{(k)}) - d(T^{(k+1)})$. If the convergence criterion is met, stop; otherwise increment k and go to step 3 for next iteration.

12.5. ELASTIC DEFORMATION-BASED REGISTRATION

Elastic deformation methods mimic a manual registration process. In the registration process, one of the two volumes is considered to be made of elastic material while the other volume serves as a rigid reference. The purpose of elastic matching is to map the elastic volume to the reference volume. The elastic volume is deformed by applying external forces such that it matches the reference model. The matching process starts in a coarse mode in which large differences are corrected first. The fine, detailed adjustments are the done later in the deformation-based mapping process. The process stops when an objective function based on the similarity measure is optimized.

There are several constraints that can be applied during the deformation for local matching. The constraints include smoothness and incompressibility. The smoothness constraint ensures that there is continuity in the deformed volume while the incompressibility constraint guarantees that there is no change in the total volume. The forces required to locally match the volumes of interest are calculated with these constraints and can be expressed by the general equation for motion of a deformable body in Lagrangian form as

$$f(r,t) = \mu \frac{\partial^2 r}{\partial t^2} + \gamma \frac{\partial r}{\partial t} + \frac{\partial \varepsilon(r)}{\partial r} \qquad (12.36)$$

where $f(r, t)$ is the force acting on a particle at the position r at time t, μ, and γ are, respectively, the mass and damping constant of the deformable body; and $\varepsilon(r)$ is the internal energy of deformation. For implementation, an image voxel can be treated as a particle for which a movement is calculated for image registration.

Let the elastic volume be represented by V_1 with the coordinate system $x = (x_1, x_2, x_3)$ and the reference volume be represented by V_2 with the coordinate system $x' = (x'_1, x'_2, x'_3)$. A relationship between the two coordinate systems can be expressed as

$$d\mathbf{r} = \frac{\partial \mathbf{r}}{\partial x_1} dx_1 + \frac{\partial \mathbf{r}}{\partial x_2} dx_2 + \frac{\partial \mathbf{r}}{\partial x_3} dx_3. \qquad (12.37)$$

The partial differential operators on a position vector r of a voxel in the registration space can be represented as

$$\vec{g}_i = \frac{\partial \mathbf{r}}{\partial x_i} \quad \text{for } i = 1,2,3. \qquad (12.38)$$

Thus Equation 12.37 can be written as

$$d\mathbf{r} = \vec{g}_i dx_i. \qquad (12.39)$$

Let u be an arbitrary vector represented by (u_1, u_2, u_3) with respect to the coordinate system such that

$$\mathbf{u} = u_1 \vec{g}_1 + u_2 \vec{g}_2 + u_3 \vec{g}_3 \qquad (12.40)$$

It can be shown that

$$u_i = (u_j \vec{g}_j) \cdot \vec{g}_i = g_{ij} u_j$$
$$\text{with } g_{ij} = \vec{g}_i \cdot \vec{g}_j \qquad (12.41)$$

where the quantities g_{ij} are components of the generalized metric tensor G_{ijk} in a 3-D coordinate system. The metric tensor G_{ijk} represents a distance measure with respect to a given coordinate system. Any transformation applied to the metric tensor generates a new metric tensor for the new coordinate system.

12.5. ELASTIC DEFORMATION-BASED REGISTRATION

Thus, considering the position vector $\boldsymbol{u}$ with respect to a point $\boldsymbol{a}$ (a_1, a_2, a_3) in the coordinate system, the metric tensor can be defined as

$$G_{ijk} = \int \frac{\partial \boldsymbol{u}}{\partial a_i} \frac{\partial \boldsymbol{u}}{\partial a_j} \frac{\partial \boldsymbol{u}}{\partial a_k}. \tag{12.42}$$

The metric tensor G_{ijk} can be considered the first-order derivative for the displacement field in the deformation process. A curvature tensor B_{ijk} can be defined to represent the second-order partial derivative form as

$$B_{ijk} = \int \frac{\partial^2 \boldsymbol{u}}{\partial a_i \partial a_j} \frac{\partial^2 \boldsymbol{u}}{\partial a_j \partial a_k} \frac{\partial^2 \boldsymbol{u}}{\partial a_k \partial a_i}. \tag{12.43}$$

The potential energy $\varepsilon(x)$ can be defined in terms of the metric tensor as

$$\varepsilon(\boldsymbol{x}) = k \sum_{ijk} (G_{ijk} - G^0_{ijk})^2 \tag{12.44}$$

where G^0_{ijk} is the resting metric tensor without any displacement field (undeformed situation) and k is a constant.

The elastic deformation function model can now be represented as

$$\varepsilon(\boldsymbol{r}) = \int_\Omega \left\| G_{ijk} - G^0_{ijk} \right\|^2 d\boldsymbol{u} \tag{12.45}$$

where Ω represents all voxels in the volume for registration.

A computational model for matching through elastic deformation can be formulated as a minimization problem of the cost function that is based on a similarity measure between the two volumes to be registered. Let $S(\boldsymbol{x}, \boldsymbol{x}')$ represent a similarity measure between the local region R centered at the location $\boldsymbol{x}$ in V_1 and the region R' centered at $\boldsymbol{x}'$ in V_2. A displacement vector $\boldsymbol{u}$ is defined as the difference between the two locations. The optimal match for R to the region R' for the displacement vector $\boldsymbol{u}$ is the one that maximizes the similarity measure $S(\boldsymbol{x}, \boldsymbol{x}')$.

A possible form of the similarity measure can be expressed in terms of metric and curvature tensors as

$$S(\boldsymbol{x}, \boldsymbol{x}') = \int_\Omega \left(\left\| G^1_{ijk} - G^2_{ijk} \right\|^2 + \left\| B^1_{ijk} - B^2_{ijk} \right\|^2 \right) da_i da_j d_k \tag{12.46}$$

where the superscripts 1 and 2 represent, respectively, the deformable volume V_1 and the reference volume V_2.

Alternately, the similarity measure $S(\boldsymbol{x}, \boldsymbol{x}')$ can be expressed in terms of differences in intensity levels or metric tensors. A cost function is defined to include the similarity measure and elastic constraints for regularization. The cost function guides the image matching process for computing the displacement vector for local regions. The optimization of the cost function provides the final mapping for image registration. For example, Christensen and Johnson (35) included a similarity measure based on the difference of intensity and a linear elastic operator L_r applied on the displacement vector $\boldsymbol{u}(\boldsymbol{x})$ in the cost function $C(g_r, R, R')$ with a mapping transformation as

328 CHAPTER 12 IMAGE REGISTRATION

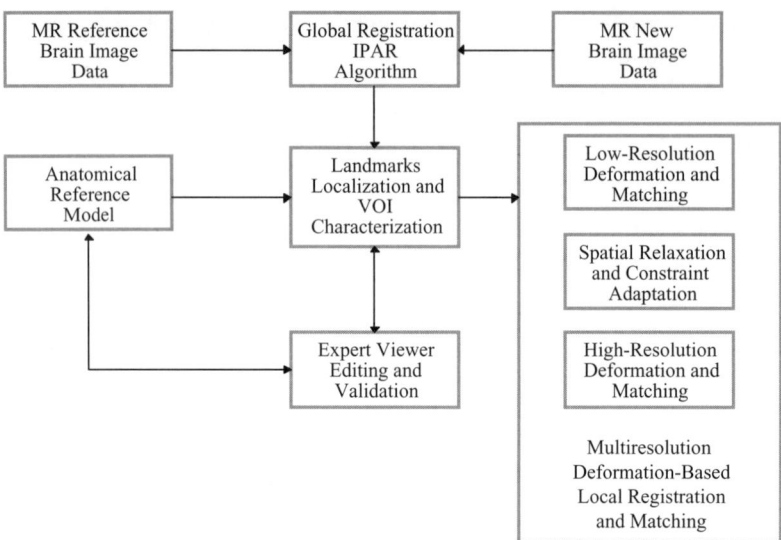

Figure 12.8 Block diagram for the MR image registration procedure.

$$C(g_r, R, R') = \int_{\Omega_R} |R(g_r(x)) - R'(x)|^2 dx + \int_{\Omega_R} \|L_r u(x)\|^2 dx$$

with $L_r u(x) = -\alpha \nabla^2 u(x) - \beta \nabla(\nabla \cdot u(x)) + \gamma u(x)$ (12.47)

where $\nabla = \left[\dfrac{\partial}{\partial x_1}, \dfrac{\partial}{\partial x_2}, \dfrac{\partial}{\partial x_3} \right]$ and $\nabla^2 = \left[\dfrac{\partial^2}{\partial x_1^2}, \dfrac{\partial^2}{\partial x_2^2}, \dfrac{\partial^2}{\partial x_3^2} \right].$ (12.48)

It can be noted that L_r is a differential operator that can cause the transformation to fold onto itself, destroying the topology. To avoid it, the Jacobian of the transformation is checked in each iteration to make sure that it is positive for all voxels in Ω_R, thus ensuring the preservation of topology.

As shown in Figure 12.8, for MR image registration, the MR-1 volume can be first registered with the MR-2 volume globally using the IPAR algorithm. The global registration improves the initial conditions for elastic deformation-based matching (36). Anatomical landmarks are then located from the globally registered volumes using an anatomical reference model with some topological knowledge of the respective anatomy. Thus, the whole 3-D volume can be localized into smaller volumes by choosing appropriate VOI. The VOI can be selected around the internal landmarks that are identified using the anatomical reference model. If necessary, user interaction may also be involved in the identification of the landmarks and related VOIs.

Once the VOIs are defined around internal landmarks, the VOIs of the elastic model are deformed through the application of external forces using a matching criterion that allows forces to change dynamically. The matching process, proceeding from coarse to fine mode, is repeated until the final match is achieved in the finest mode.

12.5. ELASTIC DEFORMATION-BASED REGISTRATION

In brief, the local matching algorithm can be described as follows:

1. Perform a global registration of the two 3-D data sets using the IPAR or a manual landmark-based registration algorithm.
2. Compute a total similarity measure for the deformable volume V_1 and the reference volume V_2 from the globally registered 3-D data sets.
3. Identify internal landmarks using anatomical reference models to determine volumes of interests (VOI$_i$s) where elastic deformation-based local registration is required.
4. For local registration:

For $i = 0$ to $n-1$ VOI$_i$s

   a. Compute similarity measures and cost function for optimization.
   b. If respective VOI$_i$ are not similar,
   c. Compute displacement vectors for voxels in the VOI$_i$ as required for elastic deformation using the constrained optimization of the cost function.
   d. Deform VOI$_i$ of the deformable volume using the displacement vectors.
   e. If deformed voxels are inconsistent with continuity or smoothness constraints, apply correction factors in the computation of displacement vectors and repeat step 4d.
   f. If all VOI$_i$s are processed and the cost function is minimized, end; otherwise go to step 4c.

5. Interpolate the entire deformed volume V_1 as required.
6. Compute the total similarity measure between the deformed volume V_1 and the reference volume V_2.
7. If the total similarity measure between the deformed volume and the reference volume is improved, stop; otherwise check the internal landmarks and go to step 3.

Figure 12.9 shows the results of elastic deformation-based registration of 3-D MR brain images. The left column shows three target images of the 3-D MR brain data set considered as the reference volume V_2. The middle column shows the images from the deformable volume V_1. The right column shows the respective registered images through elastic deformation method. It can be seen from Figure 12.9 that the elastic deformation-based registration method provided reasonably good results. However, distortions at some of the corners of the registered images are evident. To address this problem, more emphasis on the continuity constraint and a better interpolation method are required.

Image registration and localized mapping remains an area of active research as the resolution of medical imaging improves to unveil high-resolution physiological structures. Multimodality image analysis with high-resolution structural mapping continues to provide a basis for understanding metabolic activities in anatomically referenced structures.

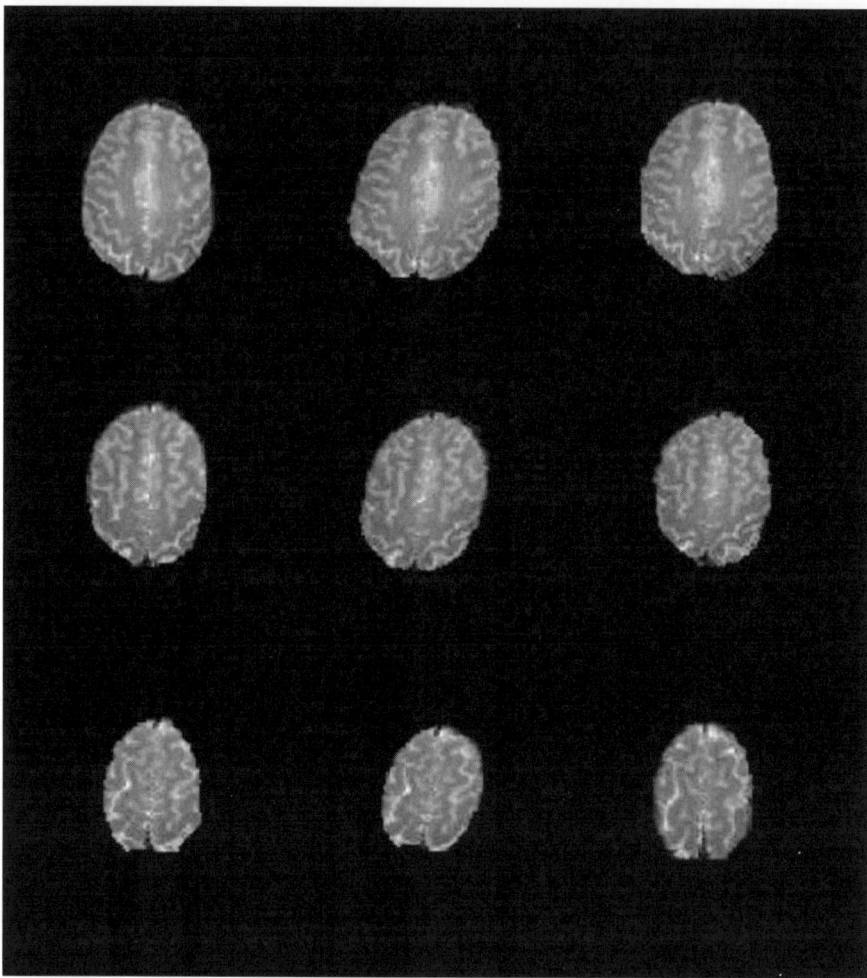

Figure 12.9 Results of the elastic deformation based registration of 3-D MR brain images: The left column shows three images of the reference volume; the middle column shows the respective images of the brain volume to be registered; and the right column shows the respective images of the registered brain volume.

12.6. EXERCISES

12.1. Define the problem of global registration of two volumes in medical imaging. Why is it important to refine global registration of multimodality medical images by local mapping and registration?

12.2. Describe the affine transformation for global image registration.

12.3. Derive mathematical expressions for the affine transformation for mapping the (x, y, z) coordinate system volume to the (x', y', z') coordinate system volume using at least using three different orders of operations. Are the final expressions same? If not, explain why.

12.4. How is a mapping relationship obtained from the eigenvalues of the rotation matrix?

12.5. What are the basic differences between the rigid-body and elastic transformation-based approaches for image registration?

12.6. Write and explain a mathematical expression for determining the displacement vector field for elastic deformation.

12.7. What are the different approaches used for external and internal landmark-based image registration?

12.8. In the MATLAB environment, extract CT images of the human brain. Using the distortion algorithm with rotation and scaling operations, obtain a second set of distorted CT images. Now use the original and distorted CT brain images for volume segmentation under the skull. Using the centroids and principal axes, apply the affine transformation to map-distorted images to the original brain images. Reslice the registered and original data sets for the three oblique cross-sections. Subtract the registered cross-section images from the respective original images to obtain residual images. Do residual images contain all zeros? Comment on the nonzero values of the residual images.

12.9. Repeat Exercise 8 for MR brain images.

12.10. Repeat Exercise 8 for PET brain images.

12.11. Register an MR brain image data set with a PET image data set of the same patient as identified in the MATLAB image database. After registration, segment the corresponding cross-section images of the registered MR and PET data sets. Use boundary detection methods to outline the ventricles and skull regions in all images. Superimpose the respective registered, segmented MR and PET images using different colors. Are the boundary segments from the respective MR and PET images aligned with each other? Comment on the registration of MR PET images with the analysis of respective boundary segment alignment.

12.7. REFERENCES

1. H. Damasio and R. Frank, "Three-dimensional in vivo mapping of brain lesions in humans," *Arch. Neurol.*, Vol. 49, pp. 137–143, 1992.
2. P.E. Roland and K. Ziles, "Brain atlases—A new research tool," *Trends Neurosci.*, Vol. 17, pp. 15–24, 1994.
3. M. Sonka, S.K. Tadikonda, and S.M. Collins, "Knowledge-based interpretation of MR brain images," *IEEE Trans. Med. Imaging*, Vol. 15, pp. 443–452, 1996.
4. K.R. Smith, K. Joarder, R.D. Bucholtz, and K.R. Smith, "Multimodality image analysis and display methods for improved tumor localization in stereotactic neurosurgery," *Proc. Annu. Int. Conf. IEEE EMBS*, Vol. 13, No. 1, p. 210, 1991.
5. A.C. Evans, C. Bell, S. Marrett, C.J. Thomson, and A. Hakim, "Anatomical-functional correlation using an adjustable MRI-based region of interest atlas with positron emission tomography," *J. Cereb. Blood Flow Metab.*, Vol. 8, No. 4, pp. 513–530, 1988.

6. A.C. Evans, S. Marrett, J. Torrescorzo, S. Ku, and L. Collins, "MRI-PET correlation in three dimensions using a volume-of-interest (VOI) atlas," *J. Cereb. Blood Flow Metab.*, Vol. 11, No. 1, pp. A69–A78, 1991.
7. M. Bergstrom, J. Boethius, L. Erikson, T. Greitz, T. Ribble, and L. Widen, "Head fixation device for reproducible position alignment in transmission CT and positron emission tomography," *J. Comput. Assist. Tomogr.*, Vol. 5, pp. 136–141, 1981.
8. P.T. Fox, J.S. Perlmutter, and M.E. Raichle, "A stereotactic method of anatomical localization for positron emission tomography," *J. Comput. Assist. Tomogr.*, Vol. 9, No. 1, pp. 141–153, 1985.
9. V. Bettinardi, R. Scardaoni, M.C. Gilardi, G. Rizzo, D. Perani, G. Striano, F. Triulzi, and F. Fazio, "Head holder for PET, CT, and MR studies," *J. Comput. Assist. Tomogr.*, Vol. 15, No. 5, pp. 886–892, 1991.
10. A.V. Levy, J.D. Brodie, J.A.G. Russell, N. D. Volkow, E. Laska, and A.P. Wolf, "The metabolic centroid method for PET brain image analysis," *J. Cereb. Blood Flow Metab.*, Vol. 9, pp. 388–397, 1989.
11. A.V. Levy, E. Laska, J.D. Brodie, N.D. Volkow, and A.P. Wolf, "The spectral signature method for the analysis of PET brain images," *J. Cereb. Blood Flow Metab.*, Vol. 11, pp. A103-A113, 1991.
12. N.M. Alpert, J.F. Bradshaw, D. Kennedy, and J.A. Correia, "The principal axes transformation: A method for image registration," *J. Nucl. Med.*, Vol. 31, No. 10, pp. 1717–1722, 1990.
13. A.V. Levy and D. Warrier, "A new composite phantom for accuracy testing of PET-MRI registration," Brookhaven National Laboratory Interim Report, Chemistry Dept., May 1992.
14. L.K. Arata, A.P. Dhawan, J.P. Broderick, M.F. Gaskil-Shipley, A. V. Levy, and N. D. Volkow, "Three-dimensional anatomical model-based segmentation of MR brain images through principal axes registration," *IEEE Trans. Biomed. Eng.*, Vol. 42, No. 11, pp. 1069–1078, 1995.
15. A.P. Dhawan, L.K. Arata, A.V. Levy, and J. Mentil, "Iterative principal axes registration method for analysis of MR-PET brain images," *IEEE Trans. Biomed. Eng.*, Vol. 42, No. 11, pp. 1079–1087, 1995.
16. C.A. Pelizzari, G.T.Y. Chen, D.R. Spelbring, R.R. Weichselbaum, and C. T. Chen, "Accurate three-dimensional registration of CT, PET and/or MR images of the brain," *J. Comput. Assist. Tomogr.*, Vol. 13, No. 1, pp. 20–26, 1989.
17. D.N. Levin, C.A. Pelizzari, G.T.Y. Chen, C.T. Chen, and M.D. Cooper, "Retrospective geometric correlation of MR, CT, and PET images," *Radiology*, Vol. 169, pp. 601–611, 1988.
18. P. Thomson and A.W. Toga, "A surface based technique for warping three-dimensional images of the brain," *IEEE Trans. Med. Imaging*, Vol. 15, pp. 402–417, 1996.
19. C.A. Davatzikos, J.L. Prince, and R.N. Bryan, "Image registration based on boundary mapping," *IEEE Trans. Med. Imaging*, Vol. 15, pp. 112–115, 1996.
20. A. Toga, *Brain Warping*, Academic Publishers, San Diego, CA, 1999.
21. S.P. Raya and J.K. Udupa, "Shape-based interpolation of multi-dimensional objects," *IEEE Trans. Med. Imaging*, Vol. 9, No. 1, pp. 32–42, 1990.
22. H. Goldstein, *Classical Mechanics*, Addison-Wesley, Reading, MA, 1980.
23. J.C. Gee, L. LeBriquer, C. Barillot, and D.R. Haynor, "Probabilistic matching of brain images," Tech. Rep. IRCS Report 95-07, The Institute for Research in Cognitive Science, April 1995.
24. J.C. Gee, L. LeBriquer, C. Barillot, D.R. Haynor, and R. Bajcsy, "Bayesian approach to the brain image matching problem," Tech Rep. IRCS Report 95-08, The Institute for Research in Cognitive Science, April 1995.
25. R. Bajcsy and S. Kovacic, "Multiresolution elastic matching," *Comput. Vis. Graph. Image Process.*, Vol. 46, No. 1, pp. 1–21, 1989.
26. D.L. Collins, T.M. Peters, and A.C. Evans, "An automated 3D non-linear image deformation procedure for determination of gross morphometric variability in human brain," *Visualization Biomed. Comput.*, SPIE Proceedings, Vol. 2359, SPIE Press, Bellingham, WA, pp. 180–190, 1994.
27. D. Terzopoulos and K. Fleischer, "Modelling inelastic deformation: Viscoelasticity, plasticity fracture," *Comput. Graph.*, Vol. 22, No. 4, pp. 269–278, 1988.
28. R. Dann, J. Holford, S. Kovacic, M. Reivich, and R. Bajcsy, "Three dimensional computerized brain atlas for elastic matching: Creation, initial evaluation," *Proc. SPIE*, Vol. 914, pp. 600–612, 1988.
29. J.C. Gee, M. Reivich, L. Bilaniuk, D. Hackney, and R. Zimmerman, "Evaluation of multiresolution elastic matching using MRI data," *Med. Imaging V: Image Process.*, Vol. 1445, pp. 226–234, 1991.

30. M.I. Miller, G.E. Christensen, Y. Amit, and U. Gerander, "Mathematical textbook of deformable neuroanatomies," *Proc. Natl. Acad. Sci. USA*, Vol. 90, pp. 11944–11948, 1993.
31. K.J. Friston, J. Ashburner, C.D. Frith, J.B. Poline, J.D. Heather, and R.S.J. Frackowiak, "Spatial registration, normalization of images," *Hum. Brain Mapp.*, Vol. 2, pp. 1–25, 1995.
32. Y. Gem, M. Fitzpatrick, B.M. Dawant, J. Bao, R.M. Kessler, and R. A. Margolin, "Accurate localization of cortical convolution in MR brain images," *IEEE Trans. Med. Imaging*, Vol. 15, pp. 418–428, 1996.
33. M. Ferrant, A. Nabavi, B. Macq, F.A. Jolsez, R. Kikinis, and S.K. Warfield, "Registration of 3-D intraoperative MR images of the brain using a finite element biomechanical model," *IEEE Trans. Med. Imaging*, Vol. 20, pp. 1384–1297, 2001.
34. K. Rohr, H.S. Stiehl, R. Sprengel, T.M. Buzug, J. Wesse, and M. H. Kahn, "Landmark based elastic registration using approximating thin-plate splines," *IEEE Trans. Med. Imaging*, Vol. 20, pp. 526–534, 2001.
35. G.E. Christensen and H.J. Johnson, "Consistent image registration," *IEEE Trans. Med. Imaging*, Vol. 20, pp. 568–582, 2001.
36. J. Park, A.A. Young, and L. Axel, "Deformable models with parameter functions for cardiac motion analysis from tagged MRI data," *IEEE Trans. Med. Imaging*, Vol. 15, pp. 278–289, 1996.
37. R.J. Althof, M.G.J. Wind, and J.T. Dobbins, "A rapid automatic image registration algorithm with subpixel accuracy," *IEEE Trans. Med. Imaging*, Vol. 16, pp. 308–316, 1997.
38. Y. Sato, M. Nakamoto, Y. Tamaki, T. Sasama, I. Sakita, Y. Nakajima, M. Monden, and S. Tamura, "Image guidance of breast cancer surgery using 3-D ultrasound images and augmented reality visualization," *IEEE Trans. Med. Imaging*, Vol. 17, pp. 681–693, 1998.
39. J.L. Herring, B.M. Dawant, C.R. Maurer, D.M. Muratore, R.L. Galloway, and J.M. Fitzpatrick, "Surface-based registration of CT images to physical space for image guided surgery of the spine," *IEEE Trans. Med. Imaging*, Vol. 17, pp. 743–752, 1998.
40. I. Bricault, G. Ferretti, and P. Cinquin, "Registration of real and CT derived virtual bronchoscopic images to assist transbronchial biopsy," *IEEE Trans. Med. Imaging*, Vol. 17, pp. 703–714, 1998.
41. J.M. Fitzpatrick, D.G. Hill, and C.R. Maurer, "Image registration," in M. Sonka and J.M. Fitzpatrick (Eds), *Handbook of Medical Imaging, Volume 2: Medical Image Processing and Analysis*, SPIE Press, Bellingham, 2000, pp. 447–514.
42. C.R. Maurer, G.B. Aboutanos, B.M. Dawant, R.J. Maciunas, and J. M. Fitzpatrick, "Registration of 3-D images using weighted geometrical features," *IEEE Trans. Med. Imaging*, Vol. 15, pp. 836–849, 1996.

CHAPTER 13

IMAGE VISUALIZATION

Visualization is an important aspect of human understanding of objects and structures. Visualization has always been an active field of research in computer image processing and graphics. In medical imaging, the visualization of internal physiological structures is the fundamental objective. However, visualization methods in medical imaging go far beyond the two-dimensional (2-D) and three-dimensional (3-D) imaging techniques. The visual observations in multidimensional medical imaging are often augmented by quantitative measurements and analysis for better understanding. Often the features extracted from analysis of medical images are incorporated in the visualization methods. For example, boundaries of a brain tumor can be superimposed on a 2-D brain image for better visualization of its local position and geometrical structure.

Recent advances in computing hardware and software capabilities have allowed the multidimensional visualization methods to incorporate multilayered representations of surface and volume structures in an interactive manner (1–5). Such methods have been found to be very useful in multimodality image fusion and visualization, allowing for better understanding of physiological structures as applied in diagnostic and intervention protocols including image-guided surgery (3–8). More recently, the multilayered image representation and visualization methods have led to a virtual reality (VR) experience where internal structures can be interactively explored, mapped, and visualized. VR provides an interactive human–computer interface that facilitates the visualization of 3-D computer-generated scenes (3). For example, virtual endoscopy has demonstrated a new role in the surgical planning system, providing adjunctive diagnostic and treatment interventional capabilities (3).

Multidimensional medical image visualization methods can be broadly categorized into four groups:

1. Feature enhanced 2-D image display methods
2. Stereo vision and semi 3-D display methods
3. Surface- and volume-based 3-D display methods
4. Interactive VR visualization methods

Medical Image Analysis, Second Edition, by Atam P. Dhawan
Copyright © 2011 by the Institute of Electrical and Electronics Engineers, Inc.

13.1. FEATURE-ENHANCED 2-D IMAGE DISPLAY METHODS

In the simplest form, 2-D gray-level images can be visualized using an appropriate medium such as radiological films (that can be put on a light box for better visualization), hard copy prints or photographs, and computer display devices. Using computerized processing, 3-D images can be visualized as a collection or stack of 2-D images that are acquired as cross-sectional images along a selected axis. For example, Figure 12.7 in Chapter 12 shows 2-D serial cross-sectional images of 3-D MR and positron emission tomography (PET) brain image data sets (7). Such a method is essentially a 2-D visualization. Specific features of an image such as edges or segmented regions can be superimposed on the same or a corresponding cross-sectional image from a different modality. Figure 9.7 shows a combined visualization of the registered magnetic resonance (MR) and PET brain images (7). In this visualization, the intensity of the combined MR–PET images is obtained from the MR images, but the color is coded using the gray values (glucose metabolism) of the corresponding PET images. The color representation can be directly mapped from the gray value histogram of the PET images. The histogram can be linearly scaled into blue (lowest partition representing low metabolism), green (middle partition representing medium metabolism), and red (highest partition representing the highest metabolism).

Figure 13.1 shows another example of a 2-D multimodality image visualization of brain images (8). The top left image of Figure 13.1 shows a T_2-weighted MR brain image. A perfusion MR image of the corresponding cross-section of the brain is shown in the top right corner. Using the multiparameter adaptive image segmentation algorithm described in Chapter 9, the segmented MR brain image is shown in the bottom left corner with color-coded segmented regions. The segmented image is superimposed onto the perfusion MR image to visualize the vascular structure in the context of segmented brain regions.

13.2. STEREO VISION AND SEMI-3-D DISPLAY METHODS

Direct 3-D visualization methods such as stereo pairs with color- or polarization-coded depth perception have been investigated in medical imaging. Through the distribution of brightness, the observer can visualize or perceive the depth in the volumetric data. With stereoscopic visualization, two views of an object are created with different viewing angles using a binocular vision approximating the same geometry. The difference in viewing angle depends on the viewing and interocular distances. The depth perception depends on the brain's interpretation of the viewing distance. The digital subtraction angiogram (DSA) data have been integrated with 3-D MR images using stereoscopic techniques of image-guided surgery (9).

Other direct display methods include motion parallax, varifocal mirror system, rotating light-emitting diode system, and holography (9–12). With motion parallax, a selection of rendered images acquired on each side of the viewing angles is

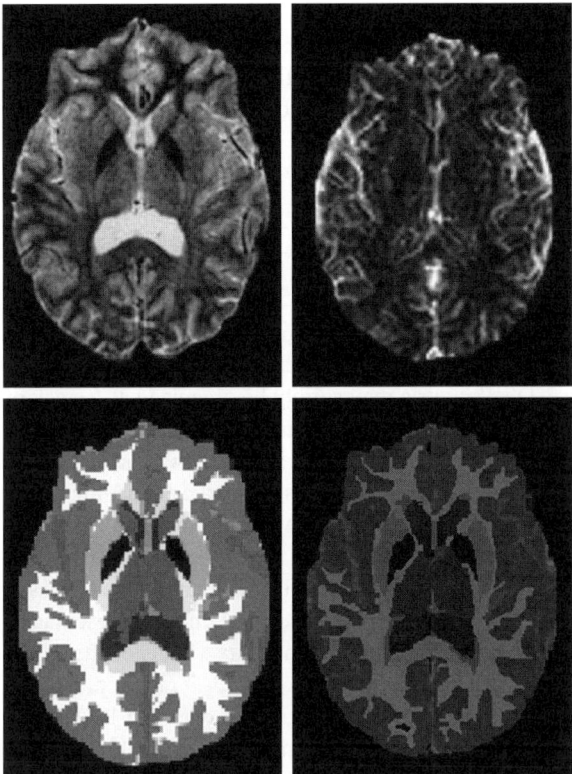

Figure 13.1 Top-left: A 2-D MR brain image; top-right: the registered MR perfusion image corresponding to the same slice position; bottom-left: the segmented MR brain image; bottom-right: superimposed perfusion image on the segmented MR brain image for composite visualization.

displayed in a sequence loop. The dithering about the central viewing axis provides the perception of depth and 3-D position. With specific hardware and numerical projection techniques, direct display methods can be used for visual interpretation to search for a desired region within the volumetric image. A more detailed visualization can then be performed in the regions of interest. A varifocal mirror system for 3-D display and analysis of tomographic volume images has been described in Harris (10). In the varifocal mirror-based display system, each plane of 3-D volumetric data is brought for visualization on a cathode ray tube (CRT) display, one at a time. The user sees the screen through a mirror reflection. The mirror is mounted in such a way that it can be moved through an assembly that is controlled by the user. As each plane of volumetric data is displayed, the mirror is displaced slightly. Thus, due to the displacement in the mirror position, the distance between the viewer's eye and display screen is changed, providing depth perception for 3-D visualization.

Holography has the potential to provide realistic 3-D displays that can be viewed from different directions (12). The best holograms are displayed using coherent light from a laser and high-resolution film. Holographic displays can also be displayed on a computer-controlled LCD monitor, but the resolution of such displays is not adequate for medical image visualization.

Although direct display methods provide interesting visualization for depth perception, they have little significance in diagnostic radiology dealing with tomographic images.

13.3. SURFACE- AND VOLUME-BASED 3-D DISPLAY METHODS

Three-dimensional volumetric data can be obtained from a 3-D medical imaging modality such as computed tomography (CT), magnetic resonance imaging (MRI), or PET. In many applications the 3-D volumetric may simply be organized as a stack of serial sections that are 2-D images of a 3-D object along a specific axis. For example, the CT, MRI, and PET scanners can acquire serial 2-D images along a specific axis to cover the 3-D object. However, recent developments in medical imaging allow direct 3-D imaging to produce 3-D volumetric data. In the representation of 3-D volumetric data in the rectangular coordinate system, a voxel is defined as a 3-D element or data point at the location (x, y, z). The visualization methods map the voxel-based 3-D representation of the volumetric data onto a pixel-based 2-D image representation that is displayed on a computer monitor. The mapped intensity values of the pixels in the image provide a visualization of a specific view of the 3-D object present in the volumetric data. The methods to visualize the volumetric data can be broadly classified into two categories: surface rendering or volume rendering methods.

In the surface rendering methods, the gray-level-based 3-D data is first converted into a binary volume representation. The 3-D binary volume is then searched for the boundary voxels that are interpolated to render a specific geometrical primitive-based 3-D surface. A surface is defined by the region that contains the boundary voxels or where the binary volume changes from the value "0" (background) to the value "1" (object). The rendered surface is shown in the image for visualization. Thus, the surface rendering-based visualization shows the geometrical shape of the surface of the object but with a loss of structural details within the volume. Usually, such visualization methods are useful in understanding the geometrical shape of the object and its variation within a group or with respect to an anatomical atlas. The binary volume-based surface visualization methods are also useful in image registration as described in Chapter 12.

Volume-rendering methods allow visualization of the structural variations within the 3-D volumetric data. A common method used in volume-rendering methods is ray tracing. In the simplest form of volumetric ray tracing, a uniform light source is placed behind the voxels of the volumetric data. For each straight-line-based ray from the light source to the corresponding point (pixel) in the image plane of the display screen, the density values and location of the voxels in the path of the ray are used to calculate the intensity value of the pixel in the corresponding image. Such a volume visualization method is based on the computed projection of the object onto the image plane with weighted intensity values based on the density and locations of the voxels along the respective rays. Using the location information of the voxels of the registered volumetric data, depth-dependent shading methods can be used to modify the intensity or color values of the image for better visualization (13–21).

13.3.1 Surface Visualization

The primary objective of surface display is to present 3-D shape information efficiently. The surface is first identified in terms of regions either manually or semi-automatically using a computer algorithm. The extracted regions are then represented as a set of contours or as a surface that reflects light from an imaginary light source (12–15). The output of the latter process is displayed through a 2-D frame buffer using the monocular depth cues of shading and motion parallax (rotation) to provide a visual interpretation of depth and shape. The surface displays provide a tool for analyzing shapes and spatial relationships through the aid of visual cues such as perspective, shading, and shadowing.

Let $f(x, y, z)$ represent a point or voxel location (x, y, z) in the 3-D volume data. A binary representation $f_b(x, y, z)$ of the 3-D volume data $f(x, y, z)$ can be obtained through a binary segmentation transform T such that

$$f_b(x,y,z) = T[f(x,y,z)] = 1 \quad \text{if } f(x,y,z) \in R$$
$$= 0 \quad \text{otherwise} \quad (13.1)$$

where R represents the range of gray values such that voxels with gray values in R belong to the object to be visualized.

Once a voxel model is obtained through the segmentation, boundary voxels are determined for surface rendering. Boundary detection algorithms search for the voxels that are connected and at the edge of the binary volume. The connectivity can be defined by setting up an adjacency criterion. For example, an 8-connected adjacency criterion can be used to identify the voxels that are adjacent to each other within a given plane. Two voxels v_1 and v_2 at locations, respectively, (x_1, y_1, z_1) and (x_2, y_2, z_2) are connected through the 8-connected adjacency criterion if

$$\text{either} \quad |x_1 - x_2| = 1 \quad \text{or} \quad |y_1 - y_2| \quad \text{and} \quad z_1 = z_2 \quad (13.2)$$

For example, Figure 13.2a shows four voxels: r, s, t, and u. The voxels r and t are adjacent to the voxel s but none is adjacent to the voxel u. Figure 13.2b shows a contour of the adjacent voxels belonging to the same z-plane. It can be noted that an 8-connected contour has at least three connected voxels that are closed, and none of the voxels are identical.

The boundary voxels are sometimes referred to points for rendering the surface for visualization. A contour is defined as the ordered sequence of boundary points. For surface visualization, the points or vertices on the boundary of the object can be sampled at random and therefore do not carry an ordered sequence. The surface is the region comprised of boundary voxels where the binary volume changes from the value "0" to "1". The simplest method of surface visualization is to connect the sampled points using the zero-order interpolation to define the faces, which are shared by voxels with differing values of the binary volume. Using a higher-order interpolation function between the sampled points, a smoother surface can be

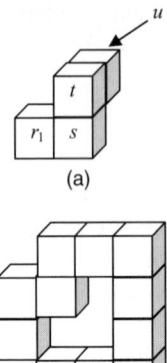

Figure 13.2 (a) Adjacent voxels r, s, and t with the 8-conneceted adjacency criterion. (b) A contour of adjacent voxels with the 8-conneceted adjacency criterion.

constructed. For example, B-splines can be used to define curved surfaces more efficiently (22, 23). Faces can also be defined through a mesh that is constructed around sampled points using a geometrical primitive to render surfaces. A mesh can be generated using a geometrical primitive such as a square or triangle (1, 2, 21). Thus, a surface visualization method connects a set of sampled points or vertices on the boundary of the object using an interpolation function or a geometrical primitive. To improve visual effects, a predefined scalar parameter such as color or brightness can be assigned to the face regions of the surface. When a continuous interpolation function is used, an iso-valued surface (or simply an iso-surface) can be defined by using a single value of the predefined scalar parameter (24–27).

If the sample points are centered at the voxels of the rendering surface, the surface passes through the sampled points and thus the zero-order interpolation method is required. However, if the voxels of the rendering surface are not centered at the sampled points of the volumetric data set (as is the case for rendering a smoother surface with higher resolution), a higher-order interpolation method is required to determine the values of a predefined scalar parameter of the voxels. Although there are a number of interpolation methods used in medical image visualization, a trilinear interpolation method, one of the most commonly used in visualization, is described here. It is the 3-D version of the popular 2-D bilinear interpolation method.

Let A, B, C, D, E, F, G, and H represent the sampled points at vertices of a hexahedron cell $ABCDEFGH$ with known values, V_a, V_b, V_c, V_d, V_e, V_f, V_g, and V_h (Fig. 13.3). Assuming the unit dimensions of the hexahedron along each direction, a value V_p of a point P at the location (x_p, y_p, z_p) inside the hexahedron can be computed linearly using the trilinear interpolation method as

$$V_p = V_a(1-x_p)(1-y_p)(1-z_p) + V_b x_p(1-y_p)(1-z_p) + \\ V_c(1-x_p)y_p(1-z_p) + V_d x_p y_p(1-z_p) + V_e(1-x_p)(1-y_p)z_p + \\ V_f x_p(1-y_p)z_p + V_g(1-x_p)y_p z_p + V_h x_p y_p z_p \quad (13.3)$$

13.3. SURFACE- AND VOLUME-BASED 3-D DISPLAY METHODS

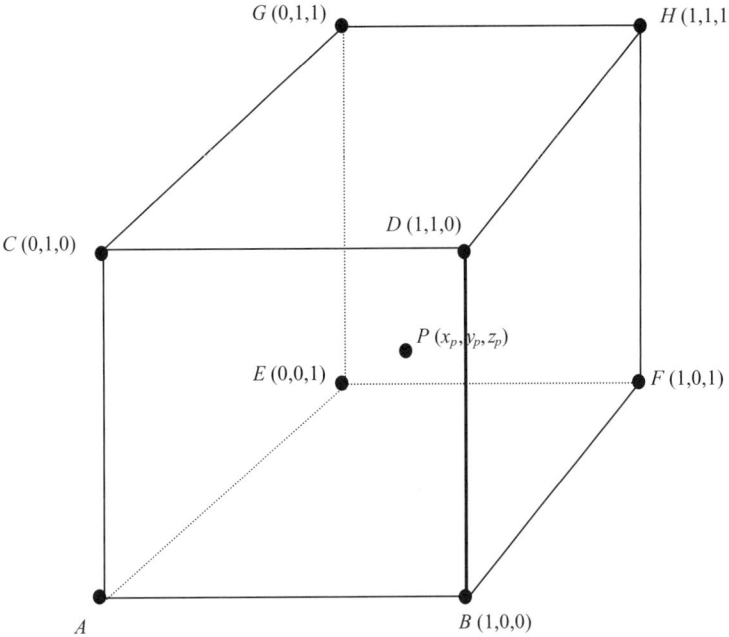

Figure 13.3 A schematic diagram of hexahedron-based sample points for trilinear interpolation method.

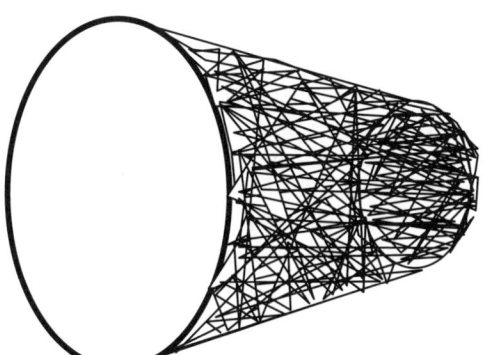

Figure 13.4 An example of rendering a mesh with triangles for surface visualization.

An example of rendering a mesh with triangles for surface visualization is shown in Figure 13.4.

Meshes generated using the sampled points in the volumetric data can be used to render iso-surfaces for visualization. A contour is defined in the 2-D space by the line path on which the value of a scalar parameter is constant. An iso-surface is the 3-D surface representing the locations of a constant scalar parameter within the volumetric data. The scalar parameter can be a raw property of the data (e.g., brightness) or a computed feature such as gradient or texture.

342 CHAPTER 13 IMAGE VISUALIZATION

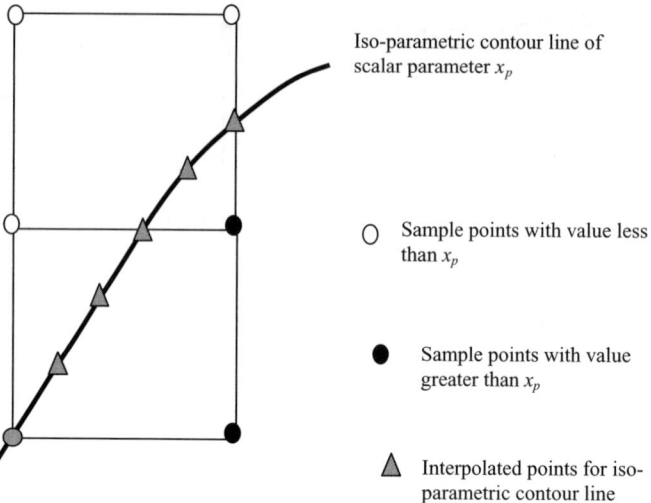

Figure 13.5 An iso-parametric contour line passing through square cells of sample points.

To compute the iso-parameteric contour line, a contour or line segment is first identified with the value of the associated scalar parameter. This can be done by setting up a look-up table of the neighboring sample points with similar values of the associated scalar parameter. Each entry in the look-up table is then followed up to define the iso-parametric contour lines. When following along the iso-parametric contour, if the value of the next sample point is the same as that of the previous point, the iso-parametric contour line is extended to include the new sample point. To improve the accuracy of the location of the iso-parametric contour lines, an interpolation function is usually required within a predefined cell of sampled points. Generally, the iso-parametric contour lines in the 2-D space are computed using a cell such as a square of vertices or sampled points. If all vertices of the cell have the values of the scalar parameter below or above the predefined value of the iso-parametric contour line, none of the vertices can be included to extend the iso-parametric contour line. If one vertex has a lower value and another has a value higher than the scalar value of the contour line, an interpolation function such as bilinear interpolation is required to determine the path of the iso-parametric contour line. As shown in Figure 13.5, additional vertices can be computed using bilinear interpolation methods to determine the path of the iso-parametric contour line between the sampled points.

Similar to the concept of the iso-parametric contour lines in the 2-D space, iso-surfaces can be computed within the 3-D volumetric data. As stated above, iso-surfaces represent the 3-D surfaces of constant values of the scalar parameter. The interpolation function required for determining iso-surfaces must interpolate in the 3-D space using a 3-D cell that may be shaped as a hexahedron or any other polygon depending on the mesh representation. If a hexahedron is used as a cell element, the eight vertices or sample points of each cell in the entire volume are searched to generate the iso-surfaces. A trilinear method (as described in Eq. 13.3) can be used as needed for interpolation to determine the path of the iso-surface. A general algorithm of generating iso-surfaces using the cubical cells in the volume is known as the "marching cube" algorithm (18). Other variants of the marching cube algorithm, such as the dividing cube algorithm, have been developed to speed up the iso-surface generation in large volumetric data sets (2). In the dividing cube algorithm, the search for the cells contributing to the iso-surface is accelerated by using a hierarchical structure of volume elements. The data is first organized using large-sized volume elements (voxels). Thus the entire volume can be searched quickly to focus the algorithm in the specific subvolumes containing the iso-surface. The subvolumes are then divided into subvoxels to improve the resolution and localization of the iso-surface.

The derivates of the volumetric data can be used to determine principal curvature direction and values to determine iso-surface directly from the voxel data (25, 26). Let C represent a curve with tangent vector t, along a section of the iso-surface S. The tangent relationship to the volume V can be expressed as

$$\nabla V \cdot t = 0 \qquad (13.4)$$

It should be noted that C is contained in a plane that contains the surface normal n. It can be shown that (25)

$$t' H t + \nabla V \cdot k n = 0 \qquad (13.5)$$

where k represents the normal curvature of C, which is the surface curvature in the direction t, and $H(V)$ is the Hessian of V as

$$H(V) = \begin{bmatrix} V_{xx} & V_{xy} & V_{xz} \\ V_{xy} & V_{yy} & V_{yz} \\ V_{xz} & V_{yz} & V_{zz} \end{bmatrix}. \qquad (13.6)$$

The principal curvatures can be obtained by optimizing k over all possible directions of t using Equation 13.5 as

$$k = -\frac{t' H t}{\|\nabla V\|}. \qquad (13.7)$$

In 3-D surface display methods, the intensity at a point to be displayed is determined using a predefined criterion such as a function of the distance between the point and the viewer or the gradient of the surface at that point. The intensity and shading of the pixels associated with the display of the rendered surface help to provide visual cues for easy 3-D perception. Color mapping can be used to help feature visualization associated with the rendered surfaces.

Figure 13.6 shows an iso-surface visualization of the brain cortical convolutions computed from MR volumetric data. Figure 13.7 shows a 3-D composite visualization of ventricles extracted and registered from brain MRI volumetric data sets of 16 subjects. Figure 13.7b shows four rotated views of the color-rendered visualization of the spatial probability distribution of the composite 3-D ventricle model. The red areas represent the minimum probability value (1/16), while the white areas indicate the maximum probability value of 1.0 (6).

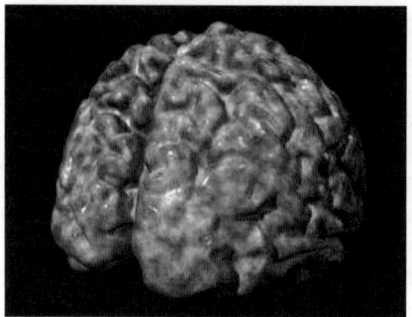

Figure 13.6   The iso-surface visualization of cortical convolutions of the human brain computed from the MRI brain volumetric data.

13.3.2   Volume Visualization

Volume rendering provides visualization of a 3-D volume through a 2-D image. Volume rendering can be implemented using an object order, image order, or a hybrid combination of these two methods (2). In object order-based volume rendering methods, an image is produced by projecting voxels of the volumetric data onto the image plane. This method is also called the forward mapping method to map volume data onto the image plane for visualization. The difficulty with this method is the likelihood of many-to-one mapping to cause ambiguous visualization. If voxels are projected onto the image plane using an arbitrary selection criterion, it is possible that two or more voxels can be mapped to the same pixel in the image. To avoid this, the voxels should be projected using one plane at a time in a sequential manner. Thus, the projections are computed slice-by-slice within the volume and row-by-row within a slice. With the mapping, distance information corresponding to the pixels in the image plane can be used to create depth information for visualization. The depth values thus obtained are used for computing 2-D discrete shading effects in the visualized image. The shading in the image can also be computed by using a combination of the 2-D depth and surface gradient information. In such methods, the 2-D depth information is passed through a gradient operator to account for the surface orientation and the distance between voxels and the light source placed in the image plane. A gradient vector at each pixel location is then estimated and used as a normal vector for computing shading and intensity values in the image for visualization.

The gradient value at a pixel location (x, y) in the image can be expressed as (2)

$$\nabla z = \left(\frac{\delta z}{\delta x}, \frac{\delta z}{\delta y}, 1 \right) \quad (13.8)$$

where $z = D(x, y)$ is the depth associated with the pixel (x, y).

In the image-order methods, a backward mapping is implemented through tracing the rays from pixels in the image to the volume data for visualization. For each pixel in the image plane, a ray is defined originating from that pixel to intersect with the objects and surfaces within the volumetric data. Two types of ray

13.3. SURFACE- AND VOLUME-BASED 3-D DISPLAY METHODS

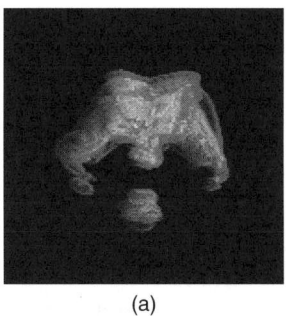

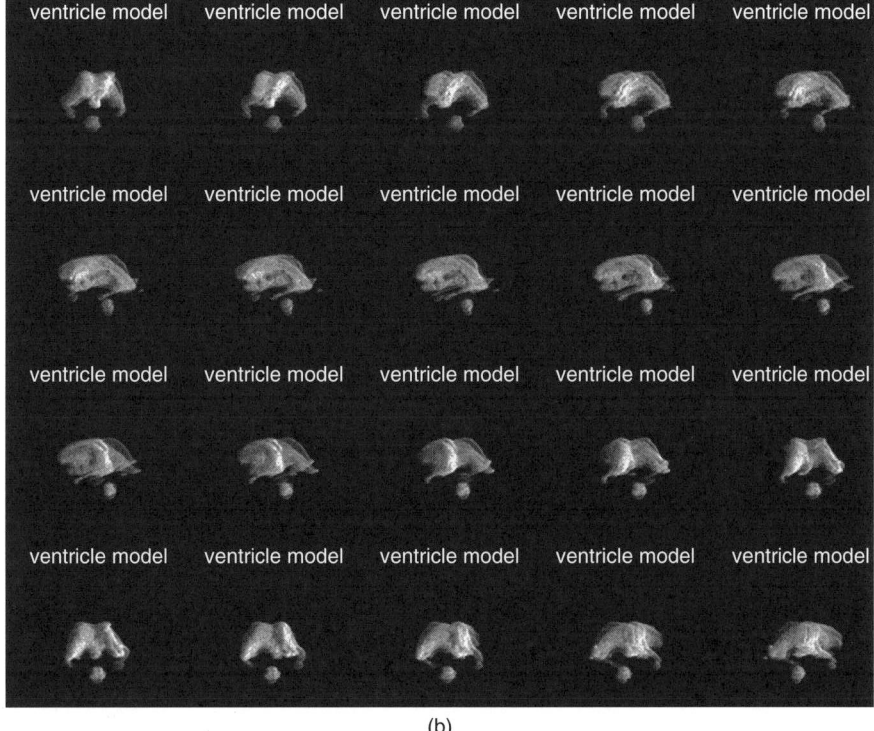

Figure 13.7 (a) Three dimensional visualization of a composite ventricle model computed from the MRI brain volumetric data of 16 subjects. (b) Four rotated views of the 3-D ventricle model.

geometries can be used: parallel beam and divergent beam. In parallel geometry, all rays are parallel to the viewing direction providing parallel projections. In divergent beam geometry, perspective projections are obtained using the rays that are cast from the eye point according to the viewing direction and the field of view (1, 2). Shading is performed at the intersections of the rays and surfaces within the volume. For each intersection, the intensity of the ray is computed using attenuation and reflection parameters for structural and shading representations. In general, the intensity of the ray from the eye point, through pixels in the image plane, and onto the volume can be expressed by

$$I = \int_{t_1}^{t_2} e^{-\tau \int_{t_1}^{t} \rho^\gamma(\lambda) d\lambda} \rho^\lambda(t)\, dt \tag{13.9}$$

where t is the location of the ray that is transversed from t_1 to t_2, $\rho^\gamma(t)$ is the accumulated density function at the location t, τ is the attenuation parameter, and γ is the parameter that controls the diffusion.

The volume visualization can also be implemented using a cell-by-cell processing method (21). In this method, each cell in the volume is traced using a ray in front-to-back order. The ray tracing and possessing starts with the plane closest to the viewpoint and continues toward the back in a plane-by-plane manner. Within each plane, the cell closed to the viewpoint is processed first. Thus the cells with the longest distance from the viewpoint are processed last. A scan line is established in the image plane to determine the pixels affected by the cell. The shading equation providing the perceived intensity $I(\lambda)$ as a function of wavelength λ can be expressed as (2)

$$I(\lambda) = \iiint_{x\,y\,z} \left[\tau(d) O(s) \left[K_a(\lambda) I_a + K_d(\lambda, M) \sum [(N \cdot L_j) I_j] \right] + (1 - \tau(d)) b(\lambda)) \right] dx\, dy\, dz \tag{13.10}$$

where I_a is the ambient intensity; $\tau(d)$ is the attenuation as a function of distance d; $O(s)$ is the opacity transfer parameter as a function of the scalar parameter s; K_a and K_d are, respectively, the ambient and diffusion coefficients; M is another parameter, such as texture, modeled to affect the diffusion; N is the normal computed from the local gradient; L_j is the position vector to the jth light source; I_j is the intensity of the jth light source; and $b(\lambda)$ is the background.

In the ray tracing method, the intensity of each ray is computed along with other parameters such as maximum value, the distance for the maximum value, and the center of gravity of the density emitters. These parameters can be used for specific color coordinates such as saturation, hue, and intensity to produce dramatic effects for color-based volume visualization. Figure 13.8 shows a volume

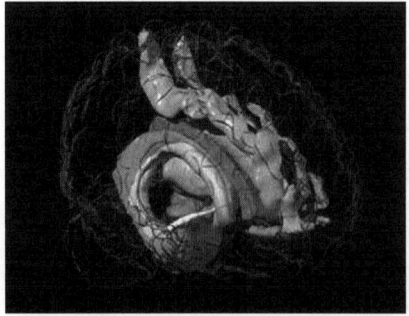

Figure 13.8 A volume visualization of MR brain volumetric data (http://www.bic.mni.mcgill.ca/).

visualization of brain structures. The density values of the cortical convolutions are assumed to be low so that the internal structures can be visualized through transparent layers.

Surface and volumetric visualization methods have been used to assist surgical planning, requiring the visualization of the location of tumors within the brain, radiation treatment planning, surgery, and other medical applications (27–37).

13.4. VR-BASED INTERACTIVE VISUALIZATION

Virtual reality is an advanced computer visualization technology that provides users with the ability to control the visualization volume. In the ideal software environment, VR allows a user to experience a synthetic world with visual scenes that mimic real-world situations. The VR environment may use extensive computer graphics, sounds, and images to reproduce electronic versions of real-world situations. In medical imaging applications, the current VR systems provide only visual experiences created by computer-assisted visualization and animation to walk through and feel the anatomical structures of an organ within a virtual human body.

From a historical perspective, a breakthrough in VR came with the development of a head-mounted display with two tiny stereoscopic screens positioned just a few inches in front of a viewer's eyes. The VR system designed by Jaron Lanier in 1989 featured a head-mounted display called the EyePhone (30, 31). Users also wear a DataGlove that generates movement and interaction in the virtual environment. The interaction and movements in the computerized virtual world or cyberspace are provided by moving the head, fingers, or entire hand through the appropriate input devices such as haptic gloves. The movements of gloves or other input devices directly control the optics in the field of vision to provide interaction and sensation in the virtual world.

The EyePhone uses a set of wide-angle optics that cover approximately 140 degrees, almost the entire horizontal field of view (31). As the user moves his or her head to look around, the images shift to create an illusion of movement. The user moves while the virtual world is standing still. The glasses also sense the user's facial expressions through embedded sensors, and that information can control the virtual version of the user's body. For example, the DataGlove, a key interface device, uses position-tracking sensors and fiber optic strands running down each finger, allowing the user to manipulate objects that exist only within the computer-simulated environment (30, 31). When the computer "senses" that the user's hand is touching a virtual object, the user "feels" the virtual object (30, 31). In VR-based systems, the user can pick up an object and do things with it just as he or she would do with a real object. VR systems have been successfully used in many simulator applications such as flying aircraft, controlling spacecrafts, and navigating and repairing instruments in space.

Recent developments in computer technology and sensory input devices have enabled VR technology to have potential use in diagnostic radiology for patient-specific dynamic interactive visualization. However, the computational issues to deal with large data sets and the complexity of physiological structures and responses

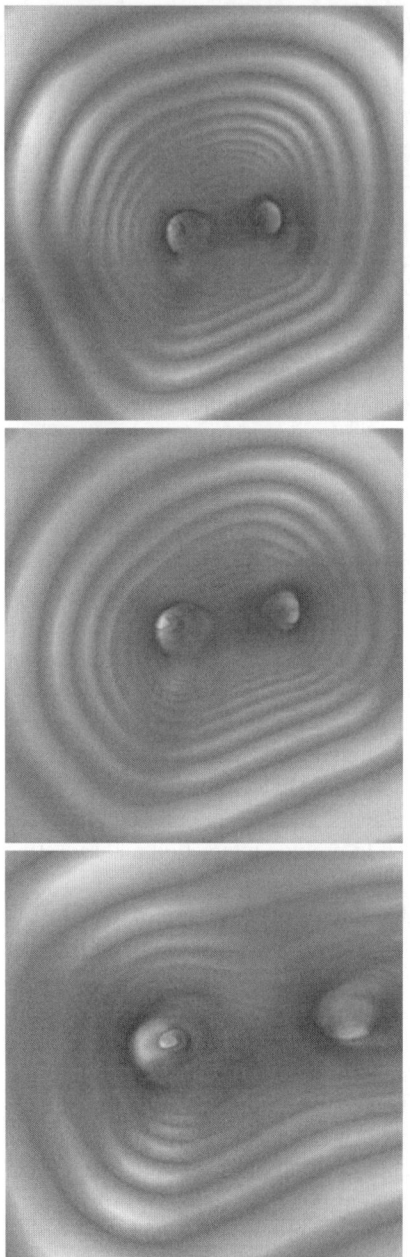

Figure 13.9 A sequence of volume-rendered images along the path through the central axis of the bronchial tube is used to produce a fly-through animation.

stjll remains as a major challenge. Recently, VR systems have been explored in medicine to simulate surgical procedures and facilitate image-guided surgery (32–34).

The major steps in developing VR-based interactive visualization are as follows:

1. Specific volumetric data sets from medical imaging scanners are segmented for regions and objects of interest.
2. Surfaces and volumes of interest are rendered in 3-D space to create sequences of 3-D scenes.
3. Specific geometrical and response models for interaction with 3-D scenes are developed and integrated with visualized data in the virtual reality modeling language (VRML) environment.
4. Interfaces to control the navigation and responses from the visual scenes are developed in the VRML environment using the appropriate input devices.
5. Navigation and interaction tutorials are developed to train the user to use the VR system.

13.4.1 Virtual Endoscopy

Recently, virtual endoscopy (VE) has been used for the visualization of bronchial airways (32, 33). The VR-based visualization technique provides a noninvasive way to examine the interior of the bronchial tubes. X-ray CT images are first segmented for airways using an adaptive thresholding method. The segmented images are used for volume rendering along the medial axis of the airways that is used as the path for animation.

The bronchial tube usually has two major skeleton branches and many smaller ones. The 3-D segmentation obtained by thresholding can provide several regional branches, making it difficult to determine a global axis through the medial axis transformation or skeletonization. A user interaction can be used to select the desired axis for fly-through animation using a VRML-based model (30). A ray-tracing method can be used with rays traveling from the user eye point into the structure for volume visualization. To visualize tube-like structures, the animation is directed toward the end of the tube. Figure 13.9 shows volume-rendered images of the bronchial tubes from a VR visualization (33).

13.5. EXERCISES

13.1. Why is 3-D visualization important in medical imaging? Explain your answer with the help of an example.

13.2. What are the different methods used in 3-D visualization in medical imaging?

13.3. What is the difference between the surface and volume visualization approaches? For brain imaging applications, which approach would you prefer and why?

13.4. What is the purpose of rendering a mesh in the volumetric data?

13.5. What type of polygon would you prefer for mesh rendering in MR brain data? Give reasons to support your answer.

13.6. What do you understand by the term iso-surface?

13.7. Explain an algorithm to generate iso-surfaces in the volumetric data. Can this algorithm be improved? If so, how would you improve the performance of this algorithm?

13.8. Why is shading important in visualization? How would you provide shading in iso-surface-based visualization of cortical structures from the MR brain volumetric data?

13.9. Segment the MR brain volumetric data for ventricles and cortical convolutions in the MATLAB environment. Display 2-D slice images in the MATLAB environment for the following

  a. Display the ventricles with boundaries outlined and superimposed on the respective 2-D slice images.

  b. Display the cortical convolutions with boundaries outlined and superimposed on the respective 2-D slice images.

13.10. Generate iso-surfaces from the MR brain volumetric data set used in Exercise 13.9. Display the extracted iso-surfaces as 2-D slice images.

13.11. Generate the 3-D iso-surface-based visualization of cortical structure segmented in Exercise 13.9. Explain the shading method used in the surface-rendered volume.

13.12. Change the opacity factor for the voxels corresponding to the cortical convolutions. Render a volume to visualize ventricles through the "see-through" cortical structure using the ray-tracing method. Comment on the quality of your visualization. How can you improve it?

13.6. REFERENCES

1. C. Bajaj (Ed.), *Data Visualization Techniques*, John Wiley and Sons, New York, 1999.
2. R.S. Gallagher (Ed.), *Computer Visualization*, CRC Press, Boca Raton, FL, 1995.
3. I.N. Bankman, *Handbook of Medical Imaging*, Academic Press, San Diego, CA, 2000.
4. A. Gueziec, "Extracting surface models of the anatomy from medical images," in M. Sonka and J.M. Fitzpatric (Eds), *Handbook of Medical Imaging*, Volume 2, SPIE Press, Bellingham, WA, 2000, pp. 343–398.
5. L.D. Harris, "Display of multidimensional biomedical image formation," in R.A. Robb (Ed.), *Three-Dimensional Biomedical Imaging*, Volume II, CRC Press, Boca Raton, FL, 1985, pp. 74–107.
6. L.K. Arata, A.P. Dhawan, J.P. Broderick, M.F. Gaskil-Shipley, A.V. Levy, and N.D. Volkow, "Three-dimensional anatomical model-based segmentation of MR brain images through principal axes registration," *IEEE Trans. Biomed. Eng.*, Vol. 42, No. 11, pp. 1069–1078, 1995.
7. A.P. Dhawan, L.K. Arata, A.V. Levy, and J. Mentil, "Iterative principal axes registration method for analysis of MR-PET brain images," *IEEE Trans. Biomed. Eng.*, Vol. 42, No. 11, pp. 1079–1087, 1995.
8. A. Zavaljevski, A.P. Dhawan, S. Holland, W. Ball, M. Giskill-Shipley, J. Johnson, and S. Dunn, "Multispectral MR brain image classification," *Comput. Med. Imaging Graph. Image Process.*, Vol. 24, pp. 87–98, 2000.

13.6. REFERENCES

9. T.M. Peters, C.J. Henri, P. Munger, A.M. Takahashi, A.C. Evans, B. Davey, and A. Olivier, "Integration of stereoscopic DSA and 3-D MRI for image-guided surgery," *Comput. Med. Imaging Graph.*, Vol. 18, pp. 289–299, 1994.
10. L.D. Harris, J.J. Camp, E.L. Ritman, and R.A. Robb, "Three-dimensional display and analysis of tomographic volume images utilizing a varifocal mirror," *IEEE Trans. Med. Imaging*, Vol. 5, pp. 67–73, 1986.
11. W. Simon, "A spinning mirror auto-stereoscopic display," *Proc. SPIE*, Vol. 120, pp. 180–185, 1977.
12. P. Greguss, "Holographic displays for computer assisted tomography," *J. Comput. Assist. Tomogr.*, Vol. 1, pp. 184–191, 1977.
13. G.T. Herman and H.K. Liu, "Three-dimensional display of human organs from computerized tomograms," *Comput. Graph. Image Proc.*, Vol. 9, pp. 1–9, 1979.
14. J.K. Udupa, "Display of 3D information in discrete 3D scenes produced by computerized tomography," *Proc. IEEE*, Vol. 71, pp. 420–431, 1983.
15. J.J. Udupa and R.J. Goncalves, "Imaging transform for visualizaing surfaces and volumes," *J. Digit. Imaging*, Vol. 6, pp. 213–236, 1993.
16. K.H. Hohne and R. Bomstein, "Shading 3D images from CT using gray-level gradients," *IEEE Trans. Med. Imaging*, Vol. MI-5, No. 1, p. 45, March 1986.
17. C.A. Pelizzari, G.T.Y. Chen, D.R. Spelbring, R.R. Weichselbaum, and C.T. Chen, "Accurate three-dimensional registration of CT, PET and/or MR images of the brain," *J. Comput. Assist. Tomogr.*, Vol. 13, No. 1, pp. 20–26, 1989.
18. W. Lorensen and H.E. Cline, "Marching cubes: A high resolution 3-D surface construction algorithm," *Proc. SIGGRAPH Comput. Graph.*, Vol. 21, pp. 163–169, 1987.
19. L. Axel, G.T. Herman, J.K. Udupa, P.A. Bottomley, and W.A. Edelstein, "Three-dimensional display of nuclear magnetic resonance (NMR) cardiovascular images," *J. Comput. Assist. Tomogr.*, Vol. 7, pp. 172–174, 1983.
20. P. Thomson and A.W. Toga, "A surface based technique for warping three-dimensional images of the brain," *IEEE Trans. Med. Imaging*, Vol. 15, pp. 402–417, 1996.
21. C. Upson and M. Keeler, "V-Buffer: Visible volume rendering," *Comput. Graph. Proc. SIGGRAPH*, pp. 59–64, 1988.
22. P. Dierckx, *Curves and Surface Fitting with Splines*, Oxford Science Publications, London, 1993.
23. T.M. Lehmann, C. Gonner, and K. Spitzer, "Addendum: B-spline interpolation in medical image processing," *IEEE Trans. Med. Imaging*, Vol. 20, pp. 660–665, 2001.
24. T.M. Lehmann, C. Gonner, and K. Spitzer, "Survey: Interpolation methods in medical image processing," *IEEE Trans. Med. Imaging*, Vol. 18, pp. 1049–1075, 1999.
25. O. Monga, S. Benayoun, and O. Faugeras, "Using third order derivatives to extract ridge lines in 3D images," Proceedings, IEEE Conference on Computer Vision and Pattern Recognition, Champaign, IL, IEEE Press, June 15–18, 1992.
26. J.P. Thirion and A. Gourdon, "Computing the differential characteristics of isointensity surfaces," *Comput. Vis. Image Underst.*, Vol. 61, pp. 190–202, 1995.
27. S.L. Hartmann and R.L. Galloway, "Depth buffer targeting for spatial accurate 3-D visualization of medical image," *IEEE Trans. Med. Imaging*, Vol. 19, pp. 1024–1031, 2000.
28. Y. Sato, M. Nakamoto, Y. Tamaki, T. Sasama, I. Sakita, Y. Nakajima, M. Monden, and S. Tamura, "Image guidance of breast cancer surgery using 3-D ultrasound images and augmented reality visualization," *IEEE Trans. Med. Imaging*, Vol. 17, pp. 681–693, 1998.
29. J.L. Herring, B.M. Dawant, C.R. Maurer, D.M. Muratore, R.L. Galloway, and J.M. Fitzpatrick, "Surface-based registration of CT images to physical space for image guided surgery of the spine," *IEEE Trans. Med. Imaging*, Vol. 17, pp. 743–752, 1998.
30. H. McLellan, "Virtual field trips: The Jason project," *VR World*, Vol. 3, pp. 49–50, 1995.
31. M. Fritz, "Eyephones, datasuits, and cyberspace," *CBT Dir.*, Vol. 28, pp. 11–17, (EJ 420 905), 1990.
32. I. Bricault, G. Ferretti, and P. Cinquin, "Registration of real and CT derived virtual bronchoscopic images to assist transbronchial biopsy," *IEEE Trans. Med. Imaging*, Vol. 17, pp. 703–714, 1998.
33. S. Loncaric and T. Markovinovic, "Web based virtual endoscopy," Proceedings, Medical Informatics Europe, Hannover, Germany, 2000.

34. J.Z. Turlington and W.E. Higgins, "New techniques for efficient sliding thin-slab volume visualization," *IEEE Trans. Med. Imaging*, Vol. 20, pp. 823–835, 2001.
35. P. St-Jean, A.F. Sadikot, L. Collins, D. Clonda, R. Kasrai, A.C. Evans, and T.M. Peters, "Automated atlas integration and interactive three-dimensional visualization tools for planning and guidance in functional neurosurgery," *IEEE Trans. Med. Imaging*, Vol. 17, pp. 672–680, 1998.
36. I. Bricault, G. Ferretti, and P. Cinquin, "Registration of real and CT-derived virtual bronchoscopic images to assist transbronchial biopsy," *IEEE Trans. Med. Imaging*, Vol. 17, pp. 703–714, 1998.
37. S. Cotin, H. Delingette, and N. Ayche, "Real-time elastic deformation of soft tissue for surgical simulations," *IEEE Trans. Vis. Comput. Graph.*, Vol. 5, pp. 62–73, 1999.

CHAPTER 14

CURRENT AND FUTURE TRENDS IN MEDICAL IMAGING AND IMAGE ANALYSIS

Recent advances in medical imaging modalities have laid the foundation for developing new methodologies to meet critical challenges in diagnostic radiology, treatment evaluation, and intervention protocols. The wide spectrum of multidisciplinary technologies that are being developed today and will continue in the future provides a better understanding of human physiology and critical diseases such as neurological disorders including Alzheimer's and Parkinson's.

14.1. MULTIPARAMETER MEDICAL IMAGING AND ANALYSIS

As described in Chapters 4–7, medical imaging modalities offer complementary information for the understanding of physiology and pathologies from molecular to organ levels. Current and future trends in functional magnetic resonance (fMR), diffusion MR, positron emission tomography (PET), ultrasound, and optical imaging are targeted toward obtaining molecular information from the cellular structure of tissue.

Future technological developments in multimodal molecular and cellular imaging should allow early detection of cellular/neurological deviations in critical diseases such as Alzheimer's, autism, or multiple sclerosis, before the first symptomatic signs. This is of great importance for better health care and prognosis. Current imaging paradigms rely on the expression of the first symptomatic signs, and then try to correlate, on an ad hoc basis, the observed signs with cellular and/or neurological deviations. The problem is that by the time the symptoms are expressed, the disease is probably already in a relatively advanced stage. Therefore, it is important that future imaging protocols are able to detect critical diseases in a presymptomatic stage for early diagnosis, treatment, evaluation, and intervention protocols.

Medical Image Analysis, Second Edition, by Atam P. Dhawan
Copyright © 2011 by the Institute of Electrical and Electronics Engineers, Inc.

Multimodality imaging and image registration have provided researchers and clinicians with important tools in diagnostic radiology. Multiparameter measurements are essential for the understanding and characterization of physiological processes. However, a multiparameter-based imaging protocol must optimize the data acquisition methods to acquire and analyze anatomical, metabolic, functional, and molecular signatures. It is important to study the variability associated with the respective structures to develop models that would further help to improve the imaging and image analysis protocols. Thus, continuous technological developments put new knowledge back into the learning cycle.

A generic paradigm for model-based medical imaging and image analysis is shown in Figure 14.1. As the computing, biochemical, and bioinstrumentation technologies continue to develop, future imaging modalities would be able to measure more parameters with higher spatial and temporal resolution. The last two decades have been largely focused on establishing the foundation of MR, single photon emission computed tomography (SPECT), PET, and ultrasound imaging modalities. Sophisticated imaging methods including perfusion, diffusion, and fMR and neuroreceptor-based fast PET have been developed to acquire more information about the physiological metabolism under specific functions (1–4). As shown in Figure 14.1, appropriate models of generalized physiological structures, imaging agents, and tissue-specific biochemical responses must be used to optimize the imaging protocols for structural and functional imaging. The model-based selection criteria would thus provide important information about the imaging parameters that can be used in a programmable way to intelligently control the imaging instrumentation. Once the data are acquired, variability models in generalized anatomical and metabolic structures can be used to improve feature selection, analysis, and interpretation.

Recent advances in MR imaging (MRI), functional MRI (fMRI), perfusion MRI (pMRI), and diffusion MRI (diffusion weighted imaging [DWI]/diffusion tensor imaging [DTI]) have provided the ability to study the functional and physiological behavior of the brain, allowing measurement of changes in blood flow and oxygenation levels for tissue characterization. While PET provides useful metabolic and receptor-site (pathophysiological) information, it lacks the ability to define anatomical details. MRI, on the other hand, provides high-resolution anatomical and physiological information. To study the physiological and functional aspects of the brain and tissue characterization, it would clearly be useful to combine PET, MRI, fMRI, pMRI, and DTI as a part of the postprocessing registration or, if possible, through simultaneous imaging.

Postprocessing image registration methods, although having the advantage of analyzing data off-line for mapping, suffer from uncertainties and errors in localization studies. This is primarily due to the small volume of interest defined for localization, limitations on resolution with different modalities, and computational inaccuracies in the postprocessing methods. For a given subject, the localized volume of interest may be small for a specific activation signal and may require submillimeter resolution. In addition, analysis of small localized volumes of interest may be needed for cellular characterization in understanding their physiological responses. Thus, accurate coregistration of the spatially distributed signals from different

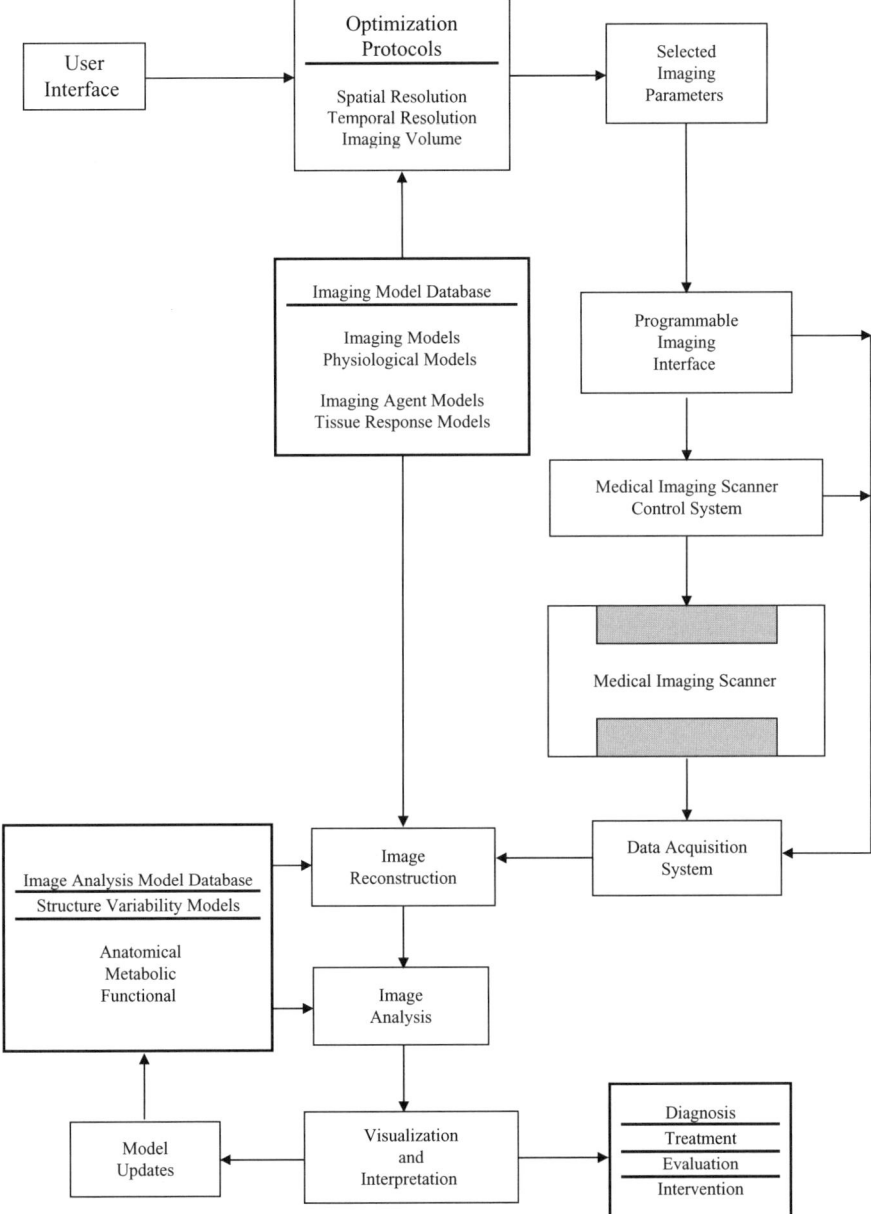

Figure 14.1 A multiparameter imaging and image analysis paradigm.

imaging modalities is an important requirement for studying physiological and functional behavior, specifically for neurological applications.

Current challenges in physiological and functional imaging include more robust and accurate imaging of cardiac motion, tissue-specific tumor imaging, and fast

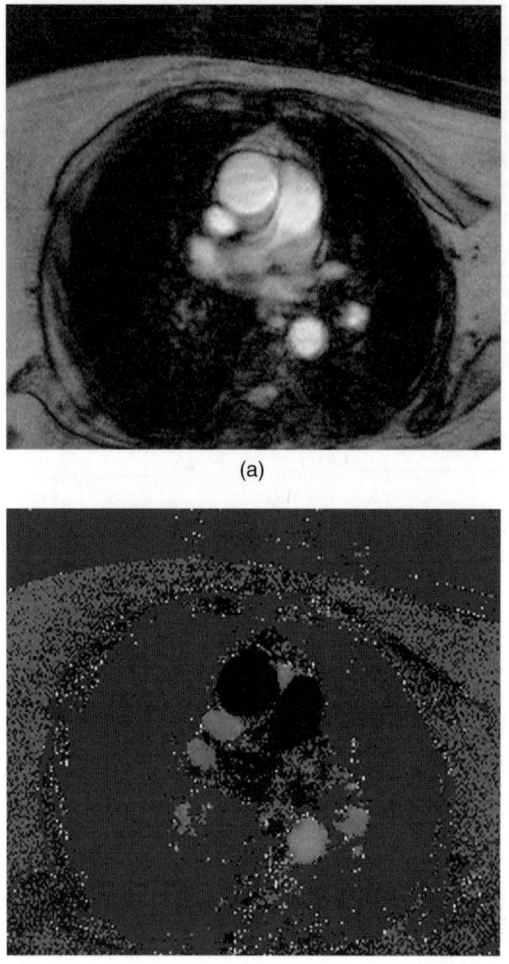

Figure 14.2 (a) The velocity encoded MR magnitude and (b) phase image of the human cardiac cavity.

neuroreceptor tagging-based imaging of the brain for cortical functional imaging. These are just examples of the challenges in diagnostic radiology and are by no means a complete representation of a large number of issues in human physiology and pathology. Recently, MRI methods have been used with magnetization transfer, tissue tagging, and phase contrast encoding methods for acquiring cine images of the beating heart (5–7). Figure 14.2 shows images of cardiac cavity with velocity-encoded MRI magnitude (Fig. 14.2a) and phase (Fig. 14.2b) information. Figure 14.2a shows the magnitude image representing the anatomical structure. The areas with blood vessels appear bright because of the high water content. Figure 14.2b represents a velocity map, in which the medium gray corresponds to stationary tissue, the darker areas correspond to negative flow, and the brighter areas correspond to positive flow.

14.2. TARGETED IMAGING

Targeted molecular imaging methods can provide a systematic investigation into a physiological process for the assessment of a specific pathology. Recent discoveries in molecular sciences and imaging contrast agents have played a significant role in designing specific biomarkers to work with medical imaging modalities such as ultrasound, PET, fMR, and optical fluorescence imaging to study molecular responses linked with the onset of a disease. Contrast agents are used to image physiology or pathology that might otherwise be difficult to distinguish from the surrounding tissue. For example, encapsulated microbubbles in ultrasound imaging can provide information about activated neutrophil, a cell involved in the inflammatory response (http://www.ImaRx.com).

The technology for a specific contrast agent for targeted imaging can also be used for better drug delivery in critical therapeutic protocols. It is expected that future diagnostic, treatment-evaluation, and therapeutic-intervention protocols will use specific multimodality targeted imaging with computerized analyses through models using molecular signatures of physiological processes. For example, tumor-induced angiogenesis is a complex process involving tumor cells, blood, and the stroma of the host tissue. Studies related to angiogenic growth factors linked with endothelial cells have shown that vascular integrin $\alpha v \beta 3$ may be a useful therapeutic target for diseases characterized by neovascularization (8). Thus, $\alpha v \beta 3$ is a prime candidate for molecular targeting and can be monitored through advanced imaging methods. Furthermore, nanoparticle-conjugated novel MRI contrast agents can be used in order to directly observe gene expression, metabolism, and neurotransmission. The advantage of these novel contrast agents is their ability to provide such information in a noninvasive fashion. This enables important cellular and metabolic processes to be observed for the first time in whole animals over repeated time periods (9).

14.3. OPTICAL IMAGING AND OTHER EMERGING MODALITIES

Several imaging modalities have recently emerged that have a potential to play a significant role in diagnostic radiology. These modalities include optical, electrical impedance, and microwave imaging. Electrical impedance tomography (EIT) has been recently used for 3-D imaging of the breast (10–12). EIT methods of breast imaging have now begun to show promise in the noninvasive detection of tumors and circumscribed masses (12).

Optical imaging systems are relatively much less expensive, are portable, noninvasive, and adaptable to acquiring physiological and functional information from microscopic to macroscopic levels. For example, optical coherence tomography (OCT) is a noninvasive imaging technique capable of producing high-resolution cross-sectional images through inhomogeneous samples. It can offer a resolution level higher than current MRI, computed tomography (CT), SPECT, PET, and ultrasound technologies. Although primary optical imaging modalities such as endoscopy have been used in clinical environments for several years, the clinical perspective of other advanced optical imaging modalities has yet to be established in diagnostic radiology. Recent advances in endoscopy, OCT, confocal microscopy, fluorescence imaging, and multispectral transillumination technologies show their great potential in becoming the mainstream diagnostic and treatment evaluation technologies of the future.

Optical imaging modalities may utilize the visible light spectrum from 400 to 700 nm of electromagnetic radiation to produce visible images in biomedical applications such as microscopy, endoscopy, and colonoscopy. However, the excitation and emission spectrum in advanced optical imaging modalities is not restricted to the visible spectrum but can be extended out on both sides into the soft ultraviolet (<400 nm) and near-infrared (NIR; >700 nm) ranges for fluorescence and multispectral imaging applications. The visible light spectrum, along with soft ultraviolet and NIR bands, follows relatively stochastic behavior in photon interaction and propagation in a heterogonous multilayered biological tissue medium. Unlike X-ray photons, optical photons do not penetrate the entire biological tissue medium with predominantly straight transmission. Electromagnetic theories of light reflection, refraction, diffusion, interference, and propagation are described in depth by Born and Wolf (13) and are also discussed in recent books (14–16).

Light radiance is characterized by the total emission or reflection within a solid angle. It is the sum of all spectral radiances at individual wavelengths. As light passes through a heterogeneous multilayered medium, it suffers from wavelength-dependent absorption and scattering events. In a multilayered heterogeneous medium such as a biological tissue, characteristic absorption and scattering coefficients determine the light radiance at a given point. Light radiance is also described by the scattering phase function, which is defined as the cosine of the angle between the incident and scattered paths. The weighted average of the scattering phase function is called the anisotropy factor. In a biological tissue, the anisotropy factor is strongly peaked in the forward direction. However, a series of scattering events in a turbid medium with a continuously changing direction of light propagation can also produce backscattered diffused radiance, which can reemerge from the surface (17, 18). Figure 14.3 shows a schematic diagram of optical reflectance, backscattered diffused reflectance, and transmission imaging modalities in a multilayered biological tissue medium. For simplicity, each layer is assigned wavelength-dependent average absorption and scattering coefficients, an anisotropy factor, and an index of refraction.

14.3.1 Optical Microscopy

Microscopic imaging modalities provide a variable magnification and depth of field for imaging a tissue in an embedded medium or in vivo. The magnification power provides the capability to image the tissue at the cellular level. The distance at which an optical system can clearly focus is known as the depth of field. Within the depth of field, objects are in focus; that is, they appear crisp and sharp. At increasing distances outside the depth of field (either closer to or further away from

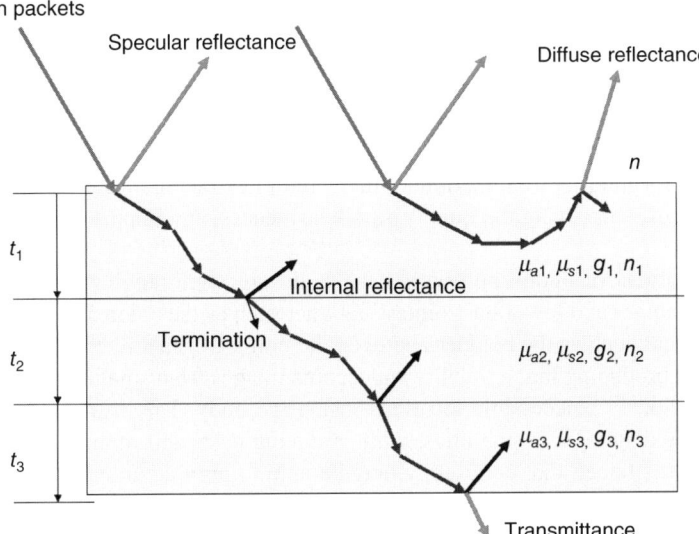

Figure 14.3 A simplified model of a biological medium with three layers. Each layer is associated with an absorption coefficient μ_a, a scattering coefficient μ_s, an anisotropic factor g, and a refractive index n.

the camera), objects gradually become more blurred. In typical photography, an image is comprised of the superposition of all the light originating from all depth planes, thus providing a wide field of view typical to what a human eye can see. For biological imaging, however, it is often desired to obtain separate images of individual depth planes. This is known as optical sectioning. In confocal microscopy, a small pinhole is used to block all out-of-focus light, therefore limiting the image to only the light reflected from objects in the focal plane. Multiphoton microscopy, on the other hand, is designed in such a way that light is emitted back only from the current point of interest. These techniques are often used to image the fluorescent light emitted from biological tissue on a slice-by-slice basis.

Fluorescence imaging uses ultraviolet light to excite fluorophores and then collect back emitted light at a higher wavelength. Fluorophores include endogenous and exogenous fluorophores. The former refers to natural fluorophores intrinsic inside tissue, such as amino acids and structural protein, and these fluorophores are typically randomly distributed. The latter usually refers to smart polymer nanoparticles targeting specific molecules such as hemoglobin. Because of its high resolution at the cellular and subcellular levels, as well as the ease of obtaining 3-D reconstructions, multiphoton microscopy is also often used for functional imaging, that is, the spatial and temporal visualization of biological processes in living cells (19). Two-photon microscopy has been applied to obtain a 3-D visualization over time of the accumulation and penetration of nanoscale drug vehicles within the skin (20), the cellular dynamics of immunology (21), mouse kidney development (22), as well as neuronal dendrite dynamics (23).

14.3.2 Optical Endoscopy

Endoscopy, as a medical tool for observation and diagnosis, is straightforward in concept and has existed since 1807 when Phillip Bozzini used candlelight and mirrors to observe the canals of the human body. Numerous developments through the decades since then have taken this technology through the initial introduction of electric light for internal illumination all the way to flexible endoscopes using fiber optics, gradually improving the quality, noninvasiveness, and impact of endoscopic procedures.

Applications of endoscopy within the body are wide-ranging, directed primarily in the upper and lower gastrointestinal tract such as the colon and esophagus, but also in areas such as the bladder and even the brain. In general, current research is focused on producing higher quality endoscopic images from smaller devices able to reach previously inaccessible locations inside the body. The primary goal is to improve early diagnostic capabilities, while reducing costs and minimizing patient discomfort. It is hoped that endoscopy may be able to provide an easy method for screening at-risk patients for signs of cancer or precancerous tissue, including dysplasia and neoplasia. It is difficult to detect dysplasia using conventional endoscopic techniques, such as white light endoscopy.

The gold standard of any endoscopic system is a histological analysis of a biopsied resection. Dysplasia can be detected through biopsy, but a suitable biopsy site needs to be selected. In addition to the typical detection of cancer and precancer in common endoscopic areas such as the upper and lower gastrointestinal tract, endoscopy has also found applications in a variety of other locations in the body, with a number of different imaging objectives. Endoscopic imaging of the brain, known as neuroendoscopy, is subjected to narrower restrictions, but still has promise to permit imaging of transventricular regions or to perform endoscope-assisted microsurgery (24, 25).

14.3.3 Optical Coherence Tomography

Optical coherence tomography was invented in early 1990s but has recently emerged as a popular 3-D imaging technology for biomedical applications (26–28). This relatively new modality makes use of the coherent properties of light. In an OCT system, light with a low coherence length is divided into two parts. One part serves as a reference while the other is directed into the tissue. When light travels in tissue, it encounters an interface with a different refractive index, and part of the light is reflected. This reflectance is subsequently mixed with the reference. Once the optical path length difference between the reference light and the reflected light is less than the coherence length, coherence occurs. By observing the coherence pattern and changing the optical path length of the reference light with a mirror, a cross-section of the tissue can be rendered. With a sufficiently low coherence length, the resolution of OCT may reach a magnitude on the micrometer scale; hence, it can disclose subtle changes in cancer tissue at the cellular level. OCT recovers the structure of interrogated tissue through a mechanism analogous to ultrasonic imaging. The latter

14.3. OPTICAL IMAGING AND OTHER EMERGING MODALITIES 361

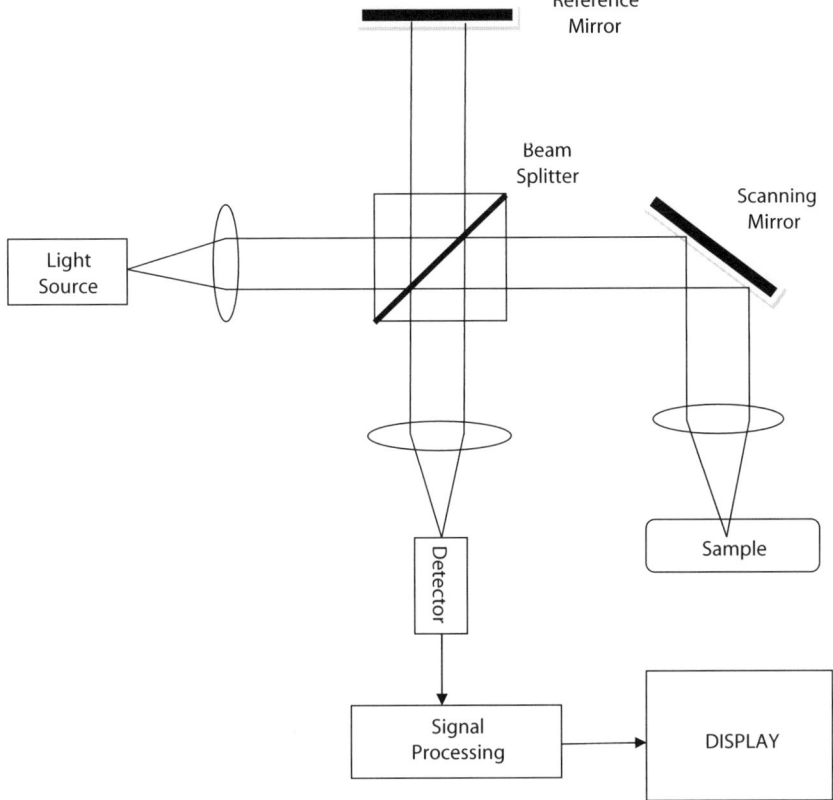

Figure 14.4 A schematic diagram of a single-point scanning-based optical coherence tomography system.

modality sends sound into tissue, which reflects when encountering an impedance-varied interface. The resolution of OCT is much higher than that of ultrasonic imaging, but it cannot penetrate as far.

There are two types of broadly classified OCT systems: a single-point scanning-based OCT system (Fig. 14.4) and a full-field OCT system (Fig. 14.5). Images can be produced in time domain OCT mode through low coherence interferometry in which the reference path length is translated longitudinally in time. A fringe pattern is obtained when the path difference lies within the coherence length of the source. In frequency domain OCT (FD-OCT), a broadband interference pattern is exploited in spectral dispersion. Spectrally separated detectors are encoded with optical frequency distribution onto a charge-coupled device (CCD) or CMOS detector array so that information about the full depth is obtained in a single shot. Alternatively, in time-encoded frequency domain OCT (TEFD-OCT, or swept source OCT), spectral dispersion on the detector is encoded in the time domain instead of with spatial separation (26–28).

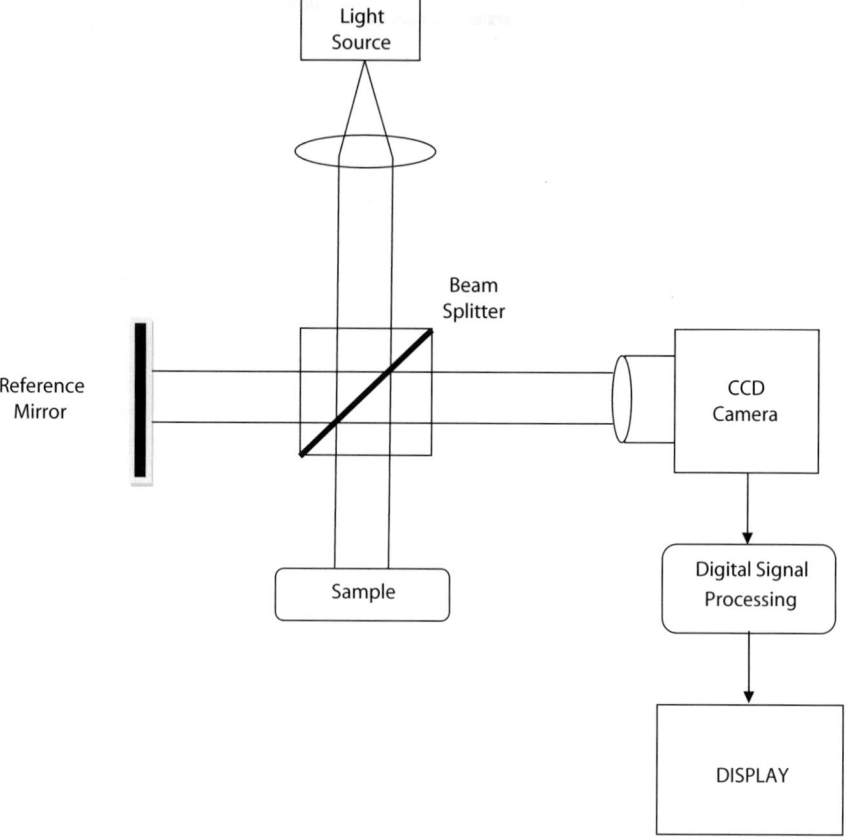

Figure 14.5 A schematic diagram of a full-field optical coherence tomography system.

14.3.4 Diffuse Reflectance and Transillumination Imaging

Diffuse reflectance images are formed by backscattered diffused light. These images represent composite information about the absorption and scattering by different chromospheres and biological structures in the medium. Although the raw images produced may be useful and may carry important diagnostic information, more significant information can be derived from the 3-D reconstruction of the biological medium from multispectral diffuse reflectance measurements.

Figure 14.6 shows a surface reflectance-based epi-illuminance light microscopy (ELM) image (left) of a malignant melanoma skin lesion and a backscattered diffuse reflectance-based transillumination image (right) obtained by the Nevoscope (29, 30). Increased absorption due to greater blood volume around the outlined lesion's boundary is evident in the transillumination image (30).

Transillumination, also known as shadowgram optical imaging or diaphanography, was first used by Cutler in 1929 to examine pathology in the breast (31). Transillumination was initially surpassed by the superiority of X-ray technology but later evolved to be a major application of visible light in medicine, particularly in

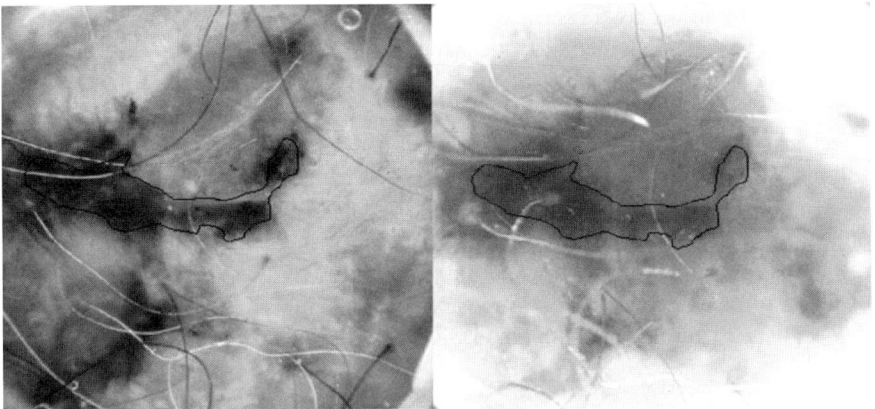

Oil Epiluminescence   Transillumination

Figure 14.6 Surface reflectance based ELM image (left) of a malignant melanoma skin lesion with a backscattered diffuse reflectance-based transillumination image (right).

aiding the early detection and diagnosis of breast cancer. Because evaluating breast cancer risk assessment with optical transillumination would avoid the need for ionized radiation through X-ray mammography, it could be safely applied more frequently to women of all ages. The parenchymal tissue density pattern is a good indicator of future breast cancer risk, and is typically obtained through mammography. As an alternative, the chromophore composition and morphology of the breast tissue, as observed though transillumination, has been used to identify women with high parenchymal density. This method may therefore provide the same odds ratio for breast cancer risk as can traditional mammography; thus, it may offer an alternative to radiation screening (32–34).

While transillumination is often performed using white visible light, infrared and ultraviolet light are also commonly used to observe interesting tissue characteristics that may not be apparent under the visible spectrum. The recent widespread availability of NIR lasers and CCDs had led to further research in optical transillumination modalities with infrared light, particularly in the last two decades. Using an NIR laser (1250 nm) for transillumination, differences in contrast and resolution were observed between normal breast tissue and cancerous breast tissue (34).

14.3.5 Photoacoustic Imaging: An Emerging Technology

Photoacoustic imaging is a fast emerging technology that utilizes the acoustic waves from the thermal expansion of an absorbing object, such as a tumor, pigmented lesion, or blood vessel, caused by the absorption of light photons. In biomedical imaging applications, light from a short pulsed laser scatters inside the target object, producing heat. The temperature is raised by a fraction of a degree, causing thermal expansion. The thermoelastic effect generates pressure transients that exactly represent the absorbing structures. These pressure transients produce ultrasonic waves that propagate to the tissue surface and are detected by an ultrasound sensor. The photoacoustic imaging methods are also known as optoacoustics, laser-induced ultrasound, or thermoacoustics imaging, and have been investigated for imaging lesions of the breast, skin, and vascular tissues. A nice overview of photoacoustic effect and imaging methods is presented in a dissertation by Niederhauser (35), and also in a tutorial paper by Wang (36). The spatial resolution of photoacoustic imaging depends on the photoacoustic emission phase. As described in (36), strong optical scattering in biological tissue causes shallow imaging depth and low spatial resolution. Because ultrasound scattering is much weaker than optical scattering, the resulting ultrasound signal from photoacoustic imaging provides better resolution than optical diffuse imaging methods for various medical imaging applications (36–40).

14.4. MODEL-BASED AND MULTISCALE ANALYSIS

The basic model-based methods for image reconstruction and analysis are described in Chapters 8–12. The trends of using more sophisticated multiparameter models in multidimensional medical image analysis will continue in the future. For example, probabilistic brain atlases incorporating specific anatomical and functional variability structures will continue to improve analysis, understanding, and visualization of brain images.

Figure 14.7 shows a visualization of cortical surfaces of a patient with a brain tumor (not shown in the image). The cortical activation due to tongue movement was measured with the fMRI and is superimposed on the cortical surface-rendered image. Figure 14.8 shows a 3-D surface-rendered image of the face and head with the cross-sectional volume visualization of MR data-based anatomical structures. The images shown in Figures 14.7 and 14.8 are just two of the many examples of multiparameter image analysis, registration, and visualization of human brain that have been explored for understanding pathologies as well as for image-guided surgery. There are still numerous challenges in this area to be addressed in the near future through the advances in multimodality multiparameter medical imaging and image analysis.

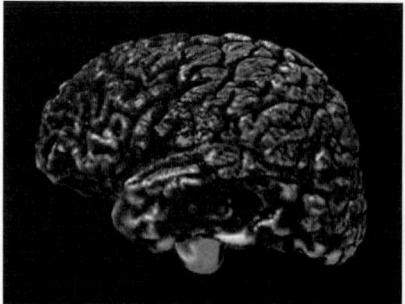

Figure 14.7 A surface visualization of cortical structure with the superposition of activation function (http://www.bic.mni.mcgill.ca/).

14.4. MODEL-BASED AND MULTISCALE ANALYSIS 365

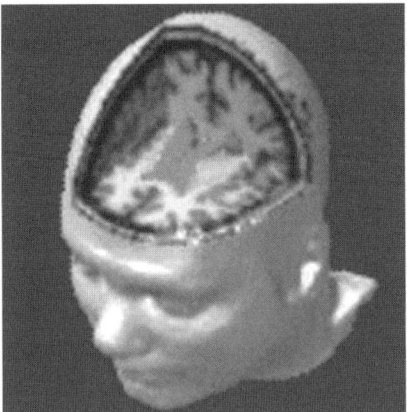

Figure 14.8 A surface visualization of human face with the volume visualization of anatomical structure of the brain (http://www.bic.mni.mcgill.ca/).

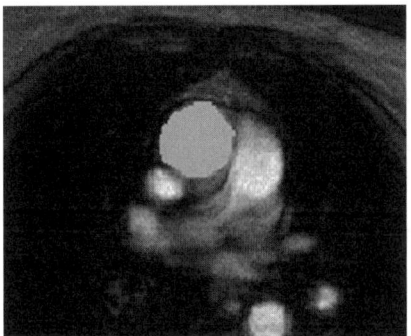

Figure 14.9 The segmentation of blood vessel shown in the magnitude and phase MR images of human cardiac cavity shown in Figure 14.2 using the wavelet-based frequency localization features.

Multiresolution-based wavelet processing methods have been used for several applications with significant improvements in tissue segmentation and characterization (41–44). Figure 14.9 shows the segmentation of a main blood vessel using wavelet processing on the magnitude and phase images shown in Figure 14.2. A training set of images was used for manual segmentation by experts to develop a signature model of the blood vessel using the wavelet processing-based frequency-localized features. Using the signature model with the nearest neighbor classifier, the blood vessel was segmented as shown in Figure 14.9.

In addition to multiparameter multiresolution image analysis, the advantage of complementary medical imaging modalities can also be realized through multi-scale imaging from cellular to tissue and organ levels. For example, while optical imaging modalities such as fluorescence microscopy and OCT can provide information at the cellular level, X-ray CT, ultrasound, MRI, fMRI, and SPECT-PET imaging modalities can provide structural and functional information at tissue and organ levels. Such multiscale analysis has been of significant interest and will continue in the future as an area of active research, specifically in neuroscience.

One of the major challenges in using multimodality multidimensional signal and imaging technologies for diagnostic and surgical applications is how to integrate information from different technological instruments. The process of information fusion requires computer processing of large data files with a common standard coordinate system so that information from different instruments can be easily read and integrated toward analysis of target areas. Large information processing, archiving, and retrieval systems such as Picture Archiving and Communication Systems (PACS) have been developed in radiological environment (45–47). Although efforts have been made in establishing common formats such as DICOM for different imaging scanners, it is a significant and challenging task to provide real-time fusion of multimodality signal and image processing features and correlate it to patient information for relevant information extraction that can be used for therapeutic and surgical intervention.

14.5. REFERENCES

1. S.L. Hartmann and R.L. Galloway, "Depth buffer targeting for spatial accurate 3-D visualization of medical image," *IEEE Trans. Med. Imaging*, Vol. 19, pp. 1024–1031, 2000.
2. M. Ferrant, A. Nabavi, B. Macq, F.A. Jolsez, R. Kikinis, and S.K. Warfield, "Registration of 3-D intraoperative MR images of the brain using a finite element biomechanical model," *IEEE Trans. Med. Imaging*, Vol. 20, pp. 1384–1297, 2001.
3. K. Rohr, H.S. Stiehl, R. Sprengel, T.M. Buzug, J. Wesse, and M.H. Kahn, "Landmark based elastic registration using approximating thin-plate splines," *IEEE Trans. Med. Imaging*, Vol. 20, pp. 526–534, 2001.
4. G.E. Christensen and H.J. Johnson, "Consistent image registration," *IEEE Trans. Med. Imaging*, Vol. 20, pp. 568–582, 2001.
5. J. Park, A.A. Young, and L. Axel, "Deformable models with parameter functions for cardiac motion analysis from tagged MRI data," *IEEE Trans. Med. Imaging*, Vol. 15, pp. 278–289, 1996.
6. G.J. Parker, H.A. Haroon, et al., "A framework for a streamline-based probabilistic index of connectivity (PICo) using a structural interpretation of MRI diffusion measurements," *J. Magn. Reson. Imaging*, Vol. 18, No. 2, pp. 242–254, 2003.
7. C.J. Baker, M.J. Hartkamp, and W.P. Mali, "Measuring blood flow by nontriggered 2D phase-contrast cine magnetic resonance imaging," *Magn. Reson. Imaging*, Vol. 14, pp. 609–614, 1996.
8. P.C. Brooks, R.A. Clark, and D.A. Cheresh, "Requirement of vascular integrin alpha v beta 3 for angiogenesis," *Science*, Vol. 264, No. 5158, pp. 569–571, 1994.
9. T. Atanasijevic, M. Shusteff, P. Fam, and A. Jasanoff, "Calcium-sensitive MRI contrast agents based on superparamagnetic iron oxide nanoparticles and calmodulin," *Proc. Natl. Acad. Sci. USA*, Vol. 103, pp. 14707–14712, 2006.
10. J. Jossinet, E. Marry, and A. Montalibet, "Electrical impedance endo-tomography: Imaging tissue from inside," *IEEE Trans. Med. Imaging*, Vol. 21, pp. 560–565, 2002.
11. T.E. Kerner, K.D. Paulsen, A. Hartov, S.K. Soho, and S.P. Poplack, "Electrical impedance spectroscopy of the breast: Clinical imaging results in 26 subjects," *IEEE Trans. Med. Imaging*, Vol. 21, pp. 638–645, 2002.
12. A.Y. Karpov, A.V. Korjenevsky, V.N. Kornienko, Y.S. Kultiasov, M.B. Ochapkin, O.V. Trochanova, and J.D. Meister, "Three-dimensional EIT imaging of breast tissues: System design and clinical testing," *IEEE Trans. Med. Imaging*, Vol. 21, pp. 662–667, 2002.
13. M. Born and E. Wolf, *Principles of Optics: Electromagnetic Theory of Propagation, Interference and Diffraction of Light*, 7th Edition, Cambridge University Press, Cambridge, UK, 1999.

14. L.V. Wang and H.-I. Wu, *Biomedical Optics: Principles and Imaging*, John Wiley & Sons, Inc, Hoboken, NJ, 2007.
15. C. Bohren and D. Huffman, *Absorption and Scattering of Light by Small Particles*, Wiley-Interscience, New York, 1983.
16. A. Ishimaru, *Wave Propagation and Scattering in Random Media*, IEEE Press, New York, 1999.
17. A.N. Bashkatov, E.A. Genina, V.I. Kochubey et al., "Optical properties of human skin, subcutaneous and mucous tissues in the wavelength range from 400 to 2000 nm," *J. Phys. D: Appl. Phys.*, Vol. 38, No. 15, pp. 2543–2555, 2005.
18. M.J.C. Van Gemert, S.L. Jacques, H.J.C.M. Sterenborg et al., "Skin optics," *IEEE Trans. Biomed. Eng.*, Vol. 36, No. 12, pp. 1146–1154, 1989.
19. M. Straub, P. Lodemann, P. Holroyd et al., "Live cell imaging by multifocal multiphoton microscopy," *Eur. J. Cell Biol.*, Vol. 79, No. 10, pp. 726–734, 2000.
20. F. Stracke, B. Weiss, C.M. Lehr et al., "Multiphoton microscopy for the investigation of dermal penetration of nanoparticle-borne drugs," *J. Invest. Dermatol.*, Vol. 126, No. 10, pp. 2224–2233, 2006.
21. M.D. Cahalan and I. Parker, "Choreography of cell motility and interaction dynamics imaged by two-photon microscopy in lymphoid organs," *Annu. Rev. Immunol.*, pp. 585–626, 2008.
22. C.L. Phillips, L.J. Arend, A.J. Filson et al., "Three-dimensional imaging of embryonic mouse kidney by two-photon microscopy," *Am. J. Pathol.*, Vol. 158, No. 1, pp. 49–55, 2001.
23. G. Duemani Reddy, K. Kelleher, R. Fink et al., "Three-dimensional random access multiphoton microscopy for functional imaging of neuronal activity," *Nat. Neurosci.*, Vol. 11, No. 6, pp. 713–720, 2008.
24. J.J.G.H.M. Bergman and G.N.J. Tytgat, "New developments in the endoscopic surveillance of Barrett's oesophagus," *Gut*, Vol. 54, No. Suppl. 1, 2005.
25. G. Cinalli, P. Cappabianca, R. de Falco et al., "Current state and future development of intracranial neuroendoscopic surgery," *Expert Rev. Med. Devices*, Vol. 2, No. 3, pp. 351–373, 2005.
26. A.F. Low, G.J. Tearney, B.E. Bouma et al., "Technology insight: Optical coherence tomography—Current status and future development," *Nat. Clin. Pract. Cardiovasc. Med.*, Vol. 3, No. 3, pp. 154–162, 2006.
27. K. Sokolov, J. Aaron, B. Hsu et al., "Optical systems for in vivo molecular imaging of cancer," *Technol. Cancer Res. Treat.*, Vol. 2, No. 6, pp. 491–504, 2003.
28. W. Drexler and J. Fujimoto, *Optical Coherence Tomography: Technology and Applications*, Springer, New York, 2008.
29. A.P. Dhawan, "Early detection of cutaneous malignant melanoma by three-dimensional Nevoscopy," *Comput. Methods Prog. Biomed.*, Vol. 21, pp. 59–68, 1985.
30. V. Terushkin, S.W. Dusza, N.A. Mullani et al., "Transillumination as a means to differentiate melanocytic lesions based upon their vascularity," *Arch. Dermatol.*, Vol. 145, No. 9, pp. 1060–1062, 2009.
31. M.D. Max, "Cutler, "Transillumination of breasts," *J. Am. Med. Assoc.*, Vol. 93, No. 21, p. 1671, 1929.
32. D.R. Leff, O.J. Warren, L.C. Enfield et al., "Diffuse optical imaging of the healthy and diseased breast: A systematic review," *Breast Cancer Res. Treat.*, Vol. 108, No. 1, pp. 9–22, 2008.
33. L.S. Fournier, D. Vanel, A. Athanasiou et al., "Dynamic optical breast imaging: A novel technique to detect and characterize tumor vessels," *Eur. J. Radiol.*, Vol. 69, No. 1, pp. 43–49, 2009.
34. M.K. Simick and L.D. Lilge, "Optical transillumination spectroscopy to quantify parenchymal tissue density: An indicator for breast cancer risk," *British J. Radiology*, Vol. 78, pp. 1009–1017, 2005.
35. J.J. Niederhauser, *Real-Time Biomedical Optoacoustic Imaging*, Swiss Federal Institute of Technology, Zürich, Switzerland, 2004.
36. L.V. Wang, "Tutorial on photoacoustic microscopy and computed tomography," *IEEE J. Sel. Top. Quantum Electron.*, Vol. 14, No. 1, pp. 171–179, 2008.
37. H.F. Zhang, K. Maslov, G. Stoica et al., "Functional photoacoustic microscopy for high-resolution and noninvasive in vivo imaging," *Nat. Biotechnol.*, Vol. 24, No. 7, pp. 848–851, 2006.
38. G. Ku, B.D. Fornage, X. Jin et al., "Thermoacoustic and photoacoustic tomography of thick biological tissues toward breast imaging," *Technol. Cancer Res. Treat.*, Vol. 4, No. 5, pp. 559–565, 2005.
39. G. Ku and L.V. Wang, "Deeply penetrating photoacoustic tomography in biological tissues enhanced with an optical contrast agent," *Opt. Lett.*, Vol. 30, No. 5, pp. 507–509, 2005.

40. X. Wang, Y. Pang, G. Ku, X. Xie, G. Stoica, and L.V. Wang, "Noninvasive laser-induced photoacoustic tomography for structural and functional *in vivo* imaging of the brain," *Nature Biotechnology*, Vol. 21, pp. 803–806, 2003.
41. S. Dippel, M. Stahl, R. Wiemker, and T. Blaffert, "Multiscale contrast enhancement for radiographies: Laplacian pyramid versus fast wavelet transform," *IEEE Trans. Med. Imaging*, Vol. 21, pp. 343–353, 2002.
42. G. Cincoti, G. Loi, and M. Pappalardo, "Frequency decomposition and compounding of ultrasound medical images with wavelet packets," *IEEE Trans. Med. Imaging*, Vol. 20, pp. 764–771, 2001.
43. X. Hao, C.J. Bruce, C. Pislaru, and J.F. Greenleaf, "Segmenting high-frequency intercardiac ultrasound images of myocardium into infracted, ischemic and normal regions," *IEEE Trans. Med. Imaging*, Vol. 20, pp. 1373–1383, 2001.
44. M. Moriyama, Y. Sato, H. Naito, M. Hanayama, T. Ueguchi, T. Harada, F. Yoshimoto, and S. Tamura, "Reconstruction of time-varying 3-D left ventricular shape multiview X-ray cineangiocardiograms," *IEEE Trans. Med. Imaging*, Vol. 21, pp. 773–785, 2002.
45. H.K. Huang, *PACS and Imaging Informatics: Principles and Applications*, John Wiley & Sons, Hoboken, NJ, 2004.
46. Z. Zhou, M.A. Gutierrez, J. Documet, L. Chan, H.K. Huang, and B.J. Liu, "The role of a data grid in worldwide imaging-based clinical trials," *J. High Speed Netw.*, Vol. 16, pp. 1–13, 2006.
47. M.Y.Y. Law, "A Model of DICOM-based electronic patient record in radiation therapy," *J. Comput. Med. Imaging Graph.*, Vol. 29, No. 2–3, pp. 125–136, 2006.

INDEX

Page numbers in *italics* refer to Figures; those in **bold** to Tables.

Accuracy, 10, 22
Acoustic imaging, 4
Affine transformation, 316
Algebraic reconstruction techniques (ART), 180–182, *181*
Alpha decay, 149
Alzheimer's disease, 353
A-mode ultrasound imaging, 166–167
Analysis, computer-aided, 2. *See also* Image analysis
Anger camera, 141
Angiography
  digital subtraction, 336
  flow imaging of contrast-enhanced, 127–128, *128*
  image from subtraction method, 204, *205*
  MR, *128*
Antiscatter grids, 84
Application domain knowledge, 2
ART. *See* algebraic reconstruction techniques
Artifacts
  motion, 6
  in MR images, 136
Atlases, computerized, 311, *312*
Attenuation
  linear coefficient for, 70, *71*
  SPECT imaging with and without, 147, *147*
Autism, 353

Backprojection method, 176–179, *179*, *180*
  ART methods compared with, 182
  of image reconstruction, 173

Backpropagation neural network (BPNN), 255–258, *256, 257*
Bandlimited filter function, *177*, 177–178
Bandlimited image signal, sampling of, 48, *49*
Barium fluoride (BaF_2), in SPECT imaging, 145
Barium sulfate, 95
Bayesian classifier, 293
Beam hardening, 96
Becquerel, Antonio Henri, 65
Becquerel (Bq), 140
Beta decay, 140
Biological tissue medium, optical reflectance in, 358, *359*
Biomedical image processing and analysis system
  components of, 11, *11*
  computer for, 12
  image acquisition system for, 12
  image display environment of, 12
  special-purpose architectures for, 13
Bismuth germinate (BGO), in SPECT imaging
Bloch, Felix, 99
Bloch's equation, 106–107
B-mode ultrasound imaging, 168, *168*
BOLD imaging sequence, 129, *130*
Boundary tracking, in image segmentation, 231–233, *233*
Brain images
  axial, sagittal, and coronal MR, *113*
  DTI, *134*
  DWI, *133*
  elastic deformation based registration of 3-D MR, 329, *330*
  endoscopic, 360
  with FDG-PET imaging, 149–150–*150*
  fMR, *130*

Medical Image Analysis, Second Edition, by Atam P. Dhawan
Copyright © 2011 by the Institute of Electrical and Electronics Engineers, Inc.

369

370 INDEX

Brain images (cont'd)
  with Fourier transform, 18, 216, *216*
  fused SPECT-CT, 152, *153*
  high-pass filtering of MR, 217, *218*
  homomorphic filtering of, 219, *219*
  hydrogen protons present in, 100, *100*
  with k-means clustering, 241, *242, 243*
  with Laplacian weight mask, 209, *209, 210*
  MAS method applied to, 254, *254*
  with median filter method, 207, *207*
  morphological operations applied to, 279, *279*
  through MR inversion recovery imaging pulse sequence, *120*
  PET-reconstructed, *193*
  proton density, *127*
  region-growing approach to, 247, *248*
  registered using IPAR method, 321, *322, 323*
  through SEPI pulse sequence, *120*
  SPECT, 147, *147*
  ^{99}Tc SPECT, 145, *145*, 152, *153*
  T_2-weighted proton density, 201, *201, 203*
  2-D multimodality image visualization of, 336, *337*
  using gray-value threshold, 235, *236, 237*
  using wavelet transform, 225, *225, 226*
  with weighted averaging mask, 206, *206*
  X-ray CT, 201, *201, 203*
Brain ventricles, composite model of, 318, 319, 343, *345*
Breast, microcalcifications of, 303–306, **305**
Breast imaging. *See also* Mammogram
  EIT methods of, 357
  radiological information for, 5
  X-ray film-screen, 357
Bremsstrahlung radiation spectrum, 81, *82*
Butterworth filters, 216

Cardiac cavity, X-ray CT image of, 92, *93*. *See also* Heart
Central slice theorem, 174–176, *175*
Cerebral artery, middle, *133*

Cesium iodide (CsI(TI), in SPECT imaging, 145
Charge-coupled devices (CCDs), 46–47, 363
Chest cavity, image analysis of, 267–268
Chest radiographs, 4, *85*
Clustering
  agglomerative method, 241
  data, 239–241
  fuzzy c-means, 242–243, 259, 260
  k-means, 241–242, *243*, 259
  partitional, 240, 241
  pixel classification through, 239–245, *243*
Coherent scattering, 67–68, 69
Collimators, 84
Comb function, 28, *29*
Compton scattering, 69
  causes of, 69
  in SPECT imaging, 147
Computed tomography (CT), 65. *See also* X-ray computed tomography
Computer technology, in medical imaging modalities, 1–2
Constrained least square filtering method, 214–215
Contrast
  improving, 266
  in MR images, 135
  in PET imaging, 150
  in SPECT imaging, 145
  in ultrasound, 170
Contrast agents
  iodine-based contrast agents, 95
  nanoparticle-conjugated, 357
  in targeted imaging, 357
Contrast enhancement processing, feature-adaptive, 13–14, *14*
Contrast-to-noise ratio (CNR), 39
  medical images characterized by, 39
  for MRI, 135
Cormack, Allen, 65, 173
Curie, Irene, 140
Curie, Jean Frederic, 140
Curie (CI), 140

Data acquisition methods, 7
DataGlove, in VR technology, 347
Daubechies filter prototypes, 303
Daubechies's db4 wavelet, 57, *59*

INDEX   **371**

Detectors
  photon detection statistics of, 182
  scintillation, 73–76, **74,** *76*
  semiconductor, 72–73
Diagnosis
  medical imaging modalities in, 1–2
  multimodality image fusion in, 151–152
Diagnostic radiology
  direct display methods, 338
  medical imaging in, 2
Diaphanography, 362
DICOM, 366
Diffuse reflectance imaging, 362, *363*
Diffusion, 354
Diffusion imaging MR, 130–135, *131–134*
Diffusion tensor imaging (DTI), 100, 130–135, *131–134,* 354
Diffusion weighted images (DWIs), 130–133, *132, 133*
Diffusion weighted imaging (DWI), 354
Digital image, for MATLAB image processing toolbox, 14–16, *16*
Digital subtraction angiogram (DSA) data, 336
Dirac delta function, 27, 28
Doppler ultrasound imaging, 169, *170*

Echo planar imaging (EPI), 119–123, *120–124*
Edge-based image segmentation, 229–230
  boundary tracking, 231–233
  edge detection operations, 230–231
  Hough transform, 233–235, *234*
Edge detection operations, in image segmentation, 230–231
Edge enhancement, 208–209
Edge-linking procedures, in image segmentation, 231
Edge map, example, 233, *233*
Elastic deformation-based registration, 325–330, *328, 330*
Electrical impedance tomography (EIT), 357
Electromagnetic (EM) radiation
  behavior of, 65–66
  components of, 66
  detection of
    ionized chambers and proportional counters for, 70–72, *71*
    scintillation detectors, 73–76, **74,** *76*
    semiconductor detectors, 72–73

  exercises, 78
  for image formation, 66–67
  interaction with matter of
    coherent or Rayleigh scattering, 67–68, 69
    Compton scattering, 69
    pair production, 69
    photoelectric absorption, 68, *68,* 69
    linear attenuation coefficient, 70, *71*
    output voltage pulse detector subsystem in, 76–77, *77*
  particle nature of, 66
Electromagnetic (EM) spectrum, 65
Emission computed tomography (ECT)
  image reconstruction for, 182
  image reconstruction in, 188–192, *191–193*
  ML-EM algorithm for, 189–190
Emission imaging methods, 139
Emission imaging principle, 4
Endoscopy
  neuroendoscopy, 360
  optical, 360
  virtual, 335, 349
Enhancement, computer-aided, 2. *See also* Image enhancement
Epi-illuminance light microscopy (ELM), 362
Estimation-model based adaptive segmentation, 249–254, *250, 254*
EyePhone, in VR technology, 347

False negative fraction (FNF), 9
False positive fraction (FPF), 9
Fast Fourier transform (FFT), 51
FCM algorithm, adaptive, 244–245
Feature classification system, 283–285
  GA-based optimization, 289–292, **291**
  linear discriminant analysis, 285–288, *286*
  PCA, 288–289
FID signal, 125–126
Field of view (FOV), in IPAR, 319–320, 321
Field programmable gate arrays (FPGA), 13
Field programmable gate arrays (FPGA) board, 77

372 INDEX

Filtering
  frequency domain, 212–213
  high-pass, 217, *218*, **224**
  homomorphic, 217–219, *218, 219*
  low-pass, 215–217, *216*, **224**
  Wiener, 200, 213–214
Filters
  Butterworth, 216
  constrained least square, 214–215
  Gaussian, 217, 219
FLASH pulse sequence, for fast MR imaging, 124–125, *125*
Flow imaging, 125–128, *126–128*
  of contrast-enhanced angiography, 127–128, *128*
  perfusion image, 127, *127*
  spin-echo sequence for, 126, *127*
Fluorescence imaging, 79
  energy source for, 5
  fluorophores in, 359
Fluorodeoxyglucose (FDG), in PET imaging, 79, 149–150, *150*
Fluorophores, 359
FMR, 354
Forward mapping method, for volume data, 344
Fourier descriptor, 273
Fourier reconstruction methods, 186
Fourier transform, 18, *18*
  discrete, 50–51
  fast (FFT), 51
  inverse, 192–193
  in medical imaging, 40
  properties of, 41–42, *42, 43*
  of radon transform, *174*, 174–176
  short-time (STFT), 52
  wavelet transform compared with, 52
Frequency domain filtering methods, 212–213
  constrained least square filtering, 214–215
  high-pass filtering, 217, *218*, **224**
  homomorphic filtering, 217–219, *218, 219*
  low-pass filtering, 215–217, *216*, **224**
  Wiener filtering, 213–214
Full width at half maximum (FWHM) measurement, 74
Functional compterized atlas (FCA), 312, *312*

Functional MRI (fMRI), 79, 100
  FCA developed from, 311
  neural activities examined by, 129–130, *130*

Gamma decay, 140
Gamma-ray emission, 67
Gaussian high-pass filter function, 217, 219
Genetic algorithms (GAs)
  best sets of features selected, 305, **305**
  optimization based on, 289–292, **291**
  sample generational cycle of, **291**
Global registration, rigid-body transformation-based, 313
Golay-type coils, 111
Gradient echo imaging, 123–125, *125*
Gray-level co-occurrence matrix (GLCM), 280–281

Heart, beating
  B-mode image of, 168, *168*
  cine images of, 356, *356, 365*
  Doppler image of, 169, *170*
  M-mode display of mitral valve leaflet of, 167, *167*
Hemoglobin
  deoxygenated (Hb), 129
  oxygenated (HbO_2), 129
High-pass filtering, 217, *218*, **224**
Histogram, in image enhancement
  histogram modification, 203–204
  transformation and equalization, *201*, 201–202, *203*
Holography, 336, 337–338
Homomorphic filtering, 217–219, *218, 219*
Hough transform, 233–235, *234*, 266
Hounsfield, Godfrey, 65, 173

Identification, computer-aided, 2
Image analysis. *See also* Image representation
  computerized, 265
  hierarchical structure of medical, 266, *267*
  multimodality multiparameter, 364
  multiparameter, 354, *355*
Image coordinate system, 24–25, *25*
  2-D image rotation in, 25–26
  3-D image rotation and translation transformation in, 26–27

Image display, in biomedical image
 processing and analysis, 12
Image enhancement, 199
 categories of, 200
 exercises, 226–227
 with frequency domain filtering,
  212–213
  constrained least square filtering,
   214–215
  high-pass filtering, 217, *218*, **224**
  homomorphic filtering, 217–219, *218*,
   219
  low-pass filtering, 215–217, *216*, **224**
  Wiener filtering, 213–214
 spatial domain methods, 200
  histogram modification, 203–204
  histogram transformation and
   equalization, *201*, 201–202, *203*
  image averaging, 204
  image subtraction, 204, *205*
  neighborhood operations, 205–212,
   205–212
 using wavelet transform, 223–226
Image formation
 basic principles of, 23
 conditional and joint probability density
  functions in, 30–31
 contrast-to-noise ratio in, 39
 discrete Fourier transform, 50–51
 electromagnetic radiation for, 66–67
 emission-based system, 32, *33*
 exercises, 60–62
 Fourier transform in, 40–42, *42, 43*
 general 3-D system, 32, *33*
 image coordinate system in, 24–27, *25*
 independent and orthogonal random
  variables in, 31–32
 linear systems, 27
 pin-hole imaging, 39–40, *40*
 point source and impulse functions in,
  27–28, *28, 29*
 probability and random variable functions
  in, 29–30
 process, 32–35, *33*
 PSF and spatial resolution, 35–37, *36, 37*
 radon transform, 44–46, *45, 46*
 sampling, 46–50, *47, 49, 50*
 signal-to-noise ratio in, 37–38
 Sinc function in, 43–44, *44*
 wavelet transform, 52–57, *54, 56, 58, 59*

Image processing
 exercises, 226–227
 wavelet transform for, 220–226,
  221–223, **224**, *225, 226*
Image Processing Interface, in MATLAB
 environment, 19
Image processing software packages, 20–21
Image reconstruction and analysis,
 model-based methods for, *364*,
 364–366, *365*. *See also*
 Reconstruction, image
Image registration. *See* Registration, image
Image representation
 classification of features for
  neural network classifiers, *296*,
   296–302, *297, 300–302*
  rule-based systems, *294*, 294–296
  statistical methods, 292–293
  support vector machine for, 302–303
 exercises, 306–308
 feature extraction
  categories of, 268
  relational features, 282–283, *284, 285*
  shape features, 270–279, *271, 272,
   275–277, 279*
  statistical pixel-level features, 268–270
  texture features, *280*, 280–282, 283
 feature selection
  for classification, 283–285
  GA-based optimization, 289–292,
   291
  linear discriminant analysis, 285–288,
   286
  PCA, 288–289
 hierarchical, *266*
 for mammographic microcalcifications,
  303–306, **305**
 nature of, 265
Images
 analog, 23
 black and white, 23, 24
 color with, 23, 24
 digital representation of, 24
 two-dimensional (2-D), 23
Image scaling, in MATLAB image
 processing toolbox, 16
Image segmentation. *See* Segmentation,
 image
Image smoothing, using wavelet transform,
 223–226

Image visualization. *See* Visualization
Imaging methods, planar, 1
Imaging modalities, radiological, 139. *See also* Medical imaging modalities
Imaging technology, 3-D, 360
Impulse function, 27, 28, *28*
Information fusion, 366
Information processing, archiving, and retrieval systems, 366
Instrumentation
  for medical imaging, 7, 35
  for MRI, 110–111, *111*
Inversion recovery imaging, *116*, 118–119, *119, 120*
Iodine-based contrast agents, 95. *See also* Contrast agents
Ionization chambers, 70–72, *71*
Ionized radiation, 3
ISH (intensity saturation hue) color representation, 23–24
Iso-parametric contour lines, 342
Iterative principal axes registration (IPAR), 319–323, *321, 322*

Laplacian, computation of, 230
Laplacian mask, 229, 230
Laplacian of Gaussian (LOG) function, 230–231, 260
Laplacian weight mask, 208–209, *209, 210*
Larmor frequency, 104, *104*, 105, *105*
Lasers, NIR, 363
Lauterbur, Paul, 99
Light radiance, 358
Linear attenuation coefficient, for EM radiation, 70, *71*
Linear discriminant analysis, 285–288, *286*
Line integral projection, of Radon transform, 45, *45*
Line spread function (LSF), 37
Log-transformation operations, in MATLAB image processing toolbox, 16
Look-up tables (LUTs), implementing, 12
Low-pass filter, 215–217, *216*, **224**

Magnetic resonance imaging (MRI), 1, 2, 65, 99, 139. *See also* functional MRI
  advantages of, 354
  basic form of, 109
  characteristics of, 136
  data produced by, 99–100, *100*
  diffusion, 354
  diffusion imaging, 130–135, *131–134*
  energy source for, 5
  general schematic of, *111*
  image reconstruction for, 192–193
  instrumentation for, 110–111, *111*
  principles of, 100–110, *101–105, 107, 108,* **110**
  pulse sequences in, 112, *113,* 114, *114*
    echo planar imaging, 119–123, *120–124*
    gradient echo imaging, 123–125, *125*
    inversion recovery imaging, *116,* 118–119, *119, 120*
    spin-echo imaging, 114–118, *115, 116*
  and relaxation process, 106–110, *107, 108,* **110**
  and spin density, 110, **110**
Magnetization transfer, MRI with, 356
Mammograms
  digitalized X-ray, 283, *283*
  gray-level scaled image, 16, *16*
  microcalcifications on, *212,* 303–306, **305**
  specific image processing operations for, 13–14, *14*
  and wavelet operations, 57, *59, 60*
Mammographic scanners, digital X-ray, 87–88, *88*
Mammography. *See also* Breast imaging
  imaging microcalcifications in, 5–6
  X-ray film-screen, 86–88, *87–89*
Mansfield, Peter, 99
MATLAB exercises, Image Processing Interface in, 19
MATLAB image processing toolbox
  basic commands, 16–18, *18, 19*
  digital image representation, 14–16, *16*
  images supported by, 18
Medical image analysis, hierarchical structure of, 266, *267*
Medical imaging
  analysis and applications, 8
  collaborative paradigm for, 2, 3
  complementary modalities, 365 (*see also* medical imaging modalities)
  data acquisition and image reconstruction in, 7–8

defined, 6
energy sources for, *3*
example of performance measures, 10–11
exercises, 21–22
instrumentation for, 7, 35
model-based, 354, *355*
multimodality multiparameter, 364
multiparameter, 353–356, *355, 356*
optical, 357–358
　diffuse reflectance images, 362, *363*
　optical coherence tomography, 360–361, *361, 362*
　optical endoscopy, 360
　optical microscopy, 358–359
　photoacoustic imaging, 363–364
　transillumination, 362–363, *363*
performance measures, *8,* 8–11, *10*
physics of, 7
physiology and imaging medium, 6
process, 199–200
research and applications, 6, *6*
targeted, 357
visualization in, 335 (*see also* Visualization, image)
Medical imaging modalities, 3–6, *4*. *See also* nuclear medicine imaging modalities
　classification of, 79
　contrast agents for, 95–96
　exercises, 96–97
　image reconstruction in, 186–194, *187, 191–193*
　magnetic resonance imaging, 99–100
　　contrast, spatial resolution, and SNR, 135–136
　　diffusion imaging, 130–135, *131–134*
　　exercises in, 137
　　flow imaging, 125–128, *126–128*
　　fMRI, 129–130, *130*
　　instrumentation for, 110–111, *111*
　　principles of, 100–110, *101–105, 107, 108,* **110**
　　pulse sequences, 112–125, *113–116, 119–125*
　for specific information, 311
　spiral X-ray CT, 92–95, *94*
　two-dimensional projection radiography, 84–86, *85*

ultrasound imaging
　A-mode, 166–167
　attenuation in, 162–163, **163**
　B-mode, 168, *168*
　contrast, spatial resolution, and SNR, 170–171
　Doppler, 169, *170*
　instrumentation, 164–166, *164–166*
　M-mode, 167, *167*
　in multilayered medium, 160–162, *162*
　propagation of sound in medium for, 157–159
　reflection and refraction in, 159–160
　reflection imaging, 163–134
X-ray CT, 88–92, *89–93*
X-ray generation, 81–84, *82, 83*
X-ray imaging, 80
X-ray mammography, 86–88, *87–89*
Mexican hat operator, 230–231
Microcalcifications, breast, 5–6, 303–306, **305**
Microscopy
　multiphoton, 359
　optical, 358–359
ML-EM algorithms, 189–190
M-mode ultrasound imaging, 167, *167*
Modulation transfer function (MTF), 37
Monte Carlo simulations, in SPECT imaging, 147
Moore-Penrose inverse, *259*
Motion artifacts, 6
Motion parallax display method, 336–337
MR spectroscopy, 100
M-script code
　for example mammogram, *16*
　for example of MR brain image, *19*
Multigrid expectation maximization (MGEM) algorithm, 190, *191,* 192, *192*
Multilevel adaptive segmentation (MAS) model, 249–250, *250*
Multiple sclerosis, 353

Nearest neighbor classifier, 293
Neighborhood operations, 205–212, *205–212*
Neural network classifiers, *296,* 296–301, *297, 300–302*

Neural networks
 arterial structure in digital subtraction, 259–261, *261*
 backpropagation network for, 255–258, *256, 257*
 image segmentation using, 254–255
 RBF, 258–259, *259*
Neuroendoscopy, 360
Neuro-fuzzy pattern classification, *296,* 296–301, *297, 300–302*
Neuron cell structure, 131, *131*
NIR lasers, 363
Nuclear magnetic resonance (NMR), 99
Nuclear medicine, 4
Nuclear medicine imaging modalities
 dual-modality SPECT-CT and PET-CT scanners, 151–154, *152, 153*
 exercises, 154–155
 PET, **148,** 148–150, *149, 150*
  contrast, spatial resolution, and SNR in, 150–151
  detectors and data acquisition systems, 150
 radioactivity and, 139–140
 SPECT, 140–142, **141**
  contrast, spatial resolution and SNR in, 145–148, *146, 147*
  detectors and data acquisition system for, 142–145, *143–146*
Nuclei, in MRI, 100–110, *101–105, 107, 108,* **110**
Nyquist criterion, 47, 50
Nyquist rate, 48, 49–50

Optical coherence tomography (OCT), 357–358, 360–361, *361, 362*
 full-field, 361, *362*
 single-point scanning-based, 361, *361*
Optical endoscopy, 360
Optical imaging systems, 357–358, *359*
Optical microscopy, 358–359
Optical sectioning, 359
Optimal global thresholding, 237–239
Optoacoustics, 364
Output signal, 13

Pair production, 69
PAR, iterative (IPAR), 319–323, *321, 322*
Perfusion, 354
Phantom, X-ray imaging, 37

Phantom images
 arterial segmentation of angiogram of pig, 260, *261*
 reconstructed, 190, *192*
Phase contrast encoding methods, MRI with, 356
Philips GEMINI TF Big Bore PET-CT imaging system, 153, *153*
Philips Gyroscan S15 scanner, 323
Philips Precedence SPECT-Xray CT scanner, 152, *152*
Photoacoustic imaging, 363–364
Photoelectric absorption, 68, *68,* 69
Photomultiplier tubes (PMTs)
 and detector subsystem output voltage pulse, 76–77, *77*
 with scintillation detectors, 73–76, *76*
Photon, in EM radiation, 66
Picture Archiving and Communication Systems (PACS), 366
Piezoelectric transducer, ultrasound beam from, 165, *165*
Pin-hole imaging method, 39–40, *40*
Pixel-by-pixel transformation, 314
Pixel classification methods, for image segmentation, 239–245, *243*
Pixel dimensions, in image formation, 24
PMT matrix, in SPECT imaging system, 143, *144*
Point spread functions (PSFs), 27
 in image formation, 27
 and spatial resolution, 35–37, *36, 37*
Poisson distribution model, 182, 183
Positive predictive value (PPV)
 measurement of, 10
Positron emission tomography (PET), 1, 4, 65, 79
 advantages of, 149–150, 354
 coincidence detection, 149, *149* 150–151
 data acquisition systems for, 150
 development of, 148
 disadvantages of, 151–154, *152, 153*
 dual-modality scanners, 151–154, *152, 153*
 FCA developed from, 311
 with FDG imaging, 149–150, *150*
 image reconstruction in, 188–192, *191–193*
 main advantage of, 149–150
 neuroreceptor-based fast, 354

Precision, defined, 22
Principal axes registration (PAR), 316
Principal axes registration, iterative (IPAR), 319–323, *321*, 322
Principal component analysis (PCA), 288–289
Probability, in image formation, 29–32
Projections, reconstructing images from, 46, *46*
Proportional counters, 70–72
Protons
 in MRI, 100–101, 100–110, *101–105, 107, 108,* **110**
 symbolic representation of, *102*
Pulse-height analyzer (PHA) circuit, in SPECT imaging, 143
Purcell, Edward, 99

Quadrature-mirror filter theory, 55
Quantum, in EM radiation, 66

Radiation, defined, 65. *See also* electromagnetic radiation
Radioactive decay, 139, 140
Radioactivity, defined, 139, 140
Radio frequency (RF) energy, with NMR imaging, 104, *104*, 105, *105*
Radiography
 digital, 86
 film-based, 86
 two-dimensional projection, 84–86, *85*
 X-ray mammography, 86–88, *87–89*
 (*see also* Mammograms)
Radiological imaging, clinical significance of, 1. *See also* Diagnostic radiology
Radionuclide imaging methods, 139
Radionuclides, positron emitter, **148,** 148–149
Radiophosphorous ^{32}P, discovery of, 140
Radon transform, 44
 and image reconstruction
  backprojection method, 176–179, *179, 180*
  central slice theorem, 174–176, *175*
  inverse radon transform, 176
 implementation of, 173
 inverse, 176
Ray geometries, 344–345
Rayleigh criterion, *36,* 36–37
Rayleigh scattering, 67–68, 69

Ray tracing method, 346
RBF network, 258–259, *259*
Receiver operating characteristic curve (ROC) analysis, 8, 8–9, *10*
Reconstruction, image, 13
 estimation methods, 182–185
 exercises, 194–195
 Fourier methods, 185–186
 iterative algebraic methods, 180–182, *181*
 in medical imaging modalities
  magnetic resonance imaging, 192–193
  nuclear emission computed tomography, 188–192
  X-ray CT, 186–188, *187*
 radon transform and
  backprojection method, 176–179, *179, 180*
  central slice theorem, 174–176, *175*
  inverse radon transform, 176
 from raw data, 173–174
 in ultrasound imaging, 193–194
Reconstruction algorithms, 7
Region-growing process, in image segmentation, 245–247, *246, 248*
Region-splitting methods, in image segmentation, 247–248, *248, 249*
Registration, image, 364
 elastic deformation-based, 325–330, *328, 330*
 exercises, 330–331
 features-based
  image landmarks and, 323–325
  weighted, 324–325
 iterative principal axes, 319–323, *321, 322*
 methods and algorithms, 312–313
 MR procedure, *328*
 multimodality brain, 313–314
 point-based, 323–324
 postprocessing methods, 311, 354
 principal axes registration, 316–318, *319*
 rigid-body transformation, 313, 314–316, *315*
 through transformation, 312–313, *313*
Reproducibility, defined, 22
Resolution
 defined, 22
 in PET imaging, 150–151

Response function, of image formation system, 33–34
RGB (red green blue) intensities, 23
Rigid-body transformation, 313, 314–316, *315*
Roentgen, Wilhelm Conrad, 65, 80
Rotating frame, with MRI imaging, 105–106
Rule-based image classification systems, *294*, 294–296

Sampling, in image formation, 46–50, *47, 49, 50*
Scanners, 13
   digital X-ray mammographic, 87–88, *88*
   dual-modality, 151–154, *152*, 153
   first commercial X-ray CT, 173
   Philips Gyroscan S15, 323
   Philips Precedence SPECT-Xray CT, 152, *152*
   in SPECT imaging, 151–154, *152*, 153
Scattering
   Compton, 69, 147
   in projection radiography, 84
   Rayleigh, 67–68, 69
Scintillation detectors, 73–76, **74**, *76*
Segmentation, image
   advanced methods, 248–249
      estimation-model based adaptive segmentation, 249–254, *250, 254*
      image segmentation using neural networks, 254–260, *256, 257, 259, 261*
   categories of, 229
   computer-aided, 2
   defined, 229
   edge-based, 229
      boundary tracking, 231–233, *233*
      edge detection operations, 230–231
      Hough transform, 233–235, *234*
   exercises, 261–262
   feature extraction following, 268
   pixel-based methods, 235–237, *236, 237*
      optimal global thresholding, 237–239
      pixel classification through clustering, 239–245, *243*
   region-based
      region-growing, 245–247, *246*, 248
      region-splitting, 247–248, *248, 249*

Semiconductor detectors, 72–73
SenoScan® digital mammography systems, 88
Sensitivity, 10, 22
SEPI. *See* spiral echo planar imaging
Shadowgram optical imaging, 362
Shape features, 270–271
   boundary encoding
      chain code, *271*, 271–173, *272*
      Fourier descriptor, 273
   shape description
      moments for, 273–274
      morphological processing for, 274–279, *275–277, 279*
Short-time Fourier Transform (STFT), 52
Signal-to-noise ratio (SNR), 100, 136
   computation of, 37–38
   defined, 37
   of MRI image, 136
   in PET imaging, 150–151
   signal averaging for enhancing, 204
   in SPECT imaging, 145–147
   in ultrasound, 170–171
   of X-ray imaging modalities, 95–96
Similarity transformation for point-based registration, 323–324
Sinc function, in image processing, 43–44, *44*
Single photon emission computed tomography (SPECT), 1, 4, 79
   with attenuation, 147, *147*
   contrast in, 145
   detectors and data acquisition system for, 142–145, *143–146*
   development of, 141
   dual-modality scanners, 151–154, *152*, 153, *153*
   FCA developed from, 311
   full-body, 5
   image reconstruction in, 188–192, *191–193*
   imaging system for, *143*, 144
   radionuclides required for, 141
   scanner, 141–142, *142*
   signal-to-noise ratio in, 145
   spatial resolution in, 145–146
Snell's law, 160
Sobel mask, 229, 230
Sobel weight mask, 208, *208*
Sodium iodide NaI(TI), in SPECT imaging, 144

Software package, 3D Slicer, 20–21
Sonar technology, 157
Sound waves, propagation of, 157–159
Spatial domain methods, 200
  histogram modification, 203–204
  histogram transformation and
     equalization, *201*, 201–202, *203*
  image averaging, 204
  image subtraction, 204, *205*
  using neighborhood operations, *205*,
     205–206, *206*
    with adaptive arithmetic mean filter,
       207–208
    adaptive processing, 209–212, *211, 212*
    image sharpening and edge
       enhancement, *208*, 208–209, *209*
    with median filter, 207, *207*
Spatial filtering methods, using
     neighborhood operations, *205*,
     205–206, *206*
  adaptive arithmetic mean filter, *207*,
     207–208
  adaptive processing, 209–212, *211, 212*
  image sharpening and edge enhancement,
     208, 208–209, *209*
  median filter, 207, *207*
Spatial resolution
  characterizing performance of, 37
  and collimator length, 372
  of photoacoustic imaging, 364
  in SPECT imaging, 145–146
  in ultrasound, 170–171
  in X-ray imaging, 95, 96
Spatial resolution performance,
     characterizing, 37
Specificity, 10, 22
SPECT-CT image, fused, 152–153, *153*
SPECT imaging
  with attenuation, 147, *147*
  full-body, 5
Spectroscopy, MR, 100
Spin-echo imaging, 114–118, *115, 116*
Spin-echo sequence, for flow imaging, 126,
     127
Spin quantum number, 101
Spiral echo planar imaging (SEPI),
     122–123, *123, 124*, 193
Spiral X-ray CT
  applications of, 92–94
  slice thickness during, 94–95

Statistical pixel-level (SPL) features,
     268–270
Storage and compression formats, for
     MATLAB program, 17
Structural computerized atlas (SCA), 312,
     312

Targeted imaging, 357
Texture features, *280*, 280–282, 283
Therapeutic evaluations, multimodality
     image fusion in, 151–152
Thermoacoustics imaging, 364
Tissue density, 6
Tissue medium, optical reflectance in, 358,
     359
Tissue tagging, MRI with, 356
Tomography. *See* Positron emission
     tomography; Single photon emission
     computed tomography; X-ray
     computed tomography
Transillumination imaging, 362–363, *363*
Treatment
  medical imaging modalities in, 1–2
  multimodality image fusion in,
     151–152
True negative fraction (TNF), 9, 10
True positive fraction (TPF), 9, 10
Tungsten, in X-ray generation, 81, *82*

Ultrasound, 1
Ultrasound, laser-induced, 364
Ultrasound imaging, 4, 65
  A-mode, 166–167
  attenuation in, 162–163, **163**
  B-mode, 168, *168*
  contrast for, 170
  Doppler, 169, *170*
  exercises in, 171–172
  image reconstruction in, 193–194
  instrumentation, 164–166, *164–166*
  M-mode, 167, *167*
  in multilayered medium, 160–162,
     162
  OCT compared with, 360–361
  propagation of sound in medium,
     157–159
  reflection and refraction, 159–160
  reflection imaging, 163–164
  SNR for, 170–171
  spatial resolution of, 170–171

Varifocal mirror system, 336, 337
Velocity map, 356, *356*
Virtual endoscopy, 335, 349
Virtual reality (VR), 335
Visualization, 335
  multidimensional methods, 335
  stereoscopic, 336
Visualization, image, 364
  3-D display methods, 338–339
    surface-based, 338, 339–343, *340–342, 344*
    volume-based, 344–347, *345*, 346
  exercises, 349–350
  feature-enhanced 2-D image display methods, 336, *337*
  semi-3-D display methods, 336–338
  VR-based interactive, 347–349
Volume of interest (VOI), 311

Wavelengths, in medical imaging applications, 159
Wavelet-based interpolation methods, of image reconstruction, 190, *191, 192*
Wavelet processing methods, multiresolution-based, 365, *365*
Wavelet transform
  application of, 57
  defined, 52
  for image processing, 220–226, *221–223*, **224**, *225, 226*
  image reconstruction, 173

linear series expansion in, 52–53
multiresolution analysis in, 53–54, *54, 56,* 56–57
multiresolution signal decomposition using, 56, *56,* 57, *58, 59*
sampling, 52
scaling and shifting in, 52, 56–57
White radiation, 81, *82*
Wiener filtering methods, 200, 213–214
WMREM algorithm, 190, *192*

X ray, invention of, 65
X-ray computed tomography (X-ray CT), 1
  basic principle of, 89, *89, 90*
  image reconstruction, 186–188, *187*
  modern scanner for, 92, *93*
  scanner geometry for, 90, *91,* 92, *92*
  spiral, 92–95, *94*
X-ray computed tomography (X-ray CT) scanner, first commercial, 173
X-ray generation
  basic principle of, 81
  for diagnostic imaging, 82–84, *83*
X-ray generation tubes, 83
X-ray imaging, 79
  medical applications of, 80
  signal-to-noise ratio of, 95–96
  spatial resolution in, 95, 96
X-ray intensifying screens, 84, *85,* 86
X rays
  as external energy source, 3
  soft, 80